Life Course Research and Social Policies

Volume 9

Life course research has been developing quickly these last decades for good reasons. Life course approaches focus on essential questions about individuals' trajectories, longitudinal analyses, cross-fertilization across disciplines like life-span psychology, developmental social psychology, sociology of the life course, social demography, socio-economics, social history. Life course is also at the crossroads of several fields of specialization like family and social relationships, migration, education, professional training and employment, and health. This Series invites academic scholars to present theoretical, methodological, and empirical advances in the analysis of the life course, and to elaborate on possible implications for society and social policies applications.

More information about this series at http://www.springer.com/series/10158

Robin Tillmann • Marieke Voorpostel
Peter Farago
Editors

Social Dynamics in Swiss Society

Empirical Studies Based on the Swiss Household Panel

Springer Open

Editors
Robin Tillmann
FORS-Swiss Centre of Expertise
in the Social Sciences
Lausanne, Switzerland

Marieke Voorpostel
FORS-Swiss Centre of Expertise
in the Social Sciences
Lausanne, Switzerland

Peter Farago
University of Lausanne
Lausanne, Switzerland

FORS
Lausanne, Switzerland

ISSN 2211-7776 ISSN 2211-7784 (electronic)
Life Course Research and Social Policies
ISBN 978-3-030-07803-4 ISBN 978-3-319-89557-4 (eBook)
https://doi.org/10.1007/978-3-319-89557-4

Printed on acid-free paper

This Springer imprint is published by the registered company Springer International Publishing AG part of Springer Nature.
The registered company address is: Gewerbestrasse 11, 6330 Cham, Switzerland

This book has been realized using the data collected by the Swiss Household Panel (SHP), which is based at the Swiss Centre of Expertise in the Social Sciences FORS. The project is supported by the Swiss National Science Foundation.

Preface

It is indeed a pleasure to write the preface to a book celebrating 20 years of the "Swiss Household Panel (SHP)." For about 20 years, I was responsible for one of SHP's twins: the German Socio-Economic Panel Study (SOEP), which is also a household panel. With each additional comparable household panel, like SHP and SOEP, researchers are able to improve their studies by making international comparisons that advance our understanding of the world.

In order to facilitate international comparative analyses, SHP was one of the first Cross-National Equivalent File (CNEF) partners. The CNEF – which originated at Syracuse University, later at Cornell University, and now based at the Ohio State University – provides access to harmonized data from a number of panel data studies. These include SHP, the Household Income and Labour Dynamics in Australia Study (HILDA), the German SOEP, the UK Household Longitudinal Study (UK HLS), and the Panel Study of Income Dynamics (PSID) in the USA. Data from the Korea Labor and Income Panel Study (KLIPS) and the Russia Longitudinal Monitoring Survey (RLMS) are also available.

The CNEF continues to expand access to data. Interesting household panel studies or cohort studies are underway in Africa and Asia, including, to name a few, the "Cape Area Panel Study (CAPS)," panel household surveys in Thailand and Vietnam (which are financed by the German Science Foundation, DFG), the "Coping with Shocks in Mongolia Household Panel Survey," and the World Bank's "LSMS Panel Surveys."

The fact that the panels in CNEF are comparable is not a lucky accident, but rather an important feature of the worldwide social and behavioral sciences research infrastructure. A concerted effort ensures that these panel studies are comparable in terms of the basic setups and the questionnaires.

The one outlier is the oldest study, the PSID, which is less comparable to the other studies. This is a surprise because, without any doubt whatsoever, the PSID was the role model for all household panel studies that followed. However, the newer studies learned from the experience of PSID. Thus, while the PSID only interviews the head of the household, all of the younger studies interview all adult household members.

The book at hand is an excellent example not just of SHP's inherent research power, but also the power of international comparisons. In this book, readers will find articles about "health, well-being, and life satisfaction," "resources, work, and living conditions," as well as "politics and attitudes." Three articles exploit international comparisons: a longitudinal analysis of cohabitation and marriage in Switzerland and Australia; an analysis of wealth, savings, and children among Swiss, German, and Australian families; and a study on home ownership and wealth in Germany and Switzerland.

Scientists use SHP's excellent data to carry out research: both local and foreign researchers focusing solely on Switzerland as well as teams of authors from multiple countries making comparative analyses. Thus, in the book at hand, readers will find papers written by authors from Australia (The University of Queensland and Queensland University of Technology), Germany (University of Mannheim and German Institute for Economic Research – DIW Berlin), Italy (Università degli Studi di Milano-Bicocca), the Netherlands (University of Amsterdam and Utrecht University), and the USA (Ohio State University and University of Colorado, Boulder).

SHP is part of a growing worldwide community of excellent researchers who analyze household panel data. These analyses make a difference in the scientific community. Many of these analyses also make a difference in local and national societies. In the future, the results of these studies will also make a difference to global society. As a member, if not a hub, of the global network of panel studies, SHP is poised to contribute significantly to science and to society.

Fellow, Max Planck Institute for Human Development
Senior Research Fellow, German Socio-Economic Panel
Study (SOEP)
Berlin, Germany

Gert G. Wagner

Introduction

Longitudinal data are indispensable for life course research. By observing individuals over time we gain insight into their life course trajectories, the events they experience, and the outcomes thereof. This edited volume bundles studies based on the Swiss Household Panel (SHP). The SHP is a longitudinal study that follows households in Switzerland on an annual basis over time since 1999. Nearly twenty years of observing Swiss households has generated a wealth of insights into the lives of people in Switzerland. Whereas a first edited volume (Zimmermann & Tillmann 2004) provided a snapshot of Swiss society at the time, this second edited volume scrutinizes changes in peoples' life courses and in society over a prolonged period, fine-tuning our conceptions and analyses of social dynamics and changes across time. In addition to the temporal dimension, also interdependencies between household members, as well as cross-country comparisons come to the foreground in this book. Longitudinal household data such as the SHP allow the study of the life course linking different life domains, and examining the interdependency of life courses within households.

This chapter first gives a more detailed description of the history and the design of the SHP, followed by a brief introduction to the studies included in this volume. A concluding paragraph shows how the studies in this book can provide insights for social policy.

The History and Design of the Swiss Household Panel

The Swiss Priority Program "Demain la Suisse" implemented the SHP as one of its key structural measures in 1999 (Budowski et al. 1998; Budowski et al. 2001; Joye & Scherpenzeel 1997). Experiences made from existing European panel surveys informed the SHP's design, notably the German Socio-Economic Panel (SOEP) (Schupp & Wagner 2007) and the British Household Panel Study (BHPS), which is now integrated into the UK Household Longitudinal Survey (UKHLS) (Buck & McFall 2011). Initially, the SHP was funded by the Swiss National Science

Foundation and hosted by the University of Neuchâtel; the Swiss Federal Statistical Office contributed matching funds. Since 2008, still mainly funded by the Swiss National Science Foundation, the SHP has been integrated into the Swiss Centre of Expertise in the Social Sciences FORS hosted by the University of Lausanne.

Two main aims guide the SHP (Farago 1996; Joye & Scherpenzeel 1997): to ensure a solid longitudinal database for social reporting on stability and changes in living arrangements and well-being in Switzerland, and to promote opportunities for quantitative social science research by making high-quality data available to Swiss social scientists and to the international social science research community.

At present, the SHP comprises three samples: the SHP_I (5,074 households and 7,799 individuals interviewed first in 1999), the SHP_II (2,538 households and 3,654 individuals interviewed first in 2004) and the SHP_III (3,989 households and 6,090 individuals interviewed first in 2013) (Voorpostel et al. 2016). All three are purely probabilistic random samples made available by the Swiss Federal Statistical Office. They are stratified by the seven major statistical regions of Switzerland. Within each major geographic region, each household (SHP_I and SHP_II) or individual (SHP_III) had the same inclusion probability, independent of the size of the household. The SHP's reference population includes all private households whose members represent the non-institutional resident population in Switzerland.

Response rates on the household level in the first wave were 64% for the first sample (1999), 65% for the second sample (2004), and 60% for the third sample (2013). On the individual level, initial response rates (conditional upon household participation) were 85%, 76%, and 81% respectively. Sample sizes in the SHP, as in most panel studies, declined over time. After eighteen waves of data collection, the number of households and individuals interviewed for the SHP_I corresponds to 52% of the initial number of households and 55% of the initial number of individuals interviewed. For the SHP_II, these figures are 49% and 51%, respectively, after thirteenth waves. SHP_III has, so far, only four waves, after which 60% of original households and 63% of original individuals remain. See Tillmann et al. (2016) for a full description of the current state of the project.

There are three types of questionnaires in the SHP: a household grid questionnaire to assess household composition, a household questionnaire, and an individual questionnaire. All household members aged 14 or older are eligible to answer the individual questionnaire. Each household has a reference person who completes the household grid and the household questionnaire. The household questionnaire includes in addition a proxy questionnaire on household members younger than 14 years, or absent for the time of the field work or unable to respond themselves due to illness or disability. The household and individual questionnaires cover a broad range of topics.[1] They are also designed to collect both objective data, such as financial resources, social position, and participation, and subjective data, such as satisfaction scores, values, and attitudes. The questionnaires constitute an operationalisation of different elements on the micro-social level: living conditions, life events, attitudes, perceptions, and lifestyles (Budowski et al. 1998).

[1] Questionnaires can be searched online, and are also available in pdf format.

The SHP allows for cross-national comparisons with other household panel studies.[2] The SHP contains measures in various domains that are comparable to those in other panels. Several contributions in this book make use of this opportunity by comparing Switzerland to Germany and Australia (chapters 1.3, 2.5 and 2.6).

The Contributions

The chapters are grouped into three topics. The first part of the book contains chapters on health, wellbeing and life satisfaction. *Lillard*'s chapter on smoking behaviour of different cohorts, linked to the context of changing regulations, the industry-government collaboration and efforts for tobacco control bring the societal context into view in which individuals shape their behaviour. *Lucchini and Della Bella* advance our understanding of the relationship between overweight and health by looking at satisfaction with health. *Hewitt, Voorpostel and Turrell* analyse the links between relationship dissolution, health and wellbeing for cohabiting and married couples in Switzerland and Australia. *Ryser and Le Goff* look into differences in attitudes and satisfaction of married and cohabiting couples and explore whether cohabiting couples who transition into marriage change their views on the family and their levels of satisfaction. The chapter by *Wernli and Zella* shows the impact of several life course events in the family domain on men and women's life satisfaction. Finally, *Potarca and Bernardi* examine whether the phenomenon of the "healthy migrant", meaning that migrants tend to report better health than the host population exists in Switzerland, and whether naturalization is of importance.

The second part of the book addresses research questions on resources, work and living conditions. *Masia, Budowski and Tillmann* focus on the relationship between individual health and financial effects on the household. Their study addresses the concept of linked lives, which is central in the life course perspective. *Gazareth, Iglesias, Crettaz and Suter* analyse trajectories of material deprivation and life course transitions. *Bühlmann*'s chapter also deals with trajectories of material poverty and vulnerability using a historical and a biographical approach to vulnerability. *Zangger, Glauser and Becker* analyse cohort differences in labour market entry and the influence of social origin on the status of the first job. The contribution by *Ravazzini and Kuhn* studies families' wealth accumulation in Switzerland, Germany and Australia, focusing especially on whether children stimulate or discourage saving and the implication for families' wealth. A second contribution on wealth, by

[2] In 2008 the SHP was included in the Cross-National Equivalent File (CNEF), which provides harmonized data from several household panel studies. To date the CNEF comprises the German SOEP, the British Understanding Society (including the former BHPS), the US Panel Study of Income Dynamics (PSID), the Canadian Survey of Labour and Income Dynamics (SLID), the Household Income and Labour Dynamics in Australia (HILDA), the Korean Labor and Income Panel Study (KLIPS) and the Russia Longitudinal Monitoring Survey (RLMS-HSE) (Frick et al. 2007).

Kuhn and Grabka, compares Germany and Switzerland on the role homeownership plays for wealth accumulation.

The third part of the book contains studies on politics and attitudes. Whereas most research on political party preferences to date looked at attitudes shaping party preferences, *Fitzgerald and Jorde* show that partisanship also shapes people's stances on key political issues in Switzerland. *Sarrasin, Kuhn and Lancee* examine the declining support for the European Union among Swiss citizens. *Pekari, Rosset and Schmid* analyse support for the Swiss welfare state. Finally, *Monsch and Passy* look at changes in general trust in people, views on gender, taxation, foreigners and environmental protection, in relation to membership in a political or civic organisation.

Outlook

With increasing diversity in life course trajectories new economic and social risks have emerged, posing important challenges for policy makers (D'Addio & Whiteford 2008). Whereas many social policies were developed to cover well-defined risks such as financial difficulties in childhood or old age or short-term unemployment, departures from the "standardized" life course require a re-evaluation of social policy in the light of new social risks. This book contributes to a better understanding of our changing society, in particular in areas that could be subject to political action. It shows trends over time as well as over the life course, and includes a multitude of life domains.

Changing life courses and new social risks are also evident in Switzerland. The contributions in this book show trends such as increasing levels of job insecurity among the youngest cohorts, the impact of life events on wellbeing and financial security, social groups facing long-term material deprivation and lower wellbeing, current levels of wealth inequality and health disparities in society, and how such group differences and life trajectories affect how individuals view the role of the welfare state. This wealth of information gathered from nearly twenty years of observing households in Switzerland provides a strong empirical basis from which fruitful directions for social policies can be developed.

FORS-Swiss Centre of Expertise in the Social Sciences
Lausanne, Switzerland
Professor emeritus, University of Lausanne,
founding director FORS
Lausanne, Switzerland

Robin Tillmann
Marieke Voorpostel
Peter Farago

References

Buck, N., & McFall, S. (2011). Understanding Society: design overview. *Longitudinal and Life Course Studies, 3*(1), 5–17.

Budowski, M., Niklowitz, M., Scherpenzeel, A., Tillmann, R., Wernli, B., & Zimmermann, E. (1998). *Aims and architecture of the Swiss Household Panel.* Neuchatel: Swiss Household Panel.

Budowski, M., Tillmann, R., Zimmermann, E., Wernli, B., Scherpenzeel, A., & Gabadinho, A. (2001). The Swiss Household Panel 1999–2003: Data for research on micro-social change. *ZUMA-Nachrichten, 50*, 100–125.

D'Addio, Anna Cristina and Peter Whiteford (2008). From separated life phases to interrelated life risks: A life course approach to social policy, in OECD, Modernising social policy for the new life course, OECD Publishing, Paris.

Farago, P. (1996). *Gesellschaftliche Dauerbeobachtung im SPP "Zukunft Schweiz/Demain la Suisse" [Swiss Priority Programme "Switzerland towards the future"].* Bern: Swiss National Science Foundation.

Frick, J. R., Jenkins, S. P., Lillard, D. R., Lipps, O., & Wooden, M. (2007). The Cross-National Equivalent File (CNEF) and its member country household panel studies. *Schmollers Jahrbuch, 127*, 627–654.

Joye, D., & Scherpenzeel, A. (1997). *Observation à long terme: Projet de panel. Programme Prioritaire Demain la Suisse*. Bern: Swiss National Science Foundation.

Schupp, J., & Wagner, G. (2007). The German Socio-Economic Panel Study (SOEP): Scope, evolution and enhancements. *Schmollers Jahrbuch, 127*(1), 139–169.

Tillmann, R., Voorpostel, M., Antal, E., Kuhn, U., Lebert, F., Ryser, V.-A.,Lipps, O., & Wernli, B. (2016). The Swiss Household Panel Study : Observing social change since 1999. *Longitudinal and Life Course Studies* 7(1), pp. 64–78.

Voorpostel, M., Tillmann, R., Lebert, F., Kuhn, U., Lipps, O., Ryser, V.-A., Schmid, F., Antal, E., & Wernli, B. (2016). *Swiss Household Panel User Guide (1999-2015), Wave 17.* Lausanne: FORS.

Zimmermann, E., & Tillmann R. (2004). *Vivre en Suisse 1999-2000/Leben in der Schweiz 1999–2000.* Bern: Peter Lang.

Contents

List of Figures

List of Tables

Part I
Health, Well-being and Life Satisfaction

Chapter 1
The Evolution of Smoking in Switzerland

Dean R. Lillard

Introduction

This chapter reviews the long history of tobacco in Switzerland and describes the smoking behavior of seven cohorts of Swiss men and women over the course of the 20th and early 21st centuries. It presents a unique window on smoking in Switzerland because it describes, for each cohort, the smoking behavior in each and every year. Most studies describe average smoking behavior for the whole population at a given point in time. The life-course perspective offers insights that are otherwise masked when researchers use population aggregates. The rest of the chapter briefly reviews some of the history of tobacco, describes the industry-government collaboration that developed during the twentieth century, and the more recent efforts at tobacco control. I describe the main sources of the data I use to construct life-course smoking histories and present those data in several innovative ways. More detailed descriptions of the data are available on request.

A Brief History of Tobacco in Switzerland

While many people know that one of the world's largest tobacco firms, Philip Morris International, has its corporate headquarters in Switzerland, fewer people know that the Swiss have cultivated and consumed tobacco since the late sixteenth century.

D. R. Lillard (✉)
Department of Human Sciences, Ohio State University, Columbus, OH, USA

Deutsches Institüt für Wirtschaftsforschung, Berlin, Germany

National Bureau of Economic Research, Cambridge, MA, USA
e-mail: lillard.13@osu.edu

R. Tillmann et al. (eds.), *Social Dynamics in Swiss Society*, Life Course Research and Social Policies 9, https://doi.org/10.1007/978-3-319-89557-4_1

Rumors suggest that tobacco arrived in Switzerland about 60 years after Christopher Columbus brought seeds from the New World. In 1559 when Hernandez de Toledo returned from Santo Domingo in the New World to Spain and Portugal, he brought tobacco with him. The same year Jean Nicot, the French ambassador to Portugal, sent tobacco to friends in France, encouraging them to partake. Hearsay accounts suggest that shortly after, in 1560, Benedictus Aretius (Marti) von Batterkinden (1505–1574) began to grow tobacco in his garden in the Berne Canton (Pignat 1981).

It is clear that, by the mid-1600s, many residents in the Swiss lands consumed tobacco because secular and religious authorities began to discourage and sometimes ban tobacco consumption. For example, Swiss Mennonites and Anabaptists adopted a set of ethical rules developed and distributed at a 1639 Mennonite council in Holland. One of the rules proclaimed that, "No one should use tobacco unnecessarily, or make it a habit, for time and money are wasted by it; and it is offensive to others…." (Eschleman 1917, p. 91). Swiss canton councils not only forbade people from consuming tobacco, they also fined and sometimes physically punished tobacco consumers.[1] In Appenzell (in 1653) and in the "Republic of the Seven Tithings" in Valais (in 1675) consumers had to pay three books when authorities caught them consuming tobacco (Grenat and de Lavallaz 1904). From 1661 through the mid-1700s authorities in Berne prohibited smoking (treating it as "adultery") and from 1670–1672 authorities in the canton of Glarus fined smokers 1 Swiss crown if they were caught smoking (MacGregor 1847).

Since the start of tobacco cultivation and until today, the lure of jobs and tobacco tax revenue has guided government policies. By 1590 the Berne Canton government protected the rights of farmers to cultivate tobacco (presumably only for trade as they continued to punish smokers) and tobacco cultivation spread during the 1600s to residents of Ticino (Pignat 1981). In 1675, the lure of state revenue led rulers of Monthey, Valais to grant one man, a gunsmith named Jacques Robert, the right to be the sole supplier of tobacco to foreigners (Grenat and de Lavallaz 1904). In 1812, domestic tobacco farmers convinced the central government to improve transportation systems to lower their costs (Grellet 1954). By 1814, when the Congress of Vienna and European powers established the boundaries of modern Switzerland, tobacco trade, cultivation, and consumption were firmly and legally part of the Swiss landscape.

---

[1]Authorities issued similar edicts in England, Persia, the Vatican (Macgregor 1847), Russia (Macgregor 1847; Lillard and Dorofeeva 2015), and Turkey (Önder 2015).

The Domestic Swiss Tobacco Industry - A Child of State Protection

The political economy of Switzerland's domestic tobacco industry survived, even thrived well into the middle of the twentieth century primarily because the Swiss government intervened.

In the first few decades of the twentieth century, competition from foreign tobacco producers almost destroyed Swiss tobacco farming. The yield in the tobacco producing cantons of Fribourg, Vaud, Ticino, Valais, and Grisons fell from an annual average of 432,200 kg in the period 1910–1914 to 150,700 kg in 1926 (Pignat 1981; Burrus 1972). In 1926, the industry almost shut down.

Two main factors allowed Swiss tobacco farming and manufacturing to survive until the 1960s. First, Swiss tobacco manufacturers and farmers formed a tightly-knit and well-organized interest group that not only acted as a cartel but that also convinced the Swiss government to protect it. The government levied lower taxes on products containing at least 50 percent domestically-grown tobacco, taxed imported tobacco and favored the domestic industry in many other ways. For example, the Swiss government issued a decree in 1938 decree that "protected" retail tobacco prices. In 1951, Swiss cigarette manufacturers agreed to limit the amount each firm could spend to advertise. They monitored and punished transgressors (Burrus 1972).

During World War II demand for Swiss tobacco increased because the war disrupted markets and trade routes of foreign suppliers. The associated chaos raised the cost of imported tobacco. Insurance premiums on shipments of imported tobacco rose during the war by 500 percent (Burrus 1972). Domestic tobacco farmers responded to the increased demand. In 1944, Swiss farmers produced almost 2 million kilos of tobacco.

The Swiss government began to eliminate its protectionist policies in the mid-1950s. In 1955, the Federal Court ruled the price regulation of tobacco to be illegal (Burrus 1972). The Swiss cigarette firms advertising restrictions slowly broke down as foreign companies entered the Swiss market (through acquisition of Swiss firms or by establishing operations in Switzerland) and advertised as they pleased.

That pressure and the Swiss government's embrace of free trade in 1960 and 1972 doomed all efforts to continue the government's interference in the tobacco industry. In 1960, Switzerland and Norway founded the European Free Trade Association and in 1972 Switzerland signed a free-trade agreement with the European Economic Community. Under the onslaught of market forces and these changes in the government's stance on free trade, the Swiss cigarette industry's agreement to limit advertising expenditures died in 1964 (Burrus 1972). Essentially, Swiss tobacco farming ended on January 1, 1965 when, as part of the free-trade agreements, Switzerland ended all differential tax treatment that had protected domestic tobacco. Today approximately 200 farmers still grow tobacco in Switzerland (Jaberg and Kern 2016).

Tobacco Control

Although the government stopped protecting the domestic tobacco industry, it continued to support the tobacco industry through its tobacco control policies. Switzerland did not enact modern tobacco control policies until the closing decades of the twentieth century - much later than most developed countries. Swiss politicians delayed enacting such policies because they feared losing the jobs, tax revenue, and benefits local economies enjoy because three major international tobacco firms, Philip Morris, British American Tobacco and Japan Tobacco International, operate in Switzerland. In 2013, those firms and the Swiss tobacco industry employed 2500 Swiss in relatively high paying jobs and generated revenues of more than 579.3 million dollars (ILO 2014). Those jobs and the taxes the firms pay, together with the lobbying efforts of various Swiss interest groups (e.g. the Swiss association representing hotels, restaurants, and cafés), help explain why the Swiss federal and canton governments have been slow to regulate tobacco (Lee and Glantz 2001).

Switzerland limits where and to whom firms can advertise tobacco products. In 1976, 1979, and 1993 Swiss interest groups tried and failed to pass initiatives that would have completely banned tobacco advertising (Isenring 1976; Swiss Federal Office of Health 2009). The industry and government agreed to a partial voluntary ban in 1978 that prohibited firms from advertising or handing out free samples at sports matches or concerts that youth under age 18 were likely to attend (Lee and Glantz 2001). Amazingly, Switzerland let firms continue to sell tobacco to youth. The 1993 initiative failed partly because the tobacco and publishing industries convinced voters that the ban would increase the price of newspapers and magazines, raise the probability that both industries would lay workers off, and restrict citizens' right to free speech (Cornuz et al. 1996).

In 2008, the Swiss prohibited smoking in enclosed public areas and places where several people work. That ban took effect on May 1, 2010. This law resembled laws that German states were adopting around the same time (Lillard and Christopoulou 2015). As in Germany, the government let patrons smoke in bars and restaurants smaller than 80 square meters and they let patrons of larger establishments smoke if owners created separate ventilated rooms for them (Rajkumar et al. 2013). Under the law, the government lets cantons impose stricter bans. Sixteen cantons have chosen to require that even small establishments ban smoking (or provide a separate, ventilated room). In 2012 Swiss voters rejected a federal referendum that would have banned smoking even in the smaller establishments previously excluded by the 2008 law (Durham et al. 2014).

Finally, the Swiss government increasingly taxes tobacco. A 1999 study estimated how various levels of cigarette taxes would affect both consumption (public health) and government revenues (Holly et al. 1999). In 2013, the Swiss government raised tobacco taxes. Switzerland levies both a specific excise tax of 118.32 Swiss francs per 1000 cigarettes and an ad valorem tax of 25 percent of the retail price. Despite the increase, the overall tax burden on tobacco is lower in Switzerland than it is in other neighboring countries. Taxes remain a key policy lever that the Swiss government may continue to use.

Smoking in the Swiss Context

Most previous research uses cross-sectional data to describe patterns of smoking in Switzerland. Such data highlight differences in participation, initiation, and cessation at a moment in time (Morabia et al. 2002) across groups of different ages and by sex (Curtin et al. 1997). Most studies find that Swiss tend to smoke at rates similar to or even lower than men and women in other European countries (WHO 2015). One observes similar smoking behavior of Swiss overall and among women who smoke before and after getting pregnant (Smedberg et al. 2014). However, a recent study compares reported smoking prevalence and aggregate sales data and concludes that true Swiss smoking prevalence may be much higher than indicated by survey smoking prevalence rates (Jakob et al. 2017).

Previous research largely relies on cross-sectional data that do not reveal some of the nuances of smoking patterns across the life-cycle of different cohorts. Cross-sectional data fail to capture how cohort differences dynamically change as social, economic and cultural conditions change. Consequently studies using cross-sectional data may miss patterns informed by the above historical events and context. Marti (2014) uses retrospectively reported data to follow individuals over longer periods but he limits his analysis to a relatively short window of 20 years. One observes different patterns when one describes smoking behavior of cohorts of men and women over longer time spans (Lillard and Christopoulou 2015). The long history of tobacco in Switzerland provides a rich setting in which to do so.

Data Sources

In what follows I plot data constructed with information from the 2007 wave of the Swiss Health Survey (SHS) and the 2011 wave of the Swiss Household Panel Study (SHP). Both surveys ask respondents about their lifetime smoking behavior - whether or not they have ever smoked, the age they started, whether they currently smoke, and the age they quit (SHP) or the number of years it has been since they smoked regularly (SHS).

I restrict the SHP part of the sample to 2011 (wave 12) respondents who provided valid responses to the smoking questions. Using the SHP and SHS data, I construct an indicator of whether or not a person smoked in each year of his or her life. For people who reported they never smoked, the smoking participation measure equals zero in every year. When a person said he currently or previously smoked, I assume he smoked in every year between the age he said he started until the age he said he quit (ex-smokers) or until the survey year (2007 for SHS, 2011 for SHP). I create a

Table 1.1 summary indicators of smoking by gender and birth year

Birth year	Sample size	Peak prevalence rate	Cigarettes per day	Years smoking	Average age at		
					Peak	Start	Quit
Males							
byr<1930	313	0.49	18	38	33	20	53
1930≤byr<1940	713	0.54	22	34	32	20	48
1940≤byr<1950	1102	0.52	21	30	26	20	42
1950≤byr<1960	1091	0.49	21	26	25	19	37
1960≤byr<1970	1209	0.43	19	20	25	19	33
1970≤byr<1980	852	0.45	17	13	26	18	29
1980≤byr<1990	571	0.49	13	7	23	17	22
Females							
byr<1930	192	0.14	10	36	40	25	56
1930≤byr<1940	475	0.21	14	32	31	23	48
1940≤byr<1950	976	0.35	15	29	32	21	42
1950≤byr<1960	1192	0.43	15	25	25	19	36
1960≤byr<1970	1344	0.40	15	20	26	19	32
1970≤byr<1980	838	0.35	12	13	25	18	27
1980≤byr<1990	569	0.37	10	6	21	17	22

Source: Swiss Health Survey 2007 and Swiss Household Panel 2011

birth year variable by subtracting age from the survey year and assign each person a birth cohort. Here I do not construct pseudo-cohorts (a common strategy when using cross-sectional data). Instead, I use the retrospective data to construct true longitudinal smoking histories of seven different (10 year) birth cohorts of Swiss men and women. The data track the actual smoking behavior of members of each cohort accurately except for the cohort of men and women who were 70 or older when they answered the survey. Christopoulou et al. (2011) show that differences in smoking-related mortality of smokers and non-smokers are trivial for cohorts who, when surveyed, were younger than 70. Although I do not weight the data, the weights will only affect the results for the oldest cohort. Table 1.1 summarizes the size of each cohort.

Cohort-Specific Smoking Prevalence Rates Over Time

Figure 1.1 plots the smoking prevalence rate of Swiss men and women born between 1909 and 1990. I group people into seven 10-year birth cohorts. On both figures, I mark three periods during which tobacco markets or consumption changed. These periods include the years of World War II, the period from 1965–1972 when Switzerland was meeting legal requirements of the free trade agreement it signed with the EEC, and the period 2008–2010 when Switzerland signed and then implemented its first public smoking ban.

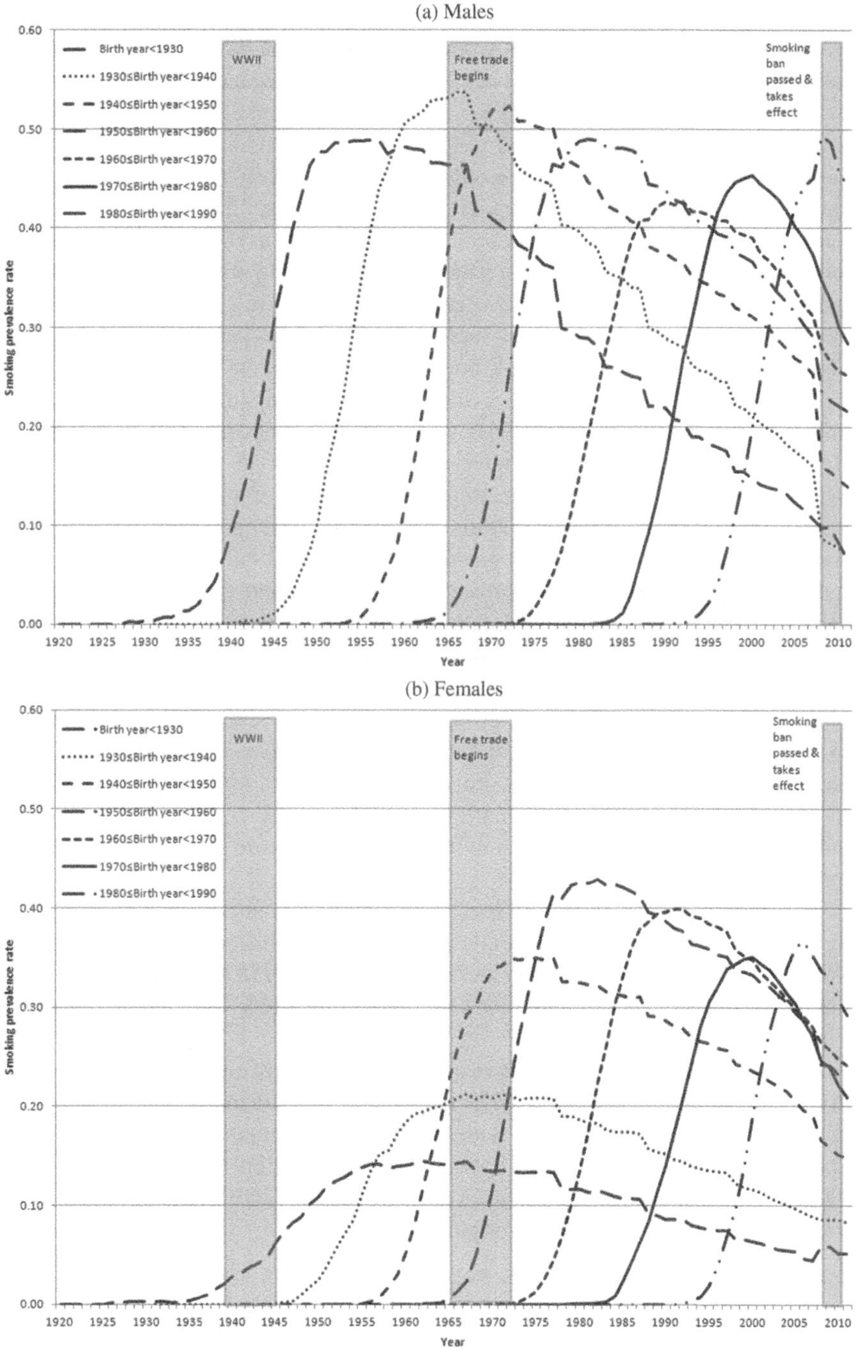

Fig. 1.1 Smoking prevalence rates over the life course by gender and birth cohort (*Source*: Swiss Health Survey 2007 and Swiss Household Panel 2011, unweighted data (see text))

Several patterns strike the eye. First, Swiss men in every cohort smoke more than the corresponding cohort of Swiss women. Second, at the peak, roughly half of the oldest cohort of Swiss men (men born before 1931) were smoking. In the next oldest cohort - those born in the 1930s - 54 percent smoked at the peak of smoking prevalence. Because smokers tend to die faster than non smokers starting around age 65, smoking prevalence in the oldest cohort was likely to have been 2–3 percentage points higher (see Christopoulou et al. 2011). Over the course of their lives men in the oldest cohort smoked at about the same rate as did men in the adjacent cohorts. For men the other striking pattern is that smoking prevalence rates first fall then rise again in the youngest two cohorts. This pattern of increasing smoking prevalence in younger cohorts of men differs from the pattern one observes in Germany, Spain, and the UK (see Lillard and Christopoulou 2015).

One observes a similar but less dramatic rise in the smoking prevalence rate among the youngest cohort of Swiss women. The bottom panel of Fig. 1.1 plots life-course smoking prevalence rates of Swiss women in the same seven birth cohorts. The most striking pattern among women is the dramatic rise in the rate of smoking across the four oldest cohorts. Among the oldest cohort of Swiss women (those born before 1930) smoking prevalence peaked in 1962 at about 14 percent of that cohort. The rate of smoking rose steadily in the next three cohorts of Swiss women, reading a peak among the cohort of women born in the 1950s.

In that cohort, 43 percent of women were smoking in 1980. Note that rates of smoking began to increase most rapidly among the cohort of women who grew up while and shortly after Switzerland began to trade more with the rest of Europe. Except for the youngest cohort, the rate of smoking prevalence steadily fell in successive cohorts. One observes similar patterns of declining rates of smoking in all developed countries as information about the health risk of smoking spread and as public health authorities convinced governments to enact stricter tobacco control laws.

The smoking behavior of both men and women were also subject to changes in cigarette prices and overall economic growth. To give historical context, Fig. 1.2 plots the average price of Swiss brand cigarettes from 1958 to 2015 and per-capita GDP from 1920 to 2015. To put these series on a comparable scale, I plot each series relative to its level in 1958.

From 1958 until the 1990s relative cigarette prices were either constant or generally falling while real per capita GDP grew much faster than the price of a pack of cigarettes. This period coincides with the increasing smoking rates among Swiss women and with their increased labor force participation rate. From 1993 until 2000, cigarette prices increased faster than per capita GDP. After 2001, cigarette prices rose at about the same rate as per capita GDP.

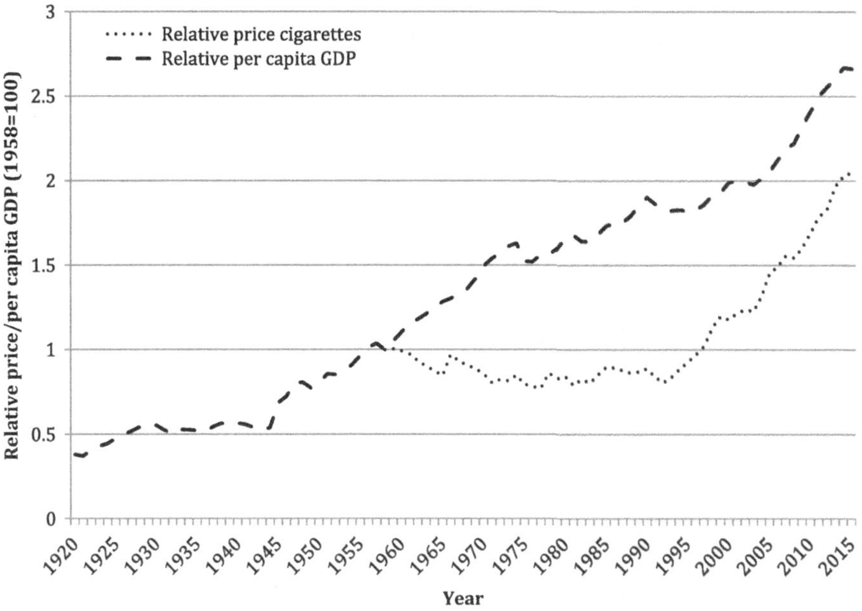

Fig. 1.2 Average cigarette price (1958–2015) and per-capita GDP (1920–2015), by year

Cohort and Gender Differences

Figure 1.3 presents these data in a way that more clearly shows that smoking patterns of men and women have been converging in successively younger cohorts. Figure 1.3 lines up each cohort's smoking prevalence rate by chronological age.

Over the course of their lives, Swiss men of different cohorts smoked in broadly similar ways at similar ages but, as noted above, the oldest cohorts of men smoked more at almost every age. Figure 1.3 shows the less obvious result that this statement is only true from about age 19 onwards. Up until age 19, the oldest cohorts of men smoked less at every age than did the men in cohorts that followed them.

The opening of Switzerland to more competition offers a plausible explanation for both the rising rate of female smoking and the increasing rates of smoking at younger ages. Recall that the signing of free trade agreements by Switzerland caused advertising of cigarettes to increase. While not a causal explanation, increased exposure to advertising is a possible factor that might explain both changes in observed smoking patterns of these cohorts.

Figure 1.3 also makes more clear the more or less monotonic reduction in smoking at every age for men and the up and down pattern of smoking participation for women. Women in the oldest cohort smoked less at every age than did women of successive cohorts. As observed above, smoking among Swiss women peaked for women in the middle cohorts. Importantly, Fig. 1.3 clearly shows that the middle cohorts smoked more than the older and younger cohorts at every age. Figure 1.3

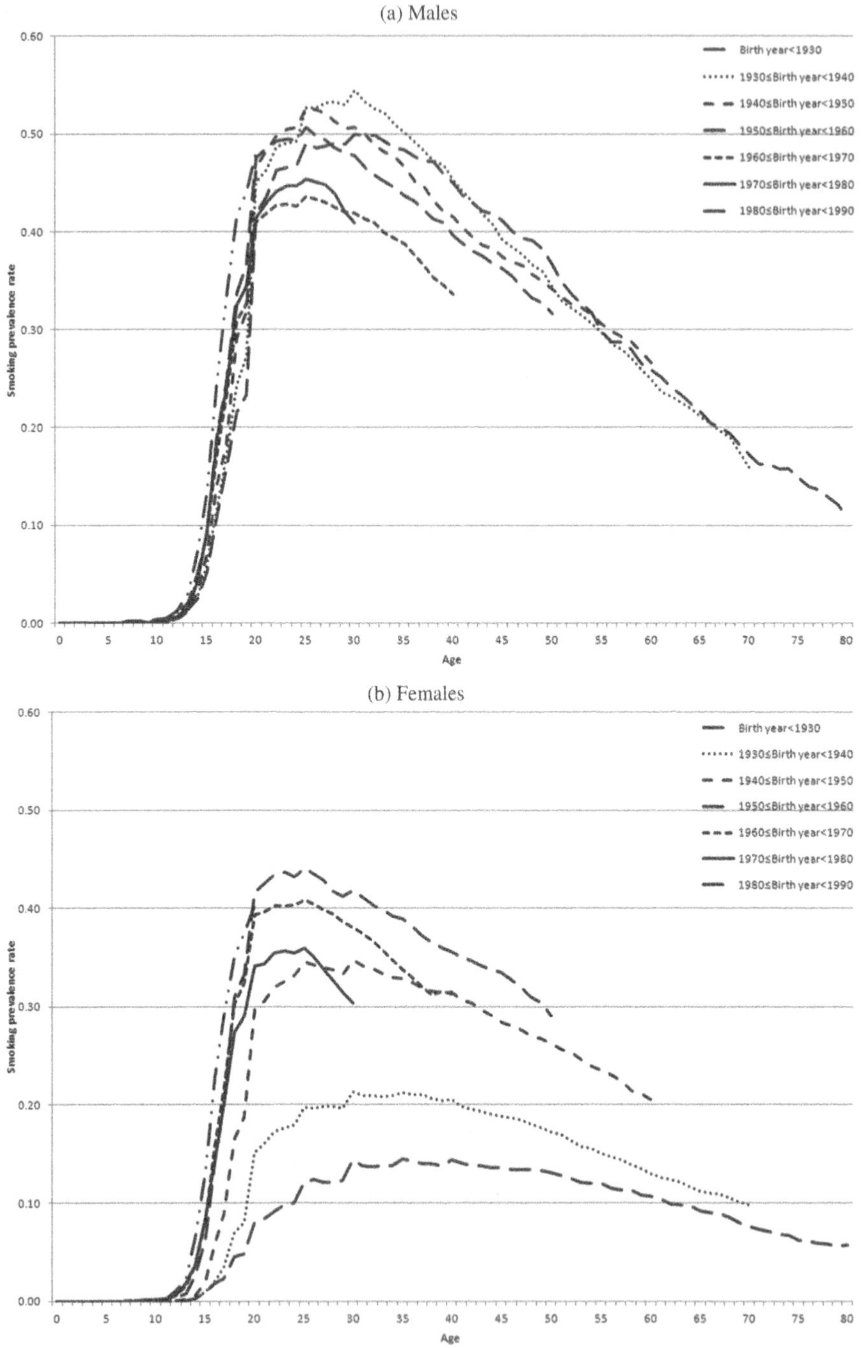

Fig. 1.3 Smoking prevalence rate by age, gender, and birth cohort (*Source*: Swiss Health Survey 2007 and Swiss Household Panel 2011)

also points to the way in which they differ because the right tail of each cohort's smoking trajectories remain more or less parallel. Because they are roughly parallel, women in each cohort were quitting smoking at about the same rate. The perhaps surprising conclusion suggests that these middle cohorts of Swiss women faced conditions that affected their initiation behavior but not their quitting behavior. Certainly, as with men, smoking became more prevalent at younger ages in successive cohorts.

In Table 1.1, I present six summary measures of smoking behavior that expose differences in smoking behavior of different cohorts that are less easy to notice in the above plot. For each gender and cohort, I list the peak smoking prevalence rate, the number of cigarettes smoked on the average day (during the time a person smoked), the number of years smoked, the age the cohort reached its peak smoking prevalence, the age current and former smokers started, and the age ex-smokers quit. One can directly compare, across gender and cohorts, the peak prevalence rate, average cigarette consumption, age at peak smoking prevalence, and the average start age. But one cannot directly compare smoking duration and quit age of men and women from a given cohort because we observe each cohort from birth until the time of interview and not from birth until death.

The comparisons reveal interesting patterns. Not only did more men smoke in the older cohorts, those who smoked also smoked more cigarettes on the average day. Consumption in the older cohorts averaged about a pack of cigarettes per day. And while a high share of men and women in the youngest cohort are smokers, they smoke the fewest cigarettes per day of any cohort. In every cohort, women were smoking fewer cigarettes per day than did their male counterparts.

One can also characterize a cohort's smoking behavior by the age at which smoking prevalence reached its peak. Peak rates of smoking occurred at older ages in the oldest cohorts (age 33 and 40 for men and women respectively). While men's age of peak smoking prevalence stabilized at around 25 or 26 in all but the youngest cohort, women's age of peak smoking prevalence declined. In the older cohorts, women started smoking at older ages than did their male counterparts.

At the same time, women's smoking patterns increasingly resembled those of men. In practically every cohort, men and women quit at similar ages and smoked for about the same number of years in every cohort. In the youngest cohort, men and women's smoking patterns are practically indistinguishable from each other.

Figure 1.4 more starkly highlights similarities and differences in smoking behavior of Swiss men and women. In each panel, I use the data reported in Table 1.1. I plot the statistic for men relative to the corresponding statistic for women. Figure 1.4 more clearly shows that men and women in each birth cohort smoked about the same number of years and quit at about the same ages. As noted before, women in older cohorts started later than their male counterparts and these older cohorts reached their peak smoking prevalence rate when they were older.

On each of these six measures of smoking behavior, younger cohorts of Swiss women increasingly behave like Swiss men. Only in two dimensions to women still differ markedly from men. Even in the younger cohorts it is still the case that more men than women smoke and they smoke more cigarettes on the average day. But the trends converge.

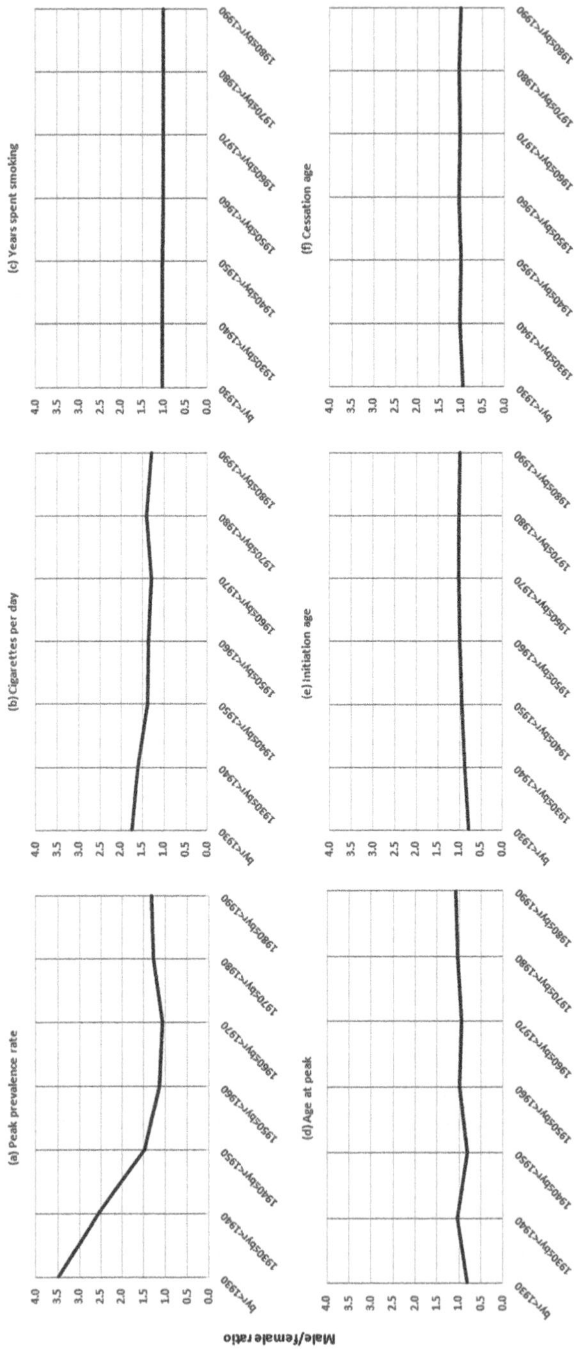

Fig. 1.4 Male/female ratio of smoking indicators, by birth years (*Source*: Swiss Health Survey 2007 and Swiss Household Panel 2011)

Conclusion

Smoking behavior of Swiss men and women resembles some of the patterns one observes in other developed economies but also follows some patterns that differ. As in the other countries, smoking patterns of Swiss men and women have converged so that smoking behavior of men and women in the youngest cohorts are increasingly the same. But the regulatory environment in Switzerland is in many ways less active than in other countries. Switzerland only recently enacted its first public smoking bans. Switzerland also has a relatively long history of collaboration between a domestic tobacco industry and the government. It may be that the patterns shown above echo some of the legacy of that history. These patterns suggest that there are systematic influences on smoking behavior that remain to be modeled to explain what caused the behavioral changes discussed in this chapter and when and how these changes occurred.

References

Burrus, L. (1972). *Le rôle du tabac en Suisse au XXe siècle. Société coopérative pour l'achat du tabac indigène (Suisse) (SOTA)*. Lausanne: SOTA.

Christopoulou, R., Han, J., Jaber, A., & Lillard, D. (2011). Dying for a smoke: How much does differential mortality of smokers affect estimated life-course smoking prevalence? *Preventive Medicine, 52*, 66–70.

Cornuz, J., Burnand, B., Kawachi, I., Gutzwiller, F., & Paccaud, F. (1996). Why did Swiss citizens refuse to ban tobacco advertising? *Tobacco Control, 5*, 149–153.

Curtin, F., Morabia, A., & Bernstein, M. (1997). Smoking behavior in a Swiss urban population: The role of gender and education. *Preventive Medicine, 26*, 658–663.

Durham, A. D., Diethelm, P., & Cornuz, J. (2014). Why did Swiss citizens refuse a comprehensive second-hand smoke ban? *Swiss Medical Weekly, 144*, w13983. http://www.smw.ch/content/smw-2014-13983/.

Eschleman, H. F. (1917). *Historic background and annals of the Swiss and German pioneer settlers of southeastern Pennsylvania, and of their remote ancestors, from the middle of the Dark Ages, down to the time of the Revolutionary War; an authentic history from original sources ... with particular reference to the German-Swiss Mennonites or Anabaptists, the Amish and other nonresistant sects*. Published 2006. Baltimore: Genealogical Publishing Company.

Grellet, P. (1954). *The Cultivation of Tobacco in Switzerland. 25th Anniversary SOTA, Co-operative Society for the Purchas of Swiss Home-Grown Tobacc, 1930–1954*. Balerna: SOTA.

Grenat, P., & de Lavallaz, J. (1904). *Histoire moderne du Valais : de 1536 à 1815*. Geneva: V. Pashe.

Holly, A., Gardiol, L., Zurn, P., & Levi F. G. (1999). *Die Beziehung(en) zwischen Tabakkonsum und Tabaksteuer - Verschiedene Szenarien. Zusammenfassung des Endberichts*. (The relationship(s) between tobacco consumption and tobacco tax - various scenarios. Summary of the final report). Lausanne: Institut d'économie et management de la santé (IEMS). Université de Lausanne; 1999.08.20.

International Labour Organization. (2014). *Employment statistical update: Tobacco sector*. Geneva: Sectoral Policies Department, International Labour Office. http://www.ilo.org/wcmsp5/groups/public/---ed_dialogue/---sector/documents/publication/wcms_329284.pdf

Isenring P. (1976). *Switzerland - Initiative by the Templerence Society for total advertising ban on alcohol and tobacco products*. Inter-office correspondence. Lausanne: Philip Morris Europe, Middle East, Africa; 1976.07.09. Accessed: 2000.01.05. Bates Number: 2024273392_3393. www.pmdocs.com/cgi-bin/rsasearch.asp

Jaberg, S, Kern, T. (2016). *Swiss tobacco fields*. Smoke Signals, swissinfo.ch accessed 10/15/2016. http://www.swissinfo.ch/eng/smoke-signals_swiss-tobacco-fields/40791130
Jakob, J., Cornuz, J., & Diethelm, P. (2017). Prevalence of tobacco smoking in Switzerland: Do reported numbers underestimate reality? *Swiss Medical Weekly, 147*, w14437. https://doi.org/10.4414/smw.2017.14437.
Lee, C., & Glantz, S. A. (2001, January). *The tobacco industry's successful efforts to control tobacco policy making in Switzerland*. Unpublished manuscript. San Francisco: University of California.
Lillard, D. R., & Christopoulou, R. (Eds.). (2015). *Life-course smoking behavior: Patterns and national context in ten countries*. Oxford: Oxford University Press.
Lillard, D. R., & Dorofeeva, Z. (2015). Smoking in Russia and Ukraine before, during, and after the Soviet Union. In D. R. Lillard & R. Christopoulou (Eds.), *Life-course smoking behavior: Patterns and National Context in ten countries* (pp. 117–140). New York: Oxford University Press.
Macgregor, J. (1847). *Commercial statistics* (Vol. III). London: Whittaker and Co.
Marti, J. (2014). The impact of tobacco control expenditures on smoking initiation and cessation. *Health Economics, 23*, 1397–1410.
Morabia, A., Costanza, M. C., Bernstein, M. S., & Rielle, J. (2002). Ages at initiation of cigarette smoking and quit attempts among women: A generation effect. *American Journal of Public Health, 92*(1), 71–74.
Önder, Z. (2015). Smoking in Turkey. In D. R. Lillard & R. Christopoulou (Eds.), *Life-course smoking behavior: Patterns and national Context in ten countries* (pp. 141–153). New York: Oxford University Press.
Pignat, R. (1981). *Le tabac dans la vallée du Rhône de 1700 à 1981*. l'Imprimerie Pillet à Martigny.
Rajkumar, S., Khanh Huynh, C., Bauer, G. F., Hoffmann, S., & Röösli, M. (2013). Impact of a smoking ban in hospitality venues on second hand smoke exposure: a comparison of exposure assessment methods. *BMC Public Health, 13*, 536. https://doi.org/10.1186/1471-2458-13-536.
Smedberg, J., Lupattelli, A., Mårdby, A., & Nordeng, H. (2014). Characteristics of women who continue smoking during pregnancy: A cross-sectional study of pregnant women and new mothers in 15 European countries. *BMC Pregnancy and Childbirth, 14*, 213. http://www.biomedcentral.com/1471-2393/14/213.
Swiss Federal Office of Health. (2009). *Passivrauchen* (in German, French, and Italian). Retrieved 29 June 2009.
World health Organization (WHO). (2015). *WHO report on the global tobacco epidemic, 2015: Raising taxes on tobacco*. Geneva, Switzerland. Available from: http://www.who.int/tobacco/global_report/2015/report/en/

Chapter 2
Body Mass Index and Satisfaction with Health in Contemporary Switzerland

Mario Lucchini and Sara Della Bella

Introduction

According to the World Health Organization (WHO 2016), worldwide the prevalence of obesity has more than doubled since 1980 and in 2014 600 million people were obese. In many countries, childhood obesity is increasing at an even higher rate than adult obesity, what would probably lead to a further increase in the prevalence of obesity, given that obese children are more likely to become obese adults (Singh et al. 2008; Reilly and Kelly 2011).

In Switzerland obesity rates are low compare to most OECD countries, but they have increased significantly in the last twenty years: in 1992, 31.3% of the Swiss population was overweight or obese, and this increased to 41,2 % in 2012 (Schneider and Venetz 2014). According to the most recent estimates of the Swiss Survey on Health, in 2012 41% of the Swiss population aged over 15 years appear to be overweight or obese (Federal Office of Public Health (FOPH) 2014).

Obesity, defined as excessive body fat and typically measured using the Body Mass Index (BMI) (WHO 2016), can impair health. There is robust evidence suggesting that obesity is an important risk factors for a set of health problems and diseases such as diabetes, cardiovascular diseases, hypertension, respiratory problems, musculoskeletal diseases and some forms of cancer (Hu 2008; WHO 2016;

M. Lucchini (✉)
Department of Sociology and Social Research, University of Milan-Bicocca, Milan, Italy

Department of Business Economics, Health and Social Care, SUPSI (University of Applied Sciences and Arts of Southern Switzerland), Manno, Switzerland
e-mail: mario.lucchini@unimib.it

S. Della Bella
Department of Business Economics, Health and Social Care, SUPSI (University of Applied Sciences and Arts of Southern Switzerland), Manno, Switzerland
e-mail: sara.dellabella@supsi.ch

R. Tillmann et al. (eds.), *Social Dynamics in Swiss Society*, Life Course Research and Social Policies 9, https://doi.org/10.1007/978-3-319-89557-4_2

Imai et al. 2008). Interestingly, the link between obesity and health has been confirmed in studies using a variety of different health indicators, such as measures of health related quality of life (Garner et al. 2011; Ford et al. 2001), measures of functional health (Ford et al. 2001; Imai et al. 2008) or self-assessed health (Cullinan and Gillespie 2016; Imai et al. 2008). Obesity has also been associated with poor mental health and depression (Ford et al. 2001; Imai et al. 2008; Luppino et al. 2010) and this is not surprising given the fact that obese person tend to suffer from prejudices and discrimination in several life domains and might suffer from low self-esteem (Puhl and Heuer 2009). Weight-related stigma seems to be particularly relevant for women, who tend to suffer the most from being obese and are more discriminated than their male counterparts (Puhl and Heuer 2009; Puhl and Brownell 2003; Hebl and Turchin 2005; Wadsworth and Pendergast 2014). These cultural reasons, together with possible physiological reasons, might explain why in some studies obesity appears to have worse health related consequences for women rather than for men (Garner et al. 2012; Wang et al. 2012).

Overweight, concof the Swiss population was overweight or obese,erning around 1,8 billion adults worldwide (WHO 2016), has also been linked to health-related conditions, but the evidence is more mixed and, in the majority of studies, overweight does not appear to increase mortality risk (rather, some studies suggested a protective role of overweight, at least in men and in the elderly) (Cullinan and Gillespie 2016; Garner et al. 2012; Lantz et al. 2010; Berrington de Gonzalez et al 2010; Flegal et al. 2007; Imai et al. 2008).

The relationship between BMI and health, hence, does not seem to be a strictly linear one. This is particularly so because several studies reported underweight to be a risk factor for health and premature mortality as well (Garner et al. 2012; Flegal et al. 2007; Imai et al. 2008; Ford et al. 2001). Again, this relationship seems to vary across age categories and gender: for instance, Garner et al. (2012) found underweight to be protective in terms of health related quality of life for young women. Despite the great deal of evidence about the link between obesity/BMI and health, the causal nature of this relationship is still disputed. There is a huge literature -comprising observational, intervention and genetic epidemiological studies using mendelian randomization (MR) - that has investigated this issue (Corbin and Timpson 2016). Every approach presents some limits in its ability to assess the causal link between obesity (or BMI) and health outcomes (confounding bias, reversed causality) and even the instrumental variable approach can be criticized because it ultimately relies on assumptions that are difficult to test (Cameron and Trivedi 2009). Moreover, results are mixed, though some MR studies (in which genetic variation is used as an instrumental variable) have found evidence of causal effects of obesity on several physical and mental health outcomes (Corbin and Timpson 2016).

This study specifically focuses on the relationship between BMI and satisfaction with health. Satisfaction with health belongs to the group of subjective measures of health that can encompass aspects of both physical and mental health, reflecting a complex process of internalized reckoning. In the health literature subjective measures of health, such as Self-Assessed Health (SAH), are widely used. Despite being a very simple measure of health, SAH is extremely powerful and appears to be related to several objective measures of health, such as morbidity and functional limitations, and it is able to predict mortality above and beyond the individual objective health status (Benyamini 2011; Benjamins et al. 2004; Idler and Benyamini 1997; Jylha 2009). The negative association between obesity and SAH has been found to hold true for adults as well as for adolescents (Imai et al. 2008; Krause and Lampert 2015; Vingilis et al. 2002), and in several countries, like Switzerland, Ireland and the USA (Cullinan and Gillespie 2016; Prosper et al. 2009; Marques-Vidal et al. 2012). However, this relationship has not been found in countries such as Portugal and Greece (Darviri et al. 2012; Marques-Vidal et al. 2012) and in specific subpopulations such as Latino immigrants living in the USA (Macmillan et al. 2011).

Moreover, the association of BMI with SAH appears to vary significantly across ages and sexes (Imai et al. 2008), although not in all studies: for instance, Cullinan and Gillespie (2016) did not find substantial differences among genders concerning the impact of obesity on SAH.

Variation in results might reflect real differences, due to the specific population under study and its cultural specificities. However, methodological shortcomings might also be partly responsible for mixed findings. Indeed, previous studies in this field have mostly used cross-sectional data and were not able to adequately control for potential confounders. One notable exception is the study by Cullinan and Gillespie (2016) who adopted the instrumental variable approach to assess the effect of obesity and overweight (underweight was not considered) on SAH in a nationally representative sample of Irish people. The authors concluded that obesity (and particularly severe obesity) negatively impacts SAH, whereas overweight does not seem to affect SAH.

The present study aimed to investigate the relationship between BMI and satisfaction with health in Switzerland, using longitudinal studies and applying panel data regression models that partly allow to control for unobserved heterogeneity.

Data and Variables

For our analysis we used data from the Swiss Household Panel (SHP), a representative longitudinal study of household and individuals, supported by the Swiss National Science Foundation, which began in 1999 with a sample of 5074 households containing 12,931 household members.[1] More precisely, we used the eleven waves from 2004 to 2014. We selected 103,861 observations nested into 22,815 individuals, aged 18–75. The dependent variable — satisfaction with health— was measured on a scale ranging from 0 (not at all satisfied) to 10 (completely satisfied). Despite its ordinal nature, following Ferrer-i-Carbonell and Frijters (2004) we considered satisfaction with health as a cardinal variable in order to facilitate

[1] http://forscenter.ch/en/our-surveys/swiss-household-panel/

interpretation of the estimated parameters. Our main focus was BMI that was coded into five categories, according to the thresholds set by the World Health Organization, as follows: underweight (BMI < 18.50), normal weight (BMI > 18.50 to 24.99), overweight (BMI >24.99 to 29.99), obesity class I (BMI >29.99 to 34.99), obesity class II and III (BMI > 34.99), also called "severe obesity". In the regression models, normal weight was the category of reference.

All models included a set of control variables, that have been proven to affect health and, in many cases, BMI as well: age, age squared, gender, a set of social relationship indicators such as civil status dummies (single, married, separated, divorced, widow), number of children in the family, size of household, death of closely related person (dummy), termination of close relationship (dummy), conflicts with or among related persons (dummy) (Umberson and Karas Montez 2010; Umberson et al. 2006); social status indicators such as the logarithm of net total annual household income, work status (employed, unemployed, not in labour force), and education dummies (less than secondary education, secondary education, tertiary education) (Marmot and Wilkinson 2006; McLaren 2007), physical activity (dummy) (Wanner et al. 2017), regional dummies (Lake Geneva, Middleland, North-West Switzerland, Zurich, East Switzerland, Central Switzerland, Ticino) (Ogna et al. 2014) and wave dummies (2004–2014). Since previous studies found gender differences in the association between self-rated health and BMI, descriptive analysis (see Table 2.1) and regression models (see Table 2.2) were carried out separately for men and women.

Table 2.1 Descriptive statistics: within and between variance of the main variables of interests (male sample: n. 7151, N.29,953; female sample: n.8142, N.35,889)

	Male			Female		
Variable		Mean	Std. Dev.		Mean	Std. Dev.
Self-assessed health	Overall	7.916419	1.669599	Overall	7.825406	1.824892
	Between		1.524697	Between		1.688332
	Within		0.9813426	Within		1.082382
BMI <18.50	Overall	0.0091811	0.0953785	Overall	0.0528853	0.2238076
	Between		0.0922419	Between		0.2174079
	Within		0.0521687	Within		0.1092517
BMI 18.50–24.99 cat.ref.	Overall	0.5115347	0.4998753	Overall	0.6416172	0.479532
	Between		0.47195	Between		0.4471349
	Within		0.2135785	Within		0.2200133
BMI 25.00–29.99	Overall	0.3804293	0.4855005	Overall	0.2185071	0.413239
	Between		0.4457702	Between		0.3687357
	Within		0.2413439	Within		0.2241873
BMI 30.00–34.99	Overall	0.0799252	0.2711819	Overall	0.0674023	0.2507209
	Between		0.245902	Between		0.224003
	Within		0.1424698	Within		0.1383976
BMI > 34.99	Overall	0.0189297	0.1362789	Overall	0.0195882	0.1385822
	Between		0.1226754	Between		0.1332532
	Within		0.065176	Within		0.066268

Table 2.2 OLS, Random (RE) and Fixed (FE) effects of BMI on satisfaction with health: results reported separately for men and women

	OLS male	OLS female	RE male	RE female	FE male	FE female
BMI 18.50–24.99 (ref. cat.)						
BMI <18.50	−0.339	−0.195*	−0.256*	−0.136*	−0.187	−0.157*
	(0.19)	(0.09)	(0.12)	(0.05)	(0.13)	(0.06)
BMI 25.00–29.99	−0.173***	−0.364***	−0.085**	−0.234***	0.015	−0.088*
	(0.04)	(0.04)	(0.03)	(0.03)	(0.04)	(0.04)
BMI 30.00–34.99	−0.438***	−0.676***	−0.332***	−0.497***	−0.087	−0.237**
	(0.07)	(0.07)	(0.05)	(0.05)	(0.07)	(0.07)
BMI > 34.99	−0.791***	−1.002***	−0.565***	−0.865***	−0.211	−0.521***
	(0.15)	(0.12)	(0.11)	(0.11)	(0.15)	(0.16)
Age	−0.078***	−0.054***	−0.061***	−0.046***	−0.083***	−0.237
	(0.01)	(0.01)	(0.01)	(0.01)	(0.02)	(0.55)
Age squared	0.001***	0.001***	0.001***	0.000***	0.000	0.000*
	(0.00)	(0.00)	(0.00)	(0.00)	(0.00)	(0.00)
Single (ref. cat)						
Married	0.076	0.140*	0.056	0.208***	−0.067	0.231**
	(0.06)	(0.06)	(0.05)	(0.05)	(0.07)	(0.07)
Separated	−0.055	0.092	−0.024	0.102	−0.143	0.226
	(0.15)	(0.14)	(0.10)	(0.10)	(0.13)	(0.13)
Divorced	−0.016	−0.100	−0.024	0.019	−0.092	0.287**
	(0.09)	(0.08)	(0.08)	(0.07)	(0.12)	(0.11)
Widower/widow	0.043	0.125	−0.049	0.110	0.053	0.100
	(0.19)	(0.11)	(0.14)	(0.10)	(0.18)	(0.16)
Family size	0.042	0.049	−0.026	0.046*	−0.089**	0.018
	(0.03)	(0.03)	(0.02)	(0.02)	(0.03)	(0.03)

(continued)

Table 2.2 (continued)

	OLS male	OLS female	RE male	RE female	FE male	FE female
n. of children	0.007	0.033	0.049	−0.024	0.079*	−0.036
	(0.04)	(0.03)	(0.03)	(0.02)	(0.03)	(0.03)
Primary educ. (ref. cat.)						
Secondary educ.	0.140*	0.247***	0.225***	0.281***	0.187**	0.113
	(0.07)	(0.06)	(0.05)	(0.05)	(0.07)	(0.07)
Tertiary educ.	0.155*	0.235**	0.298***	0.281***	0.260**	0.067
	(0.07)	(0.07)	(0.06)	(0.06)	(0.09)	(0.10)
Employed (ref.cat.)						
Unemployed	−0.340**	−0.223**	−0.016	−0.051	0.144	0.014
	(0.11)	(0.08)	(0.08)	(0.07)	(0.09)	(0.07)
Not in labor force	−0.606***	−0.375***	−0.291***	−0.168***	−0.151***	−0.077*
	(0.07)	(0.05)	(0.04)	(0.03)	(0.04)	(0.03)
Log_household_equiv_income	0.099**	0.126***	0.042	0.060**	−0.008	0.014
	(0.03)	(0.03)	(0.02)	(0.02)	(0.02)	(0.02)
Physical activity	0.418***	0.332***	0.258***	0.208***	0.195***	0.160***
	(0.04)	(0.03)	(0.02)	(0.02)	(0.03)	(0.02)
Death of closely related person	−0.117***	−0.144***	−0.064***	−0.068***	−0.054**	−0.054**
	(0.02)	(0.02)	(0.02)	(0.02)	(0.02)	(0.02)
Termination of close relationship	−0.159***	−0.225***	−0.065	−0.126***	−0.037	−0.093**
	(0.05)	(0.05)	(0.04)	(0.03)	(0.04)	(0.04)
Conflicts with or among related persons	−0.396***	−0.406***	−0.133***	−0.182***	−0.038	−0.117***
	(0.05)	(0.04)	(0.03)	(0.03)	(0.03)	(0.03)
Swiss nationality	0.089	0.275***	0.091	0.245***	−0.162	0.104
	(0.07)	(0.06)	(0.06)	(0.06)	(0.23)	(0.19)

Region						
Lake Geneva (ref.cat.)						
Middleland	0.078	0.007	0.034	0.011	−0.172	0.071
	(0.06)	(0.06)	(0.05)	(0.05)	(0.21)	(0.17)
North-west Switzerland	0.000	0.090	−0.066	0.056	−0.533*	−0.014
	(0.07)	(0.07)	(0.06)	(0.06)	(0.23)	(0.24)
Zurich	−0.058	−0.046	−0.063	−0.040	−0.432	−0.039
	(0.07)	(0.06)	(0.06)	(0.06)	(0.23)	(0.23)
East Switzerland	0.141	0.139	0.097	0.088	−0.475	0.057
	(0.07)	(0.08)	(0.06)	(0.07)	(0.25)	(0.29)
Central Switzerland	−0.005	0.065	0.025	0.114	−0.132	0.156
	(0.08)	(0.07)	(0.07)	(0.07)	(0.26)	(0.28)
Ticino	0.396***	0.196	0.259*	0.098	−0.156	−0.592*
	(0.12)	(0.13)	(0.10)	(0.11)	(0.32)	(0.27)
Constant	8.379***	7.428***	8.906***	8.131***	11.597***	16.959
	(0.42)	(0.38)	(0.28)	(0.27)	(0.51)	(22.93)
n.observations	29.923	35.852	29.923	35.852	29.923	35.852
n.of groups			7.150	8.137	7.150	8.137
R-sq: within			0.0247	0.0251	0.0292	0.0280
R-sq: between			0.0728	0.0846	0.0252	0.0234
R-sq: overall	0.0704	0.0803	0.0596	0.0728	0.0175	0.0171

* $p < 0.05$; ** $p < 0.01$
Note: All models are controlled for year dummies

Analytic Strategies

In order to investigate the existence and the nature of the relationship between health and BMI categories, we adopted different analytical strategies, with the aim of exploiting the strength of panel data and understanding to which extend unobserved individual heterogeneity could introduce a bias in the parameter estimates. More precisely, we estimated three types of regression models —pooled OLS, random effect (RE) and fixed effect (FE) models— as follows:

$$SWH_{it} = \sum_{k=1}^{K} \beta_k X_{it} + \sum_{q=1}^{Q} \gamma_q Z_{it} + \sum_{r=1}^{R} \delta_r W_i + \alpha_i + \psi_t + \varepsilon_{it}$$

Where SWH_{it} was the satisfaction with health score of respondent i at time t; X_{it} was a vector of K time-varying BMI dummies; Z_{it} and W_i represented, respectively, a vector of Q time-varying and R time-constant characteristics, that we considered as control variables. Finally, α_i was a time-invariant individual-specific effect; ψ_t corresponded to wave effects and ε_{it} was the idiosyncratic error term.

Firstly, we estimated OLS pooled regression models with clustered standard errors and subsequently random effect models (RE) that enabled us to study the effect of both time-constant and time-varying covariates. These analytical strategies allowed us to take into account differences across individuals and to control for time invariant variables. It is important to underline that since BMI is an endogenous variable, these models would give biased results, as they unrealistically assume the causal variable to be uncorrelated with the error term (Cameron and Trivedi 2009).

If variables of interest showed enough intra-individual variation, fixed effect models (FE) were also implemented. FE yields an unbiased estimate of the causal parameter by erasing the influence of time constant unobserved variables (Cameron and Trivedi 2009). This means that this estimation method allowed us to control for crucial unobservable differences in time constant individual characteristics like personality, dispositions or genetic traits that are known to be important determinants of satisfaction with health. In order to test if RE was more appropriate than FE, or vice versa, we ran a Hausman Test.

Empirical Results

Effects of BMI on satisfaction with health, obtained by applying OLS, RE and FE estimators, are reported in Table 2.2.

Overall, we could see that the sign of the coefficients were consistent and in line with the literature, although, as expected, there appeared to be a shrink in the size of estimates moving from the OLS to RE and from RE to the FE specifications.

The OLS estimates suggest that individuals with normal weight enjoyed a better health status than individuals belonging to others categories. Those with the lowest level of satisfaction with health were severely obese individuals (i.e. obesity class II and III), followed by obese individuals (obesity class I) and overweight individuals. This appeared to be true for both men and women, though these effects appeared to be more pronounced among women. Indeed, among men severe obesity reduced satisfaction with health by 0.791 points (on a 10 point-scale), among women the reduction reached 1 point.

Overweight also appeared to decrease the level of satisfaction with health, and particularly so for women. Being underweight was also associated with lower levels of satisfaction with health, but the coefficient for men did not reach statistical significance and it was only significant at the 1% level in women.

Looking at the OLS estimates for the chosen control variables, we could see that getting married (for women), secondary and tertiary education, family income, physical activity, Swiss nationality (for women) and living in Ticino (for men) were positively associated with satisfaction with health. On the contrary, ageing, getting married (for women) unemployment, inactivity, the death of a closely related person, the termination of a close relationship, the conflicts with or among related persons were negatively correlated with satisfaction with health.

RE estimates tell us roughly the same story, even though it is important to emphasize a remarkable reduction in the size of the parameter estimates. More precisely, the negative effect of obesity class II and III decreased from −0.791 to −0.565 in the male sample and from −1.002 to −0.865 in the female one. For the obesity class I the size of the effect changed from −0.438 to −0.332 for male and from −0.676 to −0.497 for female.

Finally, FE parameter estimates tell us a slightly different story. For men, the effect of the BMI categories decreased in size and lost statistical significance. For women, we observed that the size of the estimates of interest decreased, while maintaining statistical significance. This means that a change in a woman's BMI leads to a change in satisfaction with health, whereas the same conclusion does not apply to men. Women belonging to obesity class II and III showed the lowest level of satisfaction with health (0.521 point less than normal weight woman), followed by women belonging to obesity class I (−0.237), underweight (−0.157) and overweight (−0.088) women. These results might reflect the fact that weight related stigma is stronger for women and obese women tend to suffer more because of their weight status (Puhl and Heuer 2009; Puhl and Brownell 2003; Hebl and Turchin 2005; Wadsworth and Pendergast 2014) and are consistent with what has been found in some studies (Garner et al. 2012; Wang et al. 2012), albeit not in all.

A Hausman model selection test was run in order to understand whether the FE estimator was more efficient than the RE. According to this test, the FE should be preferred over the RE model in that time constant unobserved characteristics were likely to be associated with our BMI dummies.

Overall, these results suggested that, even after controlling for a range of individual, socioeconomic and lifestyle related variables, departures from normal weight had statistically significant negative impact on women's satisfaction with health. More precisely, we could see a dose-response relationship, whereby being obese had a stronger negative effect than being overweight and being severely obese had a stronger effect than being obese. The effect of underweight on women's satisfaction with health was less pronounced but still statistically significant (in line with results from Imai et al. 2008). Working on Canadian women, Garner et al. (2012) found a protective effect of underweight on women's self-assessed health, at least at younger ages, but this might reflect cultural difference in the value attributed to thinness. This difference could also be due to the fact that FE models applied in this study are not fully able to tackle the issue of reversed causality.

Conclusion

Obesity is an important risk factor for a number of diseases (cardiovascular diseases, type 2 diabetes, hypertension, some cancers, musculoskeletal disorders, etc.) and obese individuals often face discrimination and stigmatization in important domains of life and tend to report lower level of self-esteem and mental health (Hu 2008; WHO 2016; Puhl and Heuer 2009; Hebl and Turchin 2005).

Hence, the association between obesity and subjective measures of health is not surprising, since this kind of subjective measures are likely to capture aspect of both physical and mental health. However, the role of overweight and underweight is less clear and studies investigating the relationship between BMI and health have provided mixed results.

Cultural as well as methodological reasons can explain these differences. The strength of the social penalty associated with overweight and obesity can vary over population sub-groups and across societies. Moreover, previous studies in this field have not generally addressed nor taken into account the issue of endogeneity and reverse causality (with the exception of Cullinan and Gillespie 2016).

In this work, we exploited the power of panel data and appropriate analytic strategies to overcome this limitation. Working with data coming from the Swiss Household Panel (waves 2004–2015), we modelled the relationship between BMI and satisfaction with health using pooled OLS, random effects and fixed effects. Since the impact of BMI has been shown to vary between genders, we estimated separate models for women and men.

Overall, our results confirmed the non-linearity in the relationship between BMI and health.

Estimates from pool OLS and RE models showed that women and men belonging to BMI categories different from normal weight had a significantly lower level of satisfaction with health. These effects were more pronounced for women than for men.

FE estimates —that allow removing the time constant individual heterogeneity— showed that any departures from normal weight appeared to be associated with lower levels of satisfaction with health in women, but not in men. These results support previous findings showing gender differences in the association between BMI and health (Imai et al. 2008; Ford et al. 2001; Garner et al. 2012).

In every model, obese and severely obese individuals appeared to be the ones with the lowest level of satisfaction with health. Given that the prevalence of obesity is rising worldwide, these results calls for action. The pathways through which obesity impacts on health satisfaction need to be further explored. However, gender differences in empirical results suggest that stigma plays a crucial role. Interventions to tackle the stigma issue are needed together with actions to counteract the obesity epidemic.

References

Benjamins, M. R., Hummer, R. A., Eberstein, I., & Nam, C. B. (2004). Self-reported health and adult mortality risk: An analysis of cause-specific mortality. *Social Science & Medicine, 59*, 1297–1306.

Benyamini, Y. (2011). Why does self-rated health predict mortality? An update on current knowledge and a research agenda for psychologist. *Psychology & Health, 26*, 1407–1413.

Berrington de Gonzalez, A., Hartge, P., Cerhan, J. R., Flint, A. J., Hannan, L., & MacInnis, R. J. (2010). Body-mass index and mortality among 1.46 million white adults. *The New England Journal of Medicine, 363*(23), 2211–2219.

Cameron, C., & Trivedi, P. K. (2009). *Microeconometrics using stata*. College Station: Stata Press.

Corbin, L. J., & Timpson, N. J. (2016). Body mass index: Has epidemiology started to break down causal contributions to health and disease? *Obesity, 24*, 1630–1638. https://doi.org/10.1002/oby.21554.

Cullinan, J., & Gillespie, P. (2016). Does overweight and obesity impact on self-rated health? Evidence using instrumental variables ordered Probit models. *Health Economics, 25*(10), 1341–1348.

Darviri, C., Fouka, G., Gnardellis, C., Artemiadis, A. K., Tigani, X., & Alexopoulos, E. C. (2012). Determinants of self-rated health in a representative sample of a rural population: A cross-sectional study in Greece. *International Journal of Environmental Research and Public Health, 9*(3), 943–954.

Ferrer-i-Carbonell, A., & Frijters, P. (2004). How important is methodology for the estimates of the determinants of happiness? *The Economic Journal, 114*, 641–659.

Flegal, K. M., Graubard, B. I., Williamson, D. F., & Gail, M. H. (2007). Cause-specific excess deaths associated with underweight, overweight, and obesity. *The Journal of the American Medical Association, 298*(17), 2028–2037.

Ford, E. S., Moriarty, D. G., Zack, M. M., Mokdad, A. H., & Chapman, D. P. (2001). Self-reported body mass index and health-related quality of life: Findings from the behavioral risk factor surveillance system. *Obesity Research, 9*(1), 21–31.

Garner, R. E., Feeny, D. H., Thompson, A., Bernier, J., McFarland, B. H., Huguet, N., Kaplan, M. S., Orpana, H., Ross, N. A., & Blanchard, C. (2012). Bodyweight, gender, and quality of life: A population-based longitudinal study. *Quality of Life Research, 21*(5), 813–825.

Hebl, M. R., & Turchin, J. M. (2005). The stigma of obesity: What about men? *Basic Applied Social Psychology, 27*(3), 267–275.

Hu, F. B. (2008). *Obesity epidemiology*. New York: Oxford University Press.

Idler, E. L., & Benyamini, Y. (1997). Self-rated health and mortality: A review of twenty-seven community studies. *Journal of Health and Social Behavior, 38*, 21–37.

Imai, K., Gregg, E. W., Chen, Y. J., Zhang, P., de Rekeneire, N., & Williamson, D. F. (2008). The association of BMI with functional status and self-rated health in US adults. *Obesity, 16*(2), 402–408.

Jylha, M. (2009). What is self-rated health and why does it predict mortality? Towards a unified conceptual model. *Social Science and Medicine, 69*, 307–316.

Krause, L., & Lampert, T. (2015). Relation between overweight/obesity and self-rated health among adolescents in Germany. Do socio-economic status and type of school have an impact on that relation? *International Journal of Environmental Research and Public Health, 12*(2), 2262–2276.

Lantz, P. M., Golberstein, E., House, J. S., & Morenoff, J. (2010). Socioeconomic and behavioral risk factors for mortality in a national 19-year prospective study of U.S. adults. *Social Science & Medicine, 70*(10), 1558–1566.

Luppino, F. S., de Wit, L. M., Bouvy, P. F., Stijnen, T., Cuijpers, P., Penninx, B. W., & Zitman, F. G. (2010). Overweight, obesity, and depression: A systematic review and meta-analysis of longitudinal studies. *Archives of General Psychiatry, 67*(3), 220–229.

Macmillan, R., Duke, N., Oakes, J. M., & Liao, W. (2011). Trends in the association of obesity and self-reported overall health in 30 years of the integrated health interview series. *Obesity, 19*(5), 1103–1105.

Marmot, M., & Wilkinson, R. (Eds.). (2006). *Social determinants of health*. New York: Oxford University Press.

Marques-Vidal, P., Ravasco, P., & Paccaud, F. (2012). Differing trends in the association between obesity and self-reported health in Portugal and Switzerland. Data from national health surveys 1992-2007. *BMC Public Health, 12*, 588.

McLaren, L. (2007). Socioeconomic status and obesity. *Epidemiologic Reviews, 29*, 29–48.

Ogna, A., Forni Ogna, V., Bochud, M., Paccaud, F., Gabutti, L., & Burnier, M. (2014). Prevalence of obesity and overweight and associated nutritional factors in a population-based Swiss sample: An opportunity to analyze the impact of three different European cultural roots. *European Journal of Nutrition, 53*(5), 1281–1290.

Prosper, M., Moczulski, V. L., & Qureshi, A. (2009). Obesity as a predictor of self-rated health. *American Journal of Health Behavior, 33*(3), 319–329.

Puhl, R. M., & Brownell, K. D. (2003). Psychological origins of obesity stigma: Toward changing a powerful and pervasive Bias. *Obesity Reviews, 4*, 213–227.

Puhl, R. M., & Heuer, C. A. (2009). The stigma of obesity: A review and update. *Obesity, 17*(5), 941–964.

Reilly, J. J., & Kelly, J. (2011). Long-term impact of overweight and obesity in childhood and adolescence on morbidity and premature mortality in adulthood: Systematic review. *International Journal of Obesity, 35*(7), 891–898.

Schneider, H., & Venetz, W. (2014). Cost of obesity in Switzerland in 2012. Final report. Swiss Federal Office of Public Health.

Singh, A. S., Mulder, C., Twisk, J. W. R., Van Mechelen, W., & Chinapaw, M. J. M. (2008). Tracking of childhood overweight into adulthood: A systematic review of the literature. *Obesity Reviews, 9*(5), 474–488.

Umberson, D., & Karas Montez, J. (2010). Social relationships and health: A flashpoint for health policy. *Journal of Health and Social Behavior, 51*(Suppl), S54–S66.

Umberson, D., Williams, K., Powers, D., Liu, H., & Needham, B. (2006). You make me sick: Marital quality and health over the life course. *Journal of Health and Social Behavior, 47*(1), 1–16.

Vingilis, E. R., Wade, T. J., & Seeley, J. S. (2002). Predictors of adolescent self-rated health. Analysis of the National Population Health Survey. *Canadian Journal of Public Health, 93*(3), 193–197.

Wadsworth, T., & Pendergast, P. M. (2014). Obesity (sometimes) matters: The importance of context in the relationship between obesity and life satisfaction. *Journal of Health and Social Behavior, 55*(2), 196–214.

Wang, R., Wu, M. J., Ma, X. Q., Zhao, Y. F., Yan, X. Y., Gao, Q. B., & He, J. (2012). Body mass index and health-related quality of life in adults: A population based study in five cities of China. *European Journal of Public Health, 22*(4), 497–502.

Wanner, M., Richard, A., Martin, B., Faeh, D., & Rohrmann, S. (2017). Associations between self-reported and objectively measured physical activity, sedentary behavior and overweight/obesity in NHANES 2003–2006. *International Journal of Obesity, 41*(1), 186–193.
World Health Organization (WHO). (2016). *Obesity and overweight*. Fact sheet N.311 Available at http://www.who.int/mediacentre/factsheets/fs31/en/.

Chapter 3
Exploring the Cohabitation Gap in Relationship Dissolution and Health and Wellbeing: A Longitudinal Analysis of Transitions from Cohabitation and Marriage in Switzerland and Australia

Belinda Hewitt, Marieke Voorpostel, and Gavin Turrell

Introduction

A long line of research has found that being married improves health and wellbeing and that marital dissolution negatively impacts health and wellbeing (Gove and Shin 1989; Umberson et al. 2010). Yet, the institution of marriage as the bedrock of family life has declined over the last few decades. Across developed countries, divorce rates remain relatively high and unmarried cohabitation as an alternative or prelude to marriage has increased (Cherlin 2009; Kiernan 2002). The rise of cohabitation as an alternative to marriage raises questions about whether marriage confers greater benefits to health and wellbeing over cohabitation (Musick and Bumpass 2012), which also has implications for the health consequences of relationship dissolution following cohabitation and marriage. Cohabitation may provide many of the same resources as marriage in terms of social support, integration, economies of scale, and lifestyle habits and behaviours, although this may partly depend on the stability and degree of commitment in the cohabiting relationship (Seltzer 2000). Overall,

B. Hewitt (✉)
School of Social and Political Sciences, The University of Melbourne,
Parkville, VIC, Australia
e-mail: belinda.hewitt@unimelb.edu.au

M. Voorpostel
FORS-Swiss Centre of Expertise in the Social Sciences, Lausanne, Switzerland
e-mail: Marieke.voorpostel@fors.unil.ch

G. Turrell
School of Health and Social Development, Deakin University,
Melbourne, VIC, Australia
e-mail: gavin.turrell@acu.edu.au

R. Tillmann et al. (eds.), *Social Dynamics in Swiss Society*, Life Course Research and Social Policies 9, https://doi.org/10.1007/978-3-319-89557-4_3

cohabiting relationships tend to be less stable than marriage (Wiik et al. 2012; Hewitt and Baxter 2015). While a relatively large number of studies examine health differences between married and cohabiting people when they form relationships, much less attention has been paid to comparing the health impacts of relationship dissolution. In this chapter we examine gendered health differences in relationship dissolution, using longitudinal panel data from the Swiss Household Panel Study and the Household, Income and Labour Dynamics in Australia study, enabling a comparison between Switzerland and Australia, two countries that differ in health policy and outcomes as well as in relationship trajectories.

Background

Previous Findings on Union Dissolution and Health

Research consistently shows that married men and women have lower mortality rates and better psychological and physical wellbeing compared with unmarried individuals, and that health and wellbeing decline after divorce (Hewitt et al. 2011; Williams and Umberson 2004). Comparing previously married to married individuals, Hughes and Waite (2009) found that the previously married had worse physical and mental health. However, in their meta-analysis, Luhmann et al. (2012) found little effect of the legal act of divorce itself on positive and negative feelings, but were not able to look at the period preceding the divorce, in which wellbeing may already have declined.

The majority of studies that compare health in cohabiting and married couples have concentrated on health differences as individuals move into or remain in their relationships. The findings of these studies are mixed, but often no differences are found in physical and mental health (Wu et al. 2003; Horowitz and White 1998) or mortality (Lund et al. 2002) of cohabiting versus married people. Gender is at the centre of the debate about the health and wellbeing benefits of marriage. While both men and women have been found to benefit from marriage, on average men have been found to benefit more than women (Williams and Umberson 2004). Some studies on cohabitation show that cohabiting men have better health than women (Aassve et al. 2007).

Few studies have investigated what happens to health when cohabiting and marital relationships end and here the evidence is mixed as well. In a Canadian study, Wu et al. (2003) found no differences in the health consequences of separation for married and cohabiting couples. Other research using data from Britain (Blekesaune 2008) and Australia (Hewitt and Baxter 2015) suggests that the health consequences of relationship dissolution may not be as severe for cohabitants compared to married people.

Union Dissolution and Health: Why Would Cohabitation Be Different from Marriage?

The divorce literature proposes three mechanisms through which union dissolution affects health and wellbeing: a decrease in resources, a decrease in social support and separation as a stressful event (Johnson and Wu 2002). First, union dissolution tends to be accompanied by a decrease in economic resources (Aassve et al. 2007), which in turn has negative consequences for health and wellbeing through increased stress, cutting back spending on healthcare and a healthy life style and poorer housing. As couples separate, they lose economies of scale and may face additional costs. Whereas this applies to both married and cohabiting couples, the effects may be weaker for cohabiting couples as they are less likely to have shared bank accounts (Hiekel et al. 2014) or shared home ownership (Mulder and Wagner 2001).

The effect of separation on health and wellbeing may be stronger for women as they tend to experience a larger decrease in economic resources after divorce compared with men, mainly due to the fact that they have weaker attachment to the labour market and tend to be responsible for children (Bianchi et al. 1999). This gender difference may be smaller for separation from cohabitation, because in cohabiting relationships women tend to contribute a higher proportion of household income, and therefore tend to be less dependent on their partners (Kalmijn et al. 2007; Hewitt and Baxter 2015). In addition, cohabiting women are less likely to have responsibility for dependent children after relationship dissolution as cohabitors are less likely to have shared children than those who are married (Hewitt et al. 2010). Together this suggests that married women may lose the most economic resources after relationship dissolution and therefore have poorer health.

Second, union dissolution may affect health through changes in social networks and reduced social support. Marriage provides social support, social integration, love and companionship, as well as social status through entry into a recognised, socially and legally-supported institution (Gove and Shin 1989). There may be little or no difference between marriage and cohabitation for health because many of the social support benefits to marriage accrue to cohabitation, although it lacks the symbolic commitment and secure legal institutional status that comes from marriage. In terms of broader social networks, however, those in cohabiting relationships have been found to have smaller social networks than married people (Nock 1995). Also, cohabiting couples tend to have more independent social lives compared with married couples (Kalmijn and Bernasco 2001), which means that their social networks might be less affected by partnership dissolution. Changes to the social network upon divorce appear to be especially strong for men, whereas women may even benefit as they tend to increase their social networks following divorce (Kalmijn and Broese van Groenou 2005).

Finally, relationship dissolution may affect health because it is a stressful event in itself, even if it was desired, and may be accompanied by additional stressors, such as raising a child alone, a strained relationship with the former spouse, and possibly social stigma (Amato 2000). As cohabiting couples typically have been together less time, are less financially dependent on each other, less likely to have children (although there is an increase in births in cohabiting relationships), or to have joint bank accounts and homes, we might expect that separating from cohabitation may be logistically easier than marriage, and hence less detrimental to health and wellbeing. In addition, cohabiting couples tend to have less interpersonal commitment to their relationship, higher expectations that the relationship will end (Wiik et al. 2012) and lower levels of relationship quality and satisfaction (Brown 2003).

Together, the evidence on differences between cohabiting and married couples suggests that the economic, social and emotional costs of ending cohabiting relationships are lower than marriages, we therefore might expect that the health effects for ending a cohabiting relationship will be less severe.

Health Selection and Cohabitation

These arguments so far assume that being married or in a cohabiting relationship produces certain health outcomes. In addition to arguments that separation may negatively affect health, it is important to note that the causality may also go in the other direction. With regard to relationship dissolution the selection argument asserts that individuals in poorer health are more likely to separate, because poor health is associated with less a favourable economic situation, which may put more strain on the relationship. Overall, this reversed causality has received a lot less attention in the literature. The few studies that test both selection and causal processes find evidence for both processes (Monden and Uunk 2013; Johnson and Wu 2002). However, none of these previous studies consider cohabitation and marriage. Much of the prior research comparing health differences between cohabitors and married people has been cross-sectional comparing groups at a single point in time. Selection, causation and the health impact of transitions cannot be evaluated using cross-sectional data, because they do not enable pre-existing health and well-being to be accounted for (Johnson and Wu 2002).

This Study

We build on previous literature in several ways. By examining differences in health consequences of relationship dissolution between cohabitors and married couples, we contribute to a relatively understudied area. We further advance our understanding of the health effects of relationship dissolution by examining the short-term health outcomes when an individual transitions out of a marital or cohabiting relationship (Blekesaune 2008). We examine a range of health outcomes that capture changes in wellbeing with relationship dissolution including global health, and measures of negative and positive feelings. Finally, we compare and contrast experiences across two countries, Switzerland and Australia. These two countries offer an interesting comparison for two reasons. First, they differ in terms of their health policy, expenditure on health care and the overall health outcomes in each country. On average Switzerland enjoys higher levels of overall health, but spends less on health care (Shi 1997). In addition, the two countries have different marital and cohabiting trajectories. In Switzerland, cohabitations tend to be shorter in duration than in Australia and more likely to end in marriage rather than separation than in Australia (de Vaus 2004; Heuveline and Timberlake 2005). This suggests that cohabitation as a longer term alternative to marriage is less likely in Switzerland, which would suggest that separation from cohabiting relationships may have smaller health consequences in that country. Alternatively, the Swiss may also be less likely to enter into less serious cohabiting relationships, which indicates that there may be more severe consequences on average for them. By undertaking this comparison, this study will offer some interesting insights into the dynamics of different health policy and normative relationship contexts in shaping health outcomes.

Methods

Data

To examine the dynamics of health, marriage and cohabitation between Australia and Switzerland we use longitudinal data from the Household, Income and Labour Dynamics in Australia (HILDA) and the Swiss Household Panel (SHP). The panels are relatively well suited for comparison. They have been running about the same amount of time, HILDA began in 2000 and SHP in 1999, and have many design features in common. Most importantly, these longitudinal surveys that broadly cover similar topics, allow us to follow the same individuals over time as they move through different relationship statuses.

Dependent Variables

The SHP and the HILDA have a number of similar, although not identical, health and wellbeing measures. We examine three outcomes that capture overall health, negative and positive feelings. The first is a self-reported measure of general health. The question for SHP asks, *Talking about your health, how do you feel right now?* With responses on a 5 point scale including: "very well", "well", "so, so (average)", "not very well", to "not well at all". The question for HILDA asks, *In general, would you say your health is?* With responses ranging from "excellent" to "poor" on a 5 point scale. A higher score indicates poorer overall health. Self-reported health measures based on a single question are used extensively in epidemiological and general social surveys, and research has shown that they are a valid and reliable indicator of health status encompassing both psychosocial and biological aspects of health (Burstrom and Fredlund 2001; Martikainen et al. 1999). Moreover self-reported health is a valid indicator of objectively assessed adverse psychosocial and physiological morbidity, and is a strong and consistent predictor of mortality (Burstrom and Fredlund 2001). We also develop an indicator of negative feelings. There are no exactly matching measures. For the SHP the question asked was: *Do you often have negative feelings such as having the blues, being desperate, suffering from anxiety or depression, if 0 means "never" and 10 "always"?* For inclusion in the models this was scaled to range from 0–5. For HILDA, we used 3 questions: *How much of the time in the past 4 weeks: Have you been a nervous person + Have you felt so down in the dumps that nothing could cheer you up + Have you felt down.* Answers ranged from "all of the time" to "none of the time". These scores were reversed and then summed together and divided by 3 to get a scale ranging from 0–5. A higher score for both measures reflects more frequent negative feelings. Our third indicator captures positive feelings. The SHP measure the question asked: *Are you often plenty of strength, energy and optimism, if 0 means "never" and 10 "always"?* The HILDA measure combined 2 questions, *How much of the time during the past 4 weeks: Did you feel full of life? + Did you have a lot of energy?* Answers ranged from "all of the time" to "none of the time". These scores were summed together. Both scales ranged from 0 to 10, with a higher score reflecting more frequent positive feelings.

Key Independent Variable: Relationship Status and Relationship Dissolution

Our main independent measure of interest was relationship status. Each study identified people who were married, cohabiting, separated, divorced, widowed or never married. Because we are interested in relationship dissolution due to separation and divorce we exclude those who become widowed from our analyses. In addition, due to the relatively low numbers of those becoming either separated or divorced (see Table 3.1), we collapse them into one group. To take advantage of the longitudinal nature of the data we differentiated between those who remained stable in their relationship, either married or cohabiting between waves from those who became separated or divorced between waves. This enabled us to capture any changes in health and well-being in the lead up to relationship dissolution. Our final measure differentiated: married, married-transition (to become separated/divorced in the next wave), cohabiting, cohabiting-transition (to become separated/divorced/never married in the next wave), separated/divorced, or never married.

Controls

We want to assess health and wellbeing differences between marital dissolution and dissolution of a cohabiting relationship net of characteristics in which the two groups differ that are also associated with health. Cohabiting men tend to have lower levels of employment and earnings than married men (Xie et al. 2003; Kalmijn

Table 3.1 Descriptive statistics of dependent variables and controls for pooled sample, by men and women, Australia (14 waves HILDA) and Switzerland (16 waves SHP)

	Australia		Switzerland	
	Men	Women	Men	Women
	Mean(SD)/%[a]	Mean(SD)/%	Mean(SD)/%	Mean(SD)/%
Health measures:				
Self-reported general health (1–5)	3.43(0.9)	3.48(0.9)	4.10(0.6)	4.05(0.7)
Negative feelings (0–5)	0.84(0.8)	0.96(0.9)	0.81(0.9)	1.09(1.0)
Positive feelings (0–10)	6.07(2.1)	5.78(2.2)	7.44(1.7)	7.32(1.7)
Children:				
No dependent child <18 (ref)	55	51	52	53
Dependent child <18	45	49	48	47
Employment status:				
Working fulltime, 90–100% (ref)	77	36	79	20
Working part-time, 1–89%	9	55	13	41
Unemployed	3	3	1	2
Inactive	11	29	7	23
Education:				
Basic schooling (ref)	22	31	5	15
Secondary schooling	52	42	45	60
Tertiary schooling	26	28	50	25
Household (HH) income (quartiles)[b]:				
<25% HH income (1st quartile) (ref)	24	26	21	27
25%–50% HH income (2nd quartile)	25	25	25	25
50%–75% HH income (3rd quartile)	26	25	27	24
75% + HH income (4th quartile)	26	25	27	24
Person observations	55,162	60,195	25,775	31,268

[a]Mean and SD reported for continuous measures and % reported for categorical measures
[b]Household income quartiles were calculated on total household income both countries. The overall % of men and women each country vary due to women's increase likelihood of being in lower income households in both countries

et al. 2007), which may in turn improve the wellbeing of both partners. In part the better wellbeing of married people compared with those cohabiting is partly explained by differences in material resources (Soons and Kalmijn 2009). In our models we controlled for: age in years (centred around the mean), employment status (working 90–100%, working 1–89%, unemployed, inactive), level of education (primary, secondary, tertiary level of education), household income in quartiles, whether or not there is a child under 18 years old in the household, and whether the household owns or rents the home. Descriptive statistics for dependent variables and controls are presented in Table 3.1.

Analytic Approach

We estimated a series of fixed effects regression models for each dependent variable. In each case the dependent variable is treated continuously. To exploit the longitudinal nature of the data and to best capture the effect of relationship dissolution on health and wellbeing, we also included a 1-year lag for marital status, where the reference group were those participants stably married between waves. The inclusion of this lagged marital status measure enabled us to estimate the effect of transitions from married or cohabiting in the previous wave (t_{-1}) to being separated/divorced (t) on health and wellbeing in the current wave, compared to those who were stably married or cohabiting between waves. Assessing time varying covariates in this way allowed us to determine the extent to which within-person variation in a relationship status was associated with within person variation on the health outcomes. Because interpretation is not straight forward in that both the lagged and main effect for relationship status need to be taken into account, we present our results graphically showing the predicted change in health for respondents whose relationships ended compared to those who remained married or cohabiting that includes the main and lagged effect for relationship status. It should also be noted that the use of lagged predictors requires that respondents have complete data for at least 2 points in time, therefore our lagged analysis used wave 2 as the baseline observation point (Shaw and Liang 2012).

Analysis proceeded in two stages. First, we estimated a baseline model (Model 1) which included relationship status, relationship status in the previous wave and age. Second, we included the controls to Model 1 (Model 2). While there were changes in the magnitude of coefficients with Model 2, there were few changes in the overall significance and substantive interpretation of the results and we only present the results of the second model.

Results

Relationship Transitions

Table 3.2 shows how the respondents transition between relationship states from wave-to-wave. Switzerland and Australia are more similar than different with regard to relationship dissolution patterns. The most stable group were the married individuals; in more than 98% of observations respondents were married in both waves. We observe that about 1.69% of the HILDA sample and 0.73% of the SHP sample transition from married to separated between waves, and 0.10% and 0.18% transitioning from married to divorced. As indicated earlier we collapsed the separated and divorced in our analyses. As expected cohabiting relationships were much less stable than marriage. Around 81% of cohabiting individuals in both countries remained stably cohabiting between waves, 6.41% transition to never married in

Table 3.2 Separation and divorce transitions from cohabitation and marriage in Switzerland and Australia in percentages

		Current Relationship Status (t)				
Relationship status (t-1)	Country	Married	Cohabiting	Separated	Divorced	Never Married
Married	Australia	98.05	0.16	1.69	0.10	0
	Switzerland	98.91	0.18	0.73	0.18	0
Cohabiting	Australia	10.94	80.62	0.39	1.65	6.41
	Switzerland	10.26	81.89	0.40	1.87	5.59
Separated	Australia	6.64	9.72	63.22	20.42	0
	Switzerland	3.59	6.03	65.85	24.52	0
Divorced	Australia	3.19	10.73	1.42	84.66	0
	Switzerland	1.44	6.78	0.22	91.56	0
Never Married	Australia	1.66	15.65	0	0	82.58
	Switzerland	2.80	15.66	0	0	81.55

Australia and 5.59% transition to never married in Switzerland. A relatively large proportion of cohabitors also transitioned to divorced 1.65% in Australia and 1.87% in Switzerland. Overall, we find that Swiss relationships, both marriage and cohabitation, tend to be more stable than Australian relationships.

Next we discuss the results of the models, while there are a large number of possible transitions we could focus on (as shown in Table 3.2), we concentrate on the most common transitions, from married to separated/divorced and from cohabiting to never married.

Self-Rated Health

Our results for self-rated health are presented in Fig. 3.1, based on the results in the first two columns of Appendix Table A.1. Among Australian men there was no indication that separation from cohabitation or marriage has a negativse effect on SRH. Although Graph 1a shows an increase in self-rated health following separation from cohabitation, this effect is not significant. Australian women (Graph 1c), however, show a significant lower level of SRH the year prior to separation from cohabitation. No comparable effect was found for separation from marriage. Although the figures of the Swiss sample (Graphs 1b and 1d) show a decrease in SRH in the year of separation from marriage, these effects were only significant in the lagged effect for Swiss women. For SRH we did not find the expected negative association with relationship dissolution, neither did we find support for the idea that this effect would be different for separation from marriage and stronger in Switzerland compared with Australia.

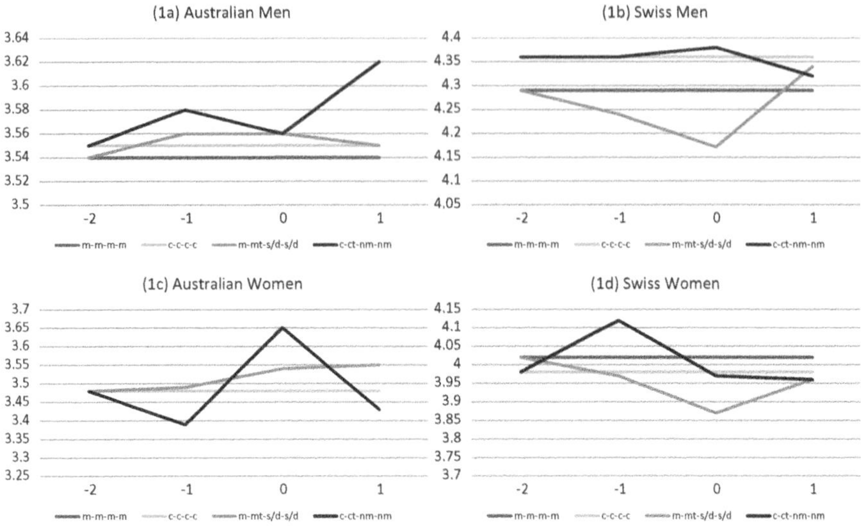

Fig. 3.1 Graphs 1a-1d, relationship dissolution and self-rated health

Negative Feelings

Our second outcome was the frequency of negative feelings, with results shown in Fig. 3.2. In the year prior to separation from marriage, there was an increase in negative feelings for all groups. Among Swiss men and Australian women this increase is still significant the year of and the year after separation. For Swiss women, these effects are significant in the lagged effect for married-transition. For Swiss men (Fig. 3.2, Graph 2b) we found that separation from cohabitation increased negative feelings, both before, during and after separation. There were no significant associations for Swiss women. Both Australian men and women were significantly more likely to have negative feelings when their cohabiting relationships ended. In sum, there is evidence that separation from both marriage and cohabitation increase the frequency of negative feelings, but separation from marriage had a stronger effect. This is similar in Switzerland and Australia.

Positive Feelings

In Fig. 3.3, we present the results of the models in the last columns of Appendix Table A.1, assessing the relationship between relationship dissolution and frequency of positive feelings. With the exception of the Swiss women, we find a decrease in the frequency of positive feelings following separation from marriage for all groups, starting the year before separation, and for Swiss men and Australian women continuing through separation and the year following the event. Whereas the pattern displayed in the Figure for Swiss women (Fig. 3.3, Graph 3d) is comparable to that

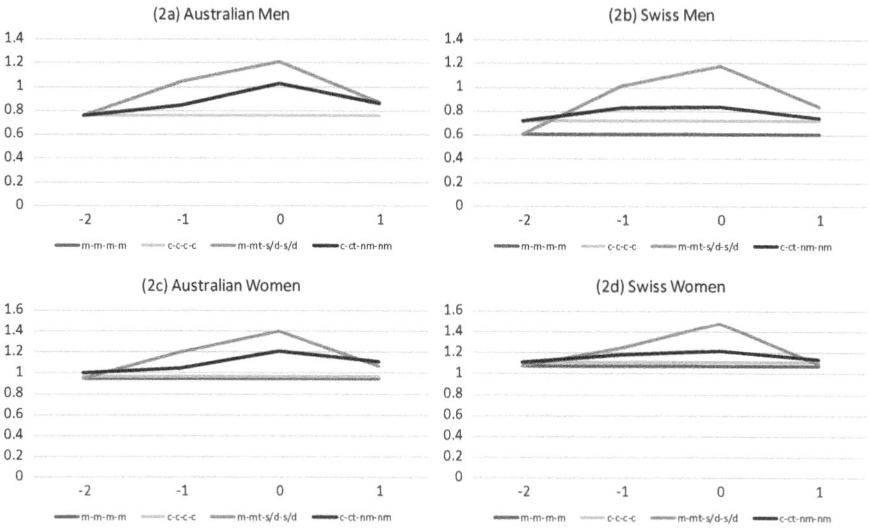

Fig. 3.2 Graphs 2a-2d, relationship dissolution and frequency of negative feelings

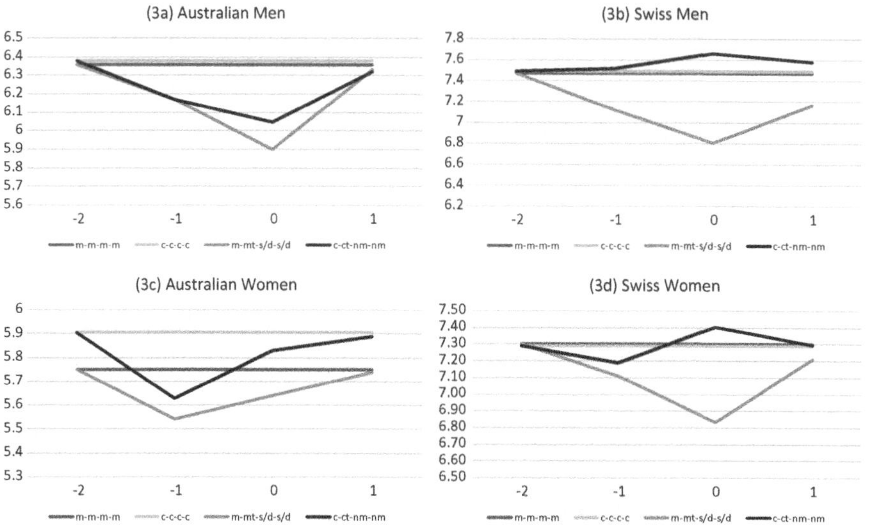

Fig. 3.3 Graphs 3a-3d relationship dissolution and frequency of positive feelings

for the Swiss men (Fig. 3.3, Graph 3b), the coefficients did not reach significance in this group. For the Australian men and women we also found a decrease in positive feelings the year before separation from cohabitation. For Australian men this persisted to the year of separation but disappeared the year after. So we find only for Australia an effect of separation from cohabitation on positive feelings, with comparable effects in Switzerland and Australia of separation from marriage.

Conclusion

In this chapter we wanted to further develop our understanding of the differences in the nature and circumstances of marriage and cohabitation by examining the health consequences or relationship dissolution. It is extensively documented that marriage breakdown negatively impacts on health and wellbeing (Umberson et al. 2010), but far less is known about relationship dissolution from cohabitation and whether and to what extent that differs from marital separation. Overall, our results suggest that relationship dissolution was associated with poorer health and wellbeing. However, the balance of evidence indicates that separation from marriage has greater consequences for health and wellbeing than from cohabitation. This is consistent with some prior research (Blekesaune 2008; Hewitt and Baxter 2015). This is also consistent with our expectations, based on the broader research literature comparing and contrasting marriage and cohabitation that finds overall cohabitors (on average) tend to have fewer legal, moral, and structural ties in their relationships, which we argued would likely reduce the health impacts of relationship dissolution for them. We also found that the patterns of associations were similar for Australia and Switzerland.

Our results also suggest differences in the importance of relationship status and relationship transitions for different health outcomes. Where self-reported general health shows the fewest significant associations, there were large and often significant changes in the frequency of negative and positive feelings. This might suggest relationships may be more important for mental well-being rather than physical health. It also indicates that examining multiple dimensions of health and wellbeing provides a more nuanced understanding of how intimate relationships are associated with health and wellbeing (Bierman et al. 2006).

There are a few notable limitations to our study. First, while the health measures available for comparison between HILDA and SHP had some similarities they were not directly comparable. Even if the measures had been identical we could not be sure that the Australian population would have understood the questions in the same way as the Swiss population. Therefore, any conclusions about the comparisons between the two countries need to take that into account. Secondly, we examine transitions from marriage or cohabitation over time, in some cases the numbers and proportions of people transitioning were small. In addition, those whose relationships breakdown have higher rates of attrition than those whose remain intact. These two factors increase the standard error and therefore increase the risk of finding non-significant results, making our results somewhat conservative.

We examined two countries, Australia and Switzerland that contrast in their family and health policy context and relationship formation and dissolution patterns (de Vaus 2004; Heuveline and Timberlake 2005; Shi 1997). Overall, our results suggest that relationship dissolution had similar associations with health in each country. There has been a generalised concern in most developed nations that the rise of cohabitation as an alternative or prelude to marriage, and the relationship instability of cohabitation, may have negative consequences for a range of life outcomes including health (Musick and Bumpass 2012). Our finding that the dissolution of cohabiting relationships were less harmful to health than marriage dissolution contributes to a growing body of evidence that cohabitation as an alternative relationship does not always compare less favourably with marriage.

Appendix Table A.1 Fixed effects models of self-reported general health, frequency of negative feelings and frequency of positive feelings for men and women in Australia and Switzerland

	Self-reported general health				Negative feelings				Positive feelings			
	Women		Men		Women		Men		Women		Men	
	b	se	b	se	b	se	b	se	b	se	b	se
	Australia											
Married (ref.)												
Married-transition	0.01	0.03	0.02	0.04	0.25***	0.04	0.28***	0.05	−0.21*	0.09	−0.19*	0.09
Cohabiting	−0.05*	0.02	−0.04	0.02	0.05*	0.02	0.04	0.02	0.01	0.06	−0.12*	0.06
Cohabiting-transition	−0.14**	0.04	−0.01	0.05	0.13*	0.05	0.13*	0.05	−0.27*	0.11	−0.33**	0.11
Separated/ Divorced	−0.02	0.04	−0.03	0.04	0.18***	0.05	0.10*	0.05	−0.26*	0.12	−0.14	0.10
Never married	−0.10*	0.05	−0.02	0.05	0.10	0.06	0.11	0.06	−0.03	0.12	−0.35**	0.12
Lagged married (ref.)												
Lagged married-transition	0.11*	0.05	0.05	0.05	0.27***	0.07	0.36***	0.07	0.02	0.14	−0.32*	0.14
Lagged cohabiting	0.05*	0.02	0.05*	0.02	−0.03	0.02	−0.04	0.02	0.15**	0.06	0.14*	0.05
Lagged cohabiting-transition	0.07	0.06	0.04	0.05	0.16*	0.06	0.16**	0.06	0.11	0.13	0.04	0.12
Lagged separated/Divorced	0.09*	0.04	0.04	0.04	−0.06	0.05	0.01	0.05	0.25*	0.10	0.11	0.09
Lagged never married	0.06	0.05	0.10*	0.05	0.06	0.06	−0.01	0.05	0.17	0.12	0.31**	0.11
Intercept	3.48***	0.04	3.54***	0.05	0.95***	0.04	0.76***	0.05	5.75***	0.08	6.36***	0.12
Person observations	46,068		40,681		46,083		40,708		46,199		40,810	

(continued)

Appendix Table A.1 (continued)

	Self-reported general health				Negative feelings				Positive feelings			
	Women		Men		Women		Men		Women		Men	
	b	se	b	se	b	se	b	se	b	se	b	se
	Switzerland											
Married (ref.)												
Married-transition	−0.05	0.04	−0.05	0.05	0.17*	0.07	0.40***	0.10	−0.19	0.11	−0.35**	0.13
Cohabiting	−0.10**	0.03	−0.03	0.03	0.07	0.05	0.15***	0.04	−0.13	0.08	−0.04	0.09
Cohabiting-transition	0.04	0.05	−0.03	0.05	0.14	0.09	0.26***	0.07	−0.23	0.15	−0.02	0.14
Separated/ Divorced	0.02	0.06	−0.12	0.07	0.06	0.09	0.46***	0.10	0.01	0.17	−0.48**	0.18
Never married	−0.08	0.07	−0.04	0.06	0.09	0.10	0.26**	0.08	0.01	0.15	0.03	0.18
Lagged married (ref.)												
Lagged married-transition	−0.17*	0.08	0.00	0.09	0.34**	0.12	0.11	0.13	−0.45*	0.21	−0.18	0.24
Lagged cohabiting	0.06	0.03	0.10***	0.03	−0.04	0.04	−0.04	0.04	0.12	0.08	0.06	0.08
Lagged cohabiting-transition	0.03	0.07	0.11	0.07	0.06	0.10	−0.03	0.09	0.10	0.17	0.16	0.18
Lagged separated/divorced	−0.04	0.06	0.19**	0.06	−0.05	0.09	−0.23*	0.09	0.10	0.17	0.26	0.17
Lagged never married	0.02	0.06	0.07	0.06	−0.02	0.09	−0.13	0.07	−0.01	0.16	0.08	0.17
Intercept	4.02***	0.07	4.29***	0.13	1.08***	0.13	0.61***	0.12	7.30***	0.23	7.47***	0.30
Person observations	25,807		20,927		25,809		20,922		25,796		20,910	

* $p < 0.05$, ** $p < 0.01$, *** $p < 0.001$ (Models controlled for age, working status, education, income quartile, children <18 in household, and home ownership)

References

Aassve, A., Betti, G., Mazzuco, S., & Menacarini, L. (2007). Marital disruption and economic well being. *Journal of the Royal Statistical Society: Series A, 170*, 781–799.

Amato, P. R. (2000). The consequences of divorce for adults and children. *Journal of Marriage and the Family, 62*(4), 1269–1287.

Bianchi, S. M., Subaiya, L., & Kahn, J. R. (1999). The gender gap in the economic well-being of nonresident fathers and custodial mothers. *Demography, 36*(2), 195–203.

Bierman, A., Fazio, E. M., & Milkie, M. (2006). A multifaceted approach to the mental health advantage of the married: Assessing how explanations vary by outcome measure and unmarried group. *Journal of Family Issues, 27*(4), 554–582.

Blekesaune, M. (2008). Partnership transitions and mental distress. *Journal of Marriage and Family, 72*, 705–725.

Brown, S. L. (2003). Relationship quality dynamics of cohabiting unions. *Journal of Family Issues, 24*(5), 583–601.

Burstrom, B., & Fredlund, P. (2001). Self rated health: Is it as good a predictor of subsequent mortality among adults in lower as well as in higher social classes? *Journal of Epidemiology and Community Health, 55*, 836–840. https://doi.org/10.1136/jech.55.11.836.

Cherlin, A. J. (2009). *The marriage-go-round. The state of marriage and family in America today*. New York: Knopf.

Gove, W. R., & Shin, H.-C. (1989). The psychological well-being of divorced and widowed men and women: An empirical analysis. *Journal of Family Issues, 10*(1), 122–144.

Heuveline, P., & Timberlake, J. (2005). The Role of cohabitation in family formation: The United States in comparative perspective. *Journal of Marriage and the Family, 66*(5), 1214–1230.

Hewitt, B., & Baxter, J. (2015). Chapter 5: Relationship dissolution. In G. Heard & D. Arunachalam (Eds.), *Family formation in 21st century Australia* (pp. 77–99). Dordrecht: Springer.

Hewitt, B., England, P., Baxter, J., & Shafer, E. F. (2010). Education and unintended pregnancies in Australia: Do differences in relationship status and age at birth explain the gradient? *Population Review, 49*(1), 36–52.

Hewitt, B., Turrell, G., & Giskes, K. (2011). Marital loss, mental health and the role of perceived social support: Findings from six waves of an Australian population based panel study. *Journal of Epidemiology and Community Health, 66*(4), 308–314. https://doi.org/10.1136/jech.2009.104893.

Hiekel, N., Liefbroer, A. C., & Poortman, A.-R. (2014). Income pooling strategies among cohabiting and married couples: A comparative perspective. *Demographic Research, 30*(55), 1527–1560. https://doi.org/10.4054/DemRes.2014.30.55.

Horowitz, A., & White, H. R. (1998). The relationship of cohabitation and mental health: A study of a young adult cohort. *Journal of Marriage and Family, 60*(2), 505–514.

Hughes, M. E., & Waite, L. J. (2009). Marital biography and health at mid-life. *Journal of Health and Social Behavior, 50*(3), 344–358.

Johnson, D. R., & Wu, J. (2002). An empirical test of crisis, social selection and role explanations of the relationship between marital disruption and psychological distress: A pooled time-series analysis of four-wave panel data. *Journal of Marriage and Family, 64*, 211–224.

Kalmijn, M., & Bernasco, W. (2001). Joint and separated lifestyles in couple relationships. *Journal of Marriage and the Family, 63*, 639–654.

Kalmijn, M., & Broese van Groenou, M. (2005). Differential effects of divorce on social integration. *Journal of Social and Personal Relationships, 22*(4), 455–476.

Kalmijn, M., Loeve, A., & Manting, D. (2007). Income dynamics in couples and the dissolution of marriage and cohabitation. *Demography, 44*(1), 159–179.

Kiernan, K. E. (2002). Cohabitation in Western Europe: Trends, issues, and implications. In A. Booth & A. C. Crouter (Eds.), *Just living together: Implications of cohabitation on families, children, and social policy*. Mahwah: Erlbaum.

Luhmann, M., Hofmann, W., Eid, M., & Lucas, R. E. (2012). Subjective well-being and adaptation to life events: A meta-analysis. *Journal of Personality and Social Psychology, 102*(3), 592–615.

Lund, R., Due, P., Modvig, J., Holstein, B. E., Damsgaard, M. T., & Andersen, P. K. (2002). Cohabitation and marital status as predictors of mortality an eight year follow-up study. *Social Science & Medicine, 55*, 673–679.
Martikainen, P., Aromaa, A., Heliovaara, M., Klaukka, T., Knekt, P., Maatela, J., et al. (1999). Reliability of perceived health by sex and age. *Social Science & Medicine, 48*(8), 1117–1122.
Monden, C. W. S., & Uunk, W. (2013). For better and for worse: The relationship between union dissolution and self-assessed health in European panel data. *European Journal of Population/ Revue Europeenne de Demographie, 29*, 103–125.
Mulder, C. H., & Wagner, M. (2001). The connections between family formation and first-time home ownership in the context of West Germany and the Netherlands. *European Journal of Population/Revue Europeenne de Demographie, 17*(2), 137–164.
Musick, K., & Bumpass, L. L. (2012). Reexamining the case for marriage: Union formation and changes in well-being. *Journal of Marriage and Family, 74*(2), 1–18.
Nock, S. L. (1995). A comparison of marriage and cohabiting relationship. *Journal of Family Issues, 16*(1), 53–76.
Seltzer, J. A. (2000). Families formed outside of marriage. *Journal of Marriage and the Family, 62*, 1247–1268.
Shaw, B., & Liang, J. (2012). Chapter 7: Growth models with multilevel regression. In J. T. Newsom, R. N. Jones, & S. M. Hofer (Eds.), *Longitudinal data analysis: A practical guide for research in aging, health and social sciences*. New York: Routledge.
Shi, L. (1997). Health care spending, delivery, and outcome in developed countries: A cross-National Comparison. *American Journal of Medical Quality, 12*(2), 83–93.
Soons, J., & Kalmijn, M. (2009). Is marriage more than cohabitation? Well-being differences in 30 European countries. *Journal of Marriage and Family, 71*, 1141–1157.
Umberson, D., Crosnoe, R., & Reczek, C. (2010). Social relationships and health behaviour across the life course. *Annual Review of Sociology, 36*, 139–157. https://doi.org/10.1146/annurev-soc-070308-120011.
de Vaus, D. A. (2004). *Diversity and change in Australian families: Statistical profiles*. Melbourne: AIFS.
Wiik, K. A., Keizer, R., & Lappegard, T. (2012). Relationship quality in marital and cohabtiing unions across Europe. *Journal of Marriage and Family, 74*, 389–398.
Williams, K., & Umberson, D. (2004). Marital status, marital transitions, and health: A gendered life course perspective. *Journal of Health & Social Behavior, 45*(1), 81–98.
Wu, Z., Penning, M. J., Pollard, M. S., & Hart, R. (2003). "In sickness and in health" : Does cohabitation count? *Journal of Family Issues, 24*(6), 811–838.
Xie, Y., Raymo, J. M., Goyette, K., & Thornton, A. (2003). Economic potential and entry into marriage and cohabitation. *Demography, 40*(2), 351–367.

Chapter 4
The Transition to Marriage for Cohabiting Couples: Does it Shape Subjective Well-being and Opinions or Attitudes Toward Family?

Valérie-Anne Ryser and Jean-Marie Le Goff

Introduction

A large body of literature describes differences between married and cohabiting couples in terms of attitudes or opinions about family and in terms of well-being, and conjugal quality (Brown 2000, 2004; Bumpass et al. 1991; Clarkberg et al. 1995; Diener et al. 2000; Jose et al. 2010; Nock 1995; Ryser and Le Goff 2015; Soons and Kalmijn 2009; van der Lippe et al. 2014; Wiik et al. 2009). Cohabitants tend to be less traditional in terms of the status and role of each partner in the family than married couples, but they also tend to be less happy. It has been argued that the lower level of well-being and the relationship instability might come from a lack of institutionalization of the cohabiting unions (Nock 1995). This lack of institutionalization leads to fewer institutional guidelines and fewer legal responsibilities for cohabitants than for married couples. Less traditional family values means that partners must discuss, and negotiate more in the relationship (Wilcox and Nock 2006). As a consequence, the relation between both partners is less peaceful than in a traditional marriage in which roles and status are well attributed (Cherlin 2004) and less likely to be objects of discussion.

In Switzerland, cohabiting is very often a prelude to marriage, which means that most couples experience the two statuses of cohabitant and spouse during their family lifecycles (Le Goff et al. 2005; Ryser and Le Goff 2011). What does it mean in regard to the general observations on traditionalism and happiness? Does it mean

V.-A. Ryser (✉)
FORS-Swiss Centre of Expertise in the Social Sciences, Lausanne, Switzerland
e-mail: Valerie-Anne.Ryser@fors.unil.ch

J.-M. Le Goff
Life course and Inequalities research Centre (Lines), University of Lausanne and National Center of Competences in Research Overcoming Vulnerability: Life course perspective (LIVES), Lausanne, Switzerland
e-mail: Jean-Marie.LeGoff@unil.ch

R. Tillmann et al. (eds.), *Social Dynamics in Swiss Society*, Life Course Research and Social Policies 9, https://doi.org/10.1007/978-3-319-89557-4_4

that the marriage as the marker of the transition from one status to the other is also a marker of the transition to more traditionalism and happiness? Or does it mean that couples share traditional values before the marriage and that the marriage is the result of a complex social mechanism of selection? To answer these questions, we will investigate Swiss Household Panel (SHP) data that concern cohabiting couples who get married. Our aim is then to compare the levels of traditionalism and life satisfaction before and after the marriage. In the following section, we review the literature in order to precise our research question and hypotheses. We then describe the data and measures we selected. We will then present the results and end with a general discussion of those results.

Married and Cohabiting Couples: To What Extent Do They Differ?

The end of the baby boom coincides with the emergence of a new demographic regime in most Western countries. This new regime can be schematically characterized by a high level of cohabiting unions, a high level of out of wedlock births, and a high level of divorces as well as late motherhood and high rates of infertility (Esping-Andersen and Billari 2015; Lesthaeghe and Surkyn 1988; van der Kaa 1987). These demographic trends indicate a context of the pluralization of unions that followed the monopoly of romantic marriage during the fifties and sixties. Long- or short-term cohabitation (Toulemon 1996), single parents, and couples who live apart coexist with the more traditional model of the conjugal couple (Regnier-Loilier et al. 2009; Villeneuve-Gokalp 1997). Nevertheless, in this new context of lifestyle pluralization, some types of union seem to be much more predominant than others, especially married couples and cohabiting couples.

In the specific case of Switzerland, cohabiting unions have quickly diffused since the early seventies. For several decades, this form of union served as a prelude to marriage (Le Goff et al. 2005; Sobotka and Toulemon 2008). In the early 1990s, 80% of union began as non-marital union (Gabadinho 1998) but 5% of children were born out of wedlock. At that time, Switzerland's situation in Europe was rather particular since northern European countries were characterized by high rates of cohabitation and out-of-wedlock children, whereas southern European countries were characterized by low rates of cohabitation and out-of-wedlock children (Le Goff et al. 2005). The situation of cohabiting unions predominantly serving as a prelude to marriage can be partly explained by the fact that married and cohabiting parents did not have the same rights (Perelli-Harris and Sánchez Gassen 2012). In addition, childbearing within cohabitation was perceived as leading to the requirement of complicated administrative procedures for men to obtain parental rights, especially by unmarried fathers (Le Goff and Ryser 2010; Ryser and Le Goff 2011).[1]

[1] Since 1 July 2014, joint parental right became the rule. Currently data available do not allow studying the changes that might be led by this institutional change.

Trends show that since the end of the nineties, there has been a slow but steady increase of non-marital births in Switzerland. In 2014, almost one birth in four was out of wedlock. Nearly all out-of-wedlock children were born to women living in cohabiting unions. Such an increase shows that cohabiting unions seem to have become, at least partly, an alternative to marriage, especially in urban areas. In addition to this trend, some institutional changes to the law on parental authority introduced in 2014 have made the recognition of parental authority easier for an unmarried father.

As mentioned in the introduction of this chapter, researchers have highlighted the differences between married couples and those living in cohabiting unions. On the one hand, cohabiting partners tend to share less traditional values, opinions, and attitudes than married partners (Clarkberg et al. 1995; Le Goff and Ryser 2013; Ryser and Le Goff 2015). On the other hand, cohabiting individuals expressed higher levels of depressive symptoms and less happiness than their married counterparts (Brown 2000; Diener et al. 2000; Soons and Kalmijn 2009). These differences are often interpreted as poorer relationship quality and lower conjugal commitment for cohabiting couples in comparison to married couples (Brown 2000; Nock 1995). However it has been shown that the degree to which cohabitation is accepted in a defined country plays a key role in the degree of well-being differences between cohabitant and married individuals (Diener et al. 2000; Soons and Kalmijn 2009). In addition Schultz Lee and Ono (2012) demonstrated that in the most gender-egalitarian countries there was no statistically significant gap in the happiness of married and cohabiting women as opposed in more traditional countries.

The SHP data show results similar to those observed in other Western countries. Less conservative values are associated with a lower level of well-being among cohabitants in comparison to married couples (Le Goff and Ryser 2013; Ryser and Le Goff 2015).

Cohabiting unions can play different roles in the life course (Manting 1996), which we can divide into two main categories. First, a cohabiting union can be a prelude to marriage, or a trial period before the couple decides to marry. Second, cohabiting unions can be alternatives to marriage due to partners' ideals or economic reasons (Perelli-Harris and Gerber 2011). Cohabitants who report that they plan to marry their current partner within two years differ much less from married individuals than cohabitants with no marriage plans. Brown (2004) adds that cohabitants with marriage plans tend to be happier than cohabitants that do not plan to marry. Such results suggest that the level of well-being is related to a process of selection of couples among those who plan to marry and those who do not. We also expect that this process of selection plays a role in traditional values, i.e., that couples who marry already shared traditional values before marriage.

The SHP allows us to further investigate this hypothesis of selection in the case of Switzerland. Rather than taking into account couples who plan to marry and comparing them with those who do not, SHP data allows us to follow cohabiting couples who got married in the 2000s and the beginning of the 2010s. Levels of traditionalism and of well-being for each partner are measured using the same protocol before and after the marriage. If the marriage results of a process of selection of conservative partners, levels of traditionalism and parallel the level of well-being should not evolve a great deal. The alternative hypothesis is that the marriage has an impact on the union and that partners become happier and more traditional. A rationale for this alternative hypothesis is that marriage might imply a reorganization of individual values and could promote conservative gendered norms and standards, which could explain the differences identified between married and cohabiting individuals in terms of beliefs, attitudes and gendered practices. This assumption is based on the fact that marriage is perceived by the individuals as the fulfillment of a strong symbolic rite that is largely related to belonging to a local community (Bozon 1992; Bozon and Héran 2006), family, or friend group. This sense of belonging to a specific group, consciously or unconsciously, could contribute to traditional norms and may subject married individuals to a certain social pressure (Théry 1998). It could push them over to traditionalism at the level of individual social representations as well as at the level of their practices.

Data, Sample and Method

Data and Sample Description

Our investigations are based on a subsample of the SHP dataset. As questions of interest have only been available since 2002, we used data starting from that year. To assess the influence of the transition to marriage, we selected individuals aged 18 to 75 who declared themselves to be cohabitants at the wave *n* and who then declared themselves to be married at waves *n + 1* and *n + 2*. The analysis was conducted on a total of 608 individuals—302 men and 306 women—who declared themselves married at some point after they began living with their partners.

Table 4.1 provides not weighted[2] information about the sociodemographic characteristics of the sample. Descriptive statistics show that the arrival of children is often linked with the transition to marriage. In addition, results demonstrate an increase in part-time work after the transition to marriage, mostly for women. This result can be explained by the fact that marriage is often linked with the transition to parenthood. During this transition, women reduce the amount of time they devote to work (Levy et al. 2006).

[2]Results have not been weighted because first, the analyses are based on a very peculiar subsample of SHP; second, because of the "experimental" dimension of our investigations: Variables are measured on each individual at two times of their life. As these two times are separated by an event, we want to see differences between these two times. In definitive, we do not have any pretention for a representative subpopulation of couples originally cohabitant that married during the period of investigation.

Table 4.1 Description of the sociodemographic characteristics of the sample before and after the transition to marriage (mean or percentage)

		Before Marriage		After Marriage	
	Range	Men	Women	Men	Women
N		302	306	302	306
Age (mean)		32.8	31.1	34.8	33
Children	0	273	281	154	157
	1	14	16	126	129
	2 or more	14	9	22	20
Education	Low	2.6	2.3	2.3	5.6
	Middle	58.3	5.6	56.0	59.2
	High	38.4	41.4	41.4	35.3
Occupation	Full time	89.1	70.9	87.4	37.9
	Part time	5.6	20.3	9.6	41.2
	At home	0.7	5.2	1.3	18.6
	Training	3.0	1.6	1.0	1.3
	Unemployed	1.0	1.3	0.7	0.3
Income (CHF) (mean)	Individual	77,693	57,166	75,946	24,259
	Household	124,019	123,090	119,243	114,780

Variables

Dependent Variables

Our different dependent variables are related on the one hand to the well-being of people and on the other hand to their degree of traditionalism in regard to the family. We selected in the SHP three repeated measures of well-being and one measure of traditionalism. All chosen indicators were initially measured using an 11-point scale from 0 to 10. We recoded these dependent variables into dummy variables in order to estimate logistic models.

Subjective Well-being We took three domains of *satisfaction* into account — satisfaction with life in general, living together, and the relationship. A t-test indicates that the transition to marriage seems to negatively impact satisfaction with the relationship ($t(352) = 2.678$, $p = 0.008$).

Family Opinion One item measures the respondent' opinion of the statement that a child suffers if he/she has a working mother on an 11-point scale ranging from 0 (completely disagree) to 10 (completely agree). A t-test shows that the transition to marriage seems to impact this statement. Individuals tend to agree less with this statement after the transition to marriage ($t(247) = 3.957$, $p = 0.000$).

Sociodemographic and Control Covariates

Education Respondent' level of education is established with a categorical variable that accounts for the highest level of education achieved. It distinguishes between low levels (e.g., incomplete compulsory school, compulsory school, elementary vocational training, domestic science courses, one-year commerce school, and general training school), middle levels (e.g., apprenticeship, technical or vocational school, full-time vocational school, vocational high school with a master's certificate, and federal certificate), and high levels (e.g., vocational high school, university, and academic high school) of education.

Income An indicator accounts for the yearly net household income (for a detailed description of the income variables, see Lipps 2010). In the analyses, we introduced the log form of the household income. A t-test indicates that the level of household income did not change before and after marriage ($t(531) = 0.414$, $p = 0.679$).

Number of Children We distinguish between zero, one, two or more children. Marriage is associated with more children than cohabiting union, as shown by the t-test: $t(606) = -19.044$, $p < 0.000$.

Age To determine any differences in the ages of the SHP-participants, we controlled for age.

Analytical Strategy

The aim of our research was to better understand to what extent the set of dependent variables might differ for individuals before and after the transition to marriage. This means that the research deals with paired outcomes. In the present case, a pair of outcomes (Y_{t1}, Y_{t2}) corresponds to a repeated dichotomized measure for one respondent, the first outcome being measured before the marriage (t_1) and the second after (t_2). We can suppose that the observations within pairs are not independent, whereas observations from different pairs are independent (Le Cessie and Van Houwelingen 1994). The potential dependence between the two outcomes in a pair of measures would be especially true for the hypothesis that there is a process of selection for the sample of cohabiting persons who marry. In order to capture this potential dependence between two outcomes, we estimated a series of *bivariate logistic models*, one for each of the pairs of dependent variables (Palmgren 1989; Yee 2010; Yee and Dirnböck 2009). The principle of that kind of model is to *simultaneously* estimate an odds ratio for each independent covariates on each outcome as well as a coefficient of association between both outcomes. This last coefficient is estimated by a new odds ratio term which corresponds to the product of probabilities to obtain the same outcome for an individual divided by the product of probabilities that the two outcomes are different. The model can be written:

$$\begin{cases} logit\left[P(Y_{t1}=1\right]=b_1+a_1X_{t1} \\ logit\left[P(Y_{t2}=1\right]=b_2+a_2X_{t2} \\ \log\left[\dfrac{P(Y_{t1}=Y_{t2}=1)P(Y_{t1}=Y_{t2}=0)}{P(Y_{t1}=1,Y_{t2}=0)P(Y_{t1}=0,Y_{t2}=1)}\right]=b_3 \end{cases}$$

where X_{t1} and X_{t2} are vectors of covariates measured before and after the marriage, respectively (level of education, age, etc.); b_1, b_2 and b_3 are intercepts to be estimated; and a_1 and a_2 are vectors of estimated coefficients attached to the covariates X_{t1} and X_{t2}. The outcome $b_3 = 0$ means that the two outcomes are independent, whereas $b_3 > 0$ means a positive dependence between them, i.e., the respondent will persist in giving a similar response after marriage. A positive association between the two outcomes would support the hypothesis of a process of selection of cohabiting couples that get married. We do not expect to observe the case of $b_3 < 0$, which would correspond to the case in which the two outcomes are negatively associated—for example, that a low level of satisfaction before marriage would be associated with a high rate of satisfaction after or *vice versa*. Models are estimated for each pair of dependent variables using the library VGAM in R-Cran (Yee 2010; Yee and Dirnböck 2009).

Results

Table 4.2 displays the results for the different measures of satisfaction with life in general, with the relationship and with living together. In each case, there is a strong association between the measure before and after the marriage (as estimated by b_3 coefficients). Such a result indicates a process of selection related to marriage.

The patterns of the results demonstrate that sometimes, covariates that play a key role before marriage do not necessarily play the same role afterward and *vice versa*. That means that in certain cases, the transition to the married status contributes to attenuating or exacerbating the way people assess their satisfaction according to their characteristics. In that sense, these results allow us to say that marriage does to some extent shape individuals' evaluation of their satisfaction.

Women tend to be more satisfied with life in general than men before the transition to marriage. In addition, highly educated individuals tend to be more satisfied with life than individuals with a middle level of education. These differences disappear after marriage.

In terms of satisfaction with the relationship, women are more satisfied with the relationship than men before as well as after the transition to marriage. Having two or more children before marriage decreases the level of satisfaction with the relationship. Differences in the level of satisfaction disappear after the marriage.

Table 4.2 Results of logistic bivariate regressions explaining the frequency of satisfaction before and after the marriage (log of odds ratio)

	Life satisfaction				Satisfaction with relationship				Satisfaction with living together			
Coefficients:	Estimate	Std. Error	z value		Estimate	Std. Error	z value		Estimate	Std. Error	z value	
Intercept												
b_1	−2.260	2.739	−0.825		4.282	3.318	1.291		−1.391	3.482	−0.400	
b_2	−4.617	3.226	−1.431		2.388	3.547	0.673		−1.430	3.695	−0.387	
b_3	1.737	0.242	7.186	***	1.266	0.246	5.142	***	1.493	0.268	5.569	***
Before marriage sex:women[a]	0.380	0.223	1.704	+	0.904	0.231	3.910	***	0.012	0.246	0.051	
After marriage sex: women[a]	0.112	0.219	0.514		0.870	0.231	3.765	***	0.037	0.231	0.161	
Before marriage:age	0.003	0.015	0.228		0.006	0.016	0.385		0.003	0.019	0.139	
After marriage: age	0.003	0.015	0.196		−0.020	0.016	−1.223		−0.039	0.017	−2.298	*
Level of education: ref. middle												
Before marriage:low[b]	0.253	0.660	0.383		−0.107	0.745	−0.144		−0.476	0.713	−0.667	
Before marriage:high[b]	0.489	0.232	2.106	*	0.239	0.240	0.998		−0.433	0.262	−1.649	+
After marriage: low[b]	0.628	0.686	0.915		−1.642	1.122	−1.464		0.368	0.798	0.461	
After marriage: high[b]	0.247	0.233	1.063		0.233	0.244	0.953		0.213	0.257	0.827	

Number of children: ref. zero child												
Before marriage:1 child[c]	−0.096	0.515	−0.187		−0.553	0.538	−1.027		−0.592	0.481	−1.232	
Before marriage: 2 or more children[c]	0.827	0.556	1.487		−2.434	0.996	−2.444	*	−0.990	0.517	−1.916	+
After marriage:1 child[c]	0.065	0.208	0.314		−0.101	0.229	−0.442		−0.578	0.232	−2.491	*
After marriage: 2 or more children[c]	0.028	0.446	0.064		0.049	0.465	0.105		−0.898	0.437	−2.054	*
Income												
Before marriage: household	0.115	0.236	0.488		−0.429	0.285	−1.508		0.238	0.304	0.783	
After marriage: household	0.348	0.280	1.241		−0.209	0.308	−0.678		0.330	0.325	1.016	
Residual deviance	887.005				840.937				822.298			
Degrees of freedom	1036				982				1135			
Log-likelihood:	−443.502				−420.468				−411.148			
Odds ratio:	5.682				3.547				4.452			

Note. + $p \leq 0.1$;* $p \leq 0.05$; *** $p \leq 0.001$
[a]ref. men
[b]ref. medium level of education
[c]ref. childless

After the transition to marriage, older individuals are less likely to express satisfaction with living together. A high level of education leads to less satisfaction with living together in comparison to a middle level of education. Finally, children play a key role in shaping the level of satisfaction with living together. Results are not significant before marriage, though the estimated coefficients before marriage are very similar to those estimated after marriage. We suppose however that this lack of significance can be related to the lack of couples having one child or more children before marriage. Having two children or more before the transition to marriage seems to be associated with a reduction of satisfaction with living together compared to having no children. After the transition to marriage, having one or more children is also linked with a decrease in satisfaction with living together. Here again, the impact of the children on the satisfaction with the relationship did differ after the transition to marriage.

Table 4.3 displays the results of the respondents' opinion of the statement that a child suffers if the mother works. As before, the general pattern is that individuals have a high probability to give the same answer before and after the transition to marriage.

Results by covariate show that women at times 1 and 2 are less likely than men to express that children with working mothers suffer before as well as after the marriage. In addition, individuals with higher levels of education are less likely to express that children with working mothers suffer. In this dimension, it seems that marriage does not shape individuals' opinion of that statement. These results thus confirm the idea of a selection effect.

Conclusion

The main aim of the present research was to explore to what extent marriage might imply more conservative values and practices (Théry 1998) and higher levels of well-being that lead to differences between married and cohabiting couples. The first hypothesis postulates that individuals who decide to get married already share more gendered values and practices that lead to the observed differences between married and cohabiting couples. Alternatively, the second hypothesis postulates that the transition to marriage could imply more gendered practices. Based on the methodology of modeling bivariate binomial responses (Yee 2010; Yee and Dirnböck 2009), the main results of our research tend to demonstrate that individuals have a high probability of responding similarly before and after the transition to marriage on measures of their well-being and values. This suggests that the differences between married and cohabiting individuals might not come from the transition to marriage *per se* but that they seem to exist before marriage. To summarize, the results tend to indicate that there is a form of selectivity among couples. Individuals who decide to get married already share more traditional perspectives on family practices and beliefs and have already made changes in their level of well-being. It might be a reason to explain why little difference between before and after marriage is observed in the study.

Table 4.3 Results of bivariate logistic regression explaining the frequency of one opinion on family, before and after the marriage (log of odds ratio)

	Child suffers with working mother			
Coefficients:				
Intercept	Estimate	Std. error	z value	
b_1	3.569	3.064	1.165	
b_2	2.270	3.966	0.572	
b_3	2.609	0.370	7.052	***
Before marriage sex:women[a]	−0.601	0.291	−2.067	*
After marriage sex: women[a]	−0.950	0.305	−3.118	**
Before marriage:age	−0.017	0.019	−0.919	
After marriage: age	−0.007	0.019	−0.364	
Level of education: ref. middle				
Before marriage:low[b]	−0.890	0.821	−1.084	
Before marriage:high[b]	−1.207	0.294	−4.114	***
After marriage: low[b]	0.075	0.927	0.081	
After marriage: high[b]	−1.594	0.314	−5.082	***
Number of children: ref. zero child				
Before marriage:1 child[c]	−0.477	0.580	−0.823	
Before marriage: 2 or more children[c]	0.257	0.723	0.355	
After marriage:1 child[c]	−0.309	0.255	−1.212	
After marriage: 2 or more children[c]	−0.058	0.586	−0.099	
Income				
Before marriage: household	−0.150	0.263	−0.569	
After marriage: household	−0.059	0.345	−0.171	
Residual deviance	505.478			
Degrees of freedom	676.000			
Log-likelihood:	−252.739			
Odds ratio:	13.590			

Note. * $p \leq 0.05$; ** $p \leq 0.01$; *** $p \leq 0.001$
[a]ref. men
[b]ref. medium level of education
[c]ref. childless

This study is of importance because it questions the origin of the highlighted differences between cohabiting and married individuals. However, it has some limitations. The first one is the relatively small numbers of married individuals included in the analyses. A larger group would lead to more robust results and allow for the study of gender differences. For the current study, the small number of men and women did not allow us to highlight these differences. A second limitation resides in the highly selective SHP subsample we investigated. The high proportion of highly educated individuals does not favor the study of dynamics for individuals with fewer resources. Despite these limitations, our study provides some results about the mechanisms that lead to the well-known differences between cohabiting and married individuals. Further research should also better tackle these questions by taking into account the heterogeneity of the cohabitation and comparing cohabitant who marry with those who do not marry (Hiekel and Castro-Martín 2014). This could become of importance in Switzerland as more and more couples decide to remain unmarried when they have children.

References

Bozon, M. (1992). Sociologie du rituel du mariage. *Population (French Edition), 47*(2), 409–433.

Bozon, M., & Héran, F. (2006). *La formation du couple - Textes essentiels pour la sociologie de la famille*. Paris: Grands Repères.

Brown, S. L. (2000). The effect of union type on psychological well-being: Depression among cohabitors versus marrieds. *Journal of Health and Social Behavior, 41*, 241–255.

Brown, S. L. (2004). Moving from cohabitation to marriage: Effects on relationship quality. *Social Science Research, 33*, 1–19. https://doi.org/10.1016/S0049-089X(03)00036-X.

Bumpass, L. L., Sweet, J. A., & Cherlin, A. (1991). The role of cohabitation in declining rates of marriage. *Journal of Marriage and the Family, 53*(4), 913–927.

Cherlin, A. J. (2004). The deinstitutionalization of american marriage. *Journal of Marriage and Family, 66*, 848–861. https://doi.org/10.1111/j.0022-2445.2004.00058.x.

Clarkberg, M., Stolzenberg, R. M., & Waite, L. J. (1995). Attitudes, values, and entrance into cohabitational versus marital unions. *Social Forces, 74*(2), 609–632.

Diener, E., Gohm, C. L., Suh, M. E., & Oishi, S. (2000). Similarity of the relations between marital status and subjective well-being across cultures. *Journal of Cross-Cultural Psychology, 31*, 419–436. https://doi.org/10.1177/0022022100031004001.

Esping-Andersen, G., & Billari, F. C. (2015). Re-theorizing family demographics. *Population and Development Review, 41*(1), 1–31.

Gabadinho, A. (1998). *L'enquête Suisse sur la famille*. Berne: Office fédéral de la statistique.

Hiekel, N., & Castro-Martín, T. (2014). Grasping the diversity of cohabitation: Fertility intentions among cohabiters across Europe. *Journal of Marriage and Family, 76*(3), 489–505.

Jose, A., O'Leary, D. K., & Moyer, A. (2010). Does premarital cohabitation predict subsequent marital stability and marital quality? A meta-analysis. *Journal of Marriage and Family, 72*, 105–116.

Le Cessie, S., & Van Houwelingen, J. (1994). Logistic regression for correlated binary data. *Applied Statistics, 43*, 95–108.

Le Goff, J.-M., & Ryser, V.-A. (2010). The meaning of marriage for men during their transition to fatherhood. The Swiss context. *Marriage & Family Review, 46*, 107–125. https://doi.org/10.1080/01494921003648654.

Le Goff, J.-M., & Ryser, V.-A. (2013). Mariage et union consensuelle avec enfant en Suisse. In D. Tabutin & B. Masquelier (Eds.), *Ralentissements, résistances et ruptures dans les transitions démographiques* (pp. 157–172). Louvain-La-Neuve: Presses universitaires de Louvain, Acte de colloque chaire de Quetelet.

Le Goff, J.-M., Sauvain-Dugerdil, C., Rossier, C., & Coenen-Huther, J. (2005). *Maternité et parcours de vie*. Berne: Peter Lang.

Lesthaeghe, R., & Surkyn, J. (1988). Cultural dynamics and economic theories of fertility change. *Population and Developpment Review, 14*(1), 1–45.

Levy, R., Gauthier, J.-A., & Widmer, E. (2006). Entre contraintes institutionnelles et domestiques : Les parcours de vie masculins et féminins en Suisse. *Canadian Journal of Sociology/Cahiers canadiens de sociologie, 31*(4), 461–489.

Lipps, O. (2010). Income imputation in the Swiss Household Panel 1999–2007. *FORS Working Paper Series*, paper 2010-1. Lausanne: FORS.

Manting, D. (1996). The changing meaning of cohabitation and marriage. *European Sociological Review, 12*(1), 53–65.

Nock, S. L. (1995). A comparison of marriages and cohabiting relationships. *Journal of Family Issues, 16*(1), 53–76. https://doi.org/10.1177/019251395016001004.

Palmgren, J. (1989). *Regression models for bivariate binary responses*. Technical Report no. 101. Seattle: University of Washington, Department of Biostatistics.
Perelli-Harris, B., & Gerber, T. P. (2011). Nonmarital childbearing in Russia: Second demographic transition or pattern of disadvantage? *Demography, 48*(1), 317–342.
Perelli-Harris, B., & Sánchez Gassen, N. (2012). How similar are cohabitation and marriage? Legal approaches to cohabitation across Western Europe. *Population and Development Review, 38*(3), 435–467.
Regnier-Loilier, A., Beaujouan, É., & Villeneuve-Gokalp, C. (2009). Neither single, nor in a couple. A study of living apart together in France. *Demographic Research, 21*(4), 75–108.
Ryser, V.-A., & Le Goff, J.-M. (2011). Le mariage en Suisse : Contrainte institutionnelle ou choix de vie. In S. Gouazé, A. Salles, & C. Prat-Erkert (Eds.), *Les enjeux démographiques en France et en Allemagne : Réalités et conséquences* (pp. 109–123). Lille: Septentrion.
Ryser, V.-A., & Le Goff, J.-M. (2015). Family attitudes and gender opinions of cohabiting and married mothers in Switzerland. *Family Science, 6*(1), 370–379.
Schultz Lee, K., & Ono, H. (2012). Marriage, cohabitation, and happiness: A cross-national analysis of 27 countries. *Journal of Marriage and Family, 74*(5), 953–972.
Sobotka, T., & Toulemon, L. (2008). Overview chapter 4: Changing family and partnership behaviour: Common trends and persistent diversity across Europe. *Demographic Research, 19*, 85–138.
Soons, J. P. M., & Kalmijn, M. (2009). Is marriage more than cohabitation? Well-being differences in 30 European countries. *Journal of Marriage and Family, 71*, 1141–1157. https://doi.org/10.1111/j.1741-3737.2009.00660.x.
Théry, I. (1998). *Couple, filiation et parenté aujourd'hui*. Paris: Odile Jacob.
Toulemon, L. (1996). La cohabitation hors mariage s' installe dans la durée. *Population (French Edition), 51*(3), 675–715.
van der Kaa, D. (1987). Europe's second demographic transition. *Population Bulletin, 42*(1), 1–59.
van der Lippe, T., Voorpostel, M., & Hewitt, B. (2014). Disagreements among cohabiting and married couples in 22 European countries. *Demographic Research, 31*(10), 247–274.
Villeneuve-Gokalp, C. (1997). Vivre en couple chacun chez soi. *Population (French Edition), 52*, 1059–1081.
Wiik, K. A., Bernhardt, E., & Noack, T. (2009). A study of commitment and relationship quality in Sweden and Norway. *Journal of Marriage and Family, 71*(3), 465–477. https://doi.org/10.1111/j.1741-3737.2009.00613.x.
Wilcox, W. B., & Nock, S. L. (2006). What's love got to do with it? Equality, equity, commitment and women's marital quality. *Social Forces, 84*(3), 1321–1345.
Yee, T. W. (2010). The VGAM package for categorical data analysis. *Journal of Statistical Software, 32*(10), 1–34.
Yee, T. W., & Dirnböck, T. (2009). Models for analysing species' presence/absence data at two time points. *Journal of Theoretical Biology, 259*(4), 684–694.

Chapter 5
Family Trajectories and Life Satisfaction: The Swiss Case

Boris Wernli and Sara Zella

Introduction

It would not be surprising to say that life has ups and downs and that its instability is caused by the events that individuals experience over time. The number of articles on happiness and well-being that appear in mainstream journals have proven a strong association between well-being and health, work career, social contacts and family episodes (Dolan et al. 2008). In this chapter, we focus on the relationship between family and happiness, which is motivated by the several changes that a family may experience and by the role that different family events may play on well-being (Vignoli et al. 2014). Expanding upon previous research on this topic, we consider five events that indicate the construction or, oppositely, the dissolution of family. The first situation is distinguished by the formation of the union, the transition from cohabitation to marriage and the birth of children. Dissolution is defined by the departure of a child from the parents' house and episodes of the divorce/separation.

Existing studies on family events and well-being support the theoretical predictions of the positive association between being in a relationship and life satisfaction (e.g. Kohler et al. 2005) and the negative impact of divorce on happiness (e.g. Kalmijn 2009). More scarce and mixed are the results of the presence of children on happiness (Aassve et al. 2012; Billari 2009; Kohler et al. 2005).

B. Wernli (✉)
Swiss Centre of Expertise in the Social Science (FORS), University of Lausanne, Lausanne, Switzerland
e-mail: boris.wernli@unil.ch

S. Zella
Swiss Centre of Expertise in the Social Science (FORS) and Oxford Institute of Population Ageing, University of Oxford, Oxford, UK
e-mail: sara.zella@ageing.ox.ac.uk

R. Tillmann et al. (eds.), *Social Dynamics in Swiss Society*, Life Course Research and Social Policies 9, https://doi.org/10.1007/978-3-319-89557-4_5

Following the mainstream research in recent years, we used a longitudinal perspective to reach a double aim. First, we did so to understand how the mentioned events are associated with changes in subjective well-being. Second, we aimed to capture the duration of this effect. Specifically, we asked whether the mentioned events have only a temporary effect on well-being or whether this impact lasts for a longer time (Anusic et al. 2013; Lucas et al. 2003; Myrskylä and Margolis 2014).

We focussed on the Swiss context and used fourteen years of the Swiss Household Panel (SHP).

Family Events and Well-Being

Across several decades, the literature has highlighted the positive effects of being part of a couple (cohabitant and married) on well-being (e.g. Kohler et al. 2005). The reasons are mainly associated with social, economic and emotional support mechanisms. Indeed, having a partner seems to help individuals cope with the difficulties of life, feel less lonely and feel less helpless (Blanchflower and Oswald 2004), and it encourages sharing resources and financial responsibility. However, a jarring challenge to the consensus of the positive effects of the creation of a couple on well-being was proposed in recent years. A rising question asks whether the level of happiness (derived from having a partner) dissipates over time, rather than remaining stable and, more generally, whether an individual can adapt to a new (expected or unforeseen) family situation.

In the literature on happiness and family, one of the first studies that answered this question was proposed by Lucas et al. (2003). They concluded that the creation of a couple only increases the life satisfaction of the partners temporarily, and typically, they revert two years after marriage to the same "baseline" level of life satisfaction that prevailed two years prior. Similarly, Lucas and Clark (2006) and Stutzer and Frey (2006) identified a sort of "honeymoon effect" in Germany, and Angeles (2010) found an analogous effects in the U.K. Angeles (2010) also underlined important differences between genders: women have a larger positive effect than men, they enjoy an anticipation effect of one year and their level of satisfaction remains statistically significant until three years after marriage (whilst for men it lasts only one year). Anusic et al. (2013) showed that Swiss individuals are not happier after marriage, but they have a higher well-being level than they would if they had remained single.

Following the previous findings, we hypothesize that unions are positively associated with life satisfaction, both for Swiss women and for Swiss men; however, we expect to find a "honeymoon effect". Therefore, the year before and the years during the union may be characterised by the highest level of life satisfaction, which may tend to decrease a few years afterwards, but it presumably remains higher than before this event (Zimmermann and Easterlin 2006).

The adaptation approach has also been used in the studies on divorce, separation and widowhood. There has been the general consensus that these events (divorce in particular) have a negative effect on one's well-being (e.g. Williams and Umberson 2004; Kalmijn and Monden 2009). Nevertheless, results were conflicting when using the longitudinal approach. For example, Amato and Booth (1991) found that people can adapt to situations of divorce, whilst Johnson and Wu (2002), using the same data, contradicted these results and concluded that divorce was associated with permanent changes in levels of distress. Lucas (2005) showed that an individual's satisfaction drops as one approaches divorce, then it gradually rebounds over time, but the return to baseline is not complete. Finally, Clark et al. (2008) found that habituation to divorce is rapid and complete, and they proved that both men and women who are divorced for more than four years are currently significantly more satisfied with their lives.

We expect similar behaviour in dealing with the divorce of Swiss couples: large losses in happiness and a strong anticipation effect. We hypothesize that the initial fall in happiness will disappear after few years, but that individuals will not reach their pre-divorce level of happiness (Lucas 2005). In addition, differences between genders may exist. Men probably suffer more than women at the time of the break (Angeles 2010), but they might recover faster than females.

Whilst the creation of a couple and its disintegration have straightforward effects on life satisfaction, more contradicted are the results on the transition to parenthood (Aassve et al. 2012; Billari 2009; Kohler et al. 2005). Psychological studies suggest negative consequences are associated with childbearing, as parents experience stress that is related to increased financial responsibilities (Zimmermann and Easterlin 2006) and reduce their leisure time, and the quality of the couple's relationship also tends to decrease (Lavee et al. 1996). In the opposite direction is the fertility theory, which suggests a positive link between life satisfaction and parenthood. Billari (2009) suggested that fertility is positively correlated with happiness, but is mediated by the policy environment. In another study, Angeles (2010) found that the birth of a child brings important happiness to women, with an anticipation effect of one year and a similar large effect at the time of birth. For men, there is an anticipation effect (though smaller than that of women), but there is an absence of such an effect at the time of birth.

Since trajectories capture not only the effect of birth but the broader process of childbearing (Myrskylä and Margolis 2014), we expect that happiness increases before a birth. In particular, Swiss women may gain more in happiness in expectation and right after a birth than Swiss men, but they may experience steeper drops the following years (Clark et al. 2008). Part of the stronger dip may be due to a larger anticipation effect, but it may also be due to the fact that women are more socially isolated after childbirth, as they have often taken leave from the labour force and act as the primary caregiver, particularly when the child is young (Della Giusta et al. 2011; Simon 1992).

Last, we consider the departure of children from their parents' home. Despite strikingly less attention being devoted to this event in the literature (Bouchard 2014), it is of great concern to researchers for two main reasons. First, because an empty nest engenders complex emotions for parents, both positive and negative (Beaupré et al. 2006; Dare 2011). Second, understanding the conditions under which couples can experience a more positive transition constitutes one of the first steps in promoting well-being among couples. Two perspectives have been developed in recent years: the role loss perspective and the role strain (relief) perspective. The first perspective predicts a decrease of parents' well-being as a consequence of a child's departure. In sharp contrast to the hypothesis of a loss, the role of strain relief perspective suggests that the empty-nest stage leads to improved parental well-being, since children at home increase exposure to stressors, such as daily demands and work–family conflicts (Erickson et al. 2010; Umberson et al. 2010; White and Edwards 1990). Notwithstanding, research has been slightly incoherent regarding the impact of the departure of a child from home, and the majority of studies published in recent decades have painted a more optimistic picture. They underline that only the absence of alternative roles in which to continue building an identity (after children leave home) explains the negative effects of children's departure on parents' well-being (e.g. Raup and Myers 1989). Looking at longitudinal studies in North America and Europe, we hypothesize that in Switzerland, the positive effect of the empty nest on parental well-being also appears to be stronger immediately after the children take their leave (White and Edwards 1990); it then decreases and tends to disappear after few years (Harkins 1978).

Data

The different subsamples of SHP (Tillmann et al. 2016) participants who completed the individual questionnaire are defined differently depending on the transition under study. For each transition, individuals were followed from wave 3 (2001) until wave 16 (2014). The first two waves are not included in our study due to the late inclusion of some indicators in the questionnaire. The composition of the different samples is explained in the follow section.

Formation of the Union At the beginning of our observation window, only single individuals were included. They could live with a partner (or not) in subsequent waves. Cases with children or with other persons living together were not considered to decontaminate this transition from other potential influences. Our sample comprises 3241 persons (1903 women and 1338 men) who fulfil the abovementioned conditions and who have validly completed the individual questionnaire on all the considered variables (complete cases). In total, 17,188 valid[1] observations were considered during this analysis.

From Cohabitation to Marriage We ran analyses for two different samples. The first sample includes only partners living in a two-person household, excluding individuals living with children or other persons (parents, etc.). At the start of our observation window, all these individuals were not married (they can be single, divorced

[1] With non-missing values for every variable included in the model.

or widowed[2]). In total, 2035 individuals (1064 women and 971 men) fulfilled these conditions, corresponding with 7197 complete cases. In the second sample, we did not impose restrictions on the household size. Therefore, children or other persons were possibly in the household before, during and after this transition. As before, selected individuals were living together with a partner at the start of the period under review and could get married (or not) during the subsequent waves. The sample comprised 2700 individuals (1421 women and 1279 men), who were followed during 12,507 complete observations.

Birth of Children In total, 15,013 individuals were considered (8034 women and 6979 men), for a total of 94,205 full observations, without an age limit or any restrictions concerning the composition of the households. Even individuals without partners were considered here, although their chances to experience this transition were low.

Dissolution of the Union We considered the persons living with a partner at the beginning of their period under review. The sample consisted of 9742 individuals (5155 women and 4587 men), all followed during 61,115 complete periods.

Departure of Children The initial sample included individuals living with a partner and one or more children. In addition, the couple remained together even after the departure of the child. In total, 5403 parents (2875 women and 2528 men) were followed, corresponding to 36,002 complete episodes.

Variables

Our dependent variable is life satisfaction, measured at each wave on an 11-point scale ranging from 0 to 10, with 5 as a neutral position.[3]

The transitions under study are defined as changes from the initial status in the interval of two successive waves. We studied their impact on the mid-term and therefore did not focus only on the observation just after the transition; rather, we it took into consideration two years before and after the event. Therefore, we constructed five dichotomous variables, indicating the two years before (t-2, t-1), the year of the transition (t0) and the two following two years (t + 1, t + 2). The reference category is any year (before or after) which is not included in the five-year string surrounding the abovementioned transitions. Transitions occurring when a wave was skipped were not taken into consideration, given the difficulty of timing events precisely and building accurate measurements.

As control variables, we include the *wave of the survey* to control for the potential effects of the period. The *ages* of the respondents were introduced as a set of

[2] To get potentially married at the subsequent wave.

[3] "In general, how satisfied are you with your life if 0 means 'not at all satisfied' and 10 means 'completely satisfied'?"

dichotomous variables, given their potential nonlinear impact: less than 30 years, 30 to 44 years, 45 thru 64 years and 65 years and older, the latter being the reference category. *Education* was introduced as a continuous scale, ranging from 0 to 10, representing the standardized levels of education in the Swiss system; its linear effect on our dependent variable was verified beforehand. *Working time* is expressed as a percentage of full-time work, and *net yearly household income* (in 10,000 Swiss Fr) was also considered, with missing values imputed (10% to 15%, depending on the wave) using the Little and Su procedure (Lipps 2010). Two parameters of *health* were considered. First, satisfaction with health status[4] was considered as a proxy of health. Second, we used a variable related to health impediments in everyday activities.[5] *Financial satisfaction* was taken into account and was evaluated on a scale of 0–10, using 0 for "not satisfied" and 10 for "very satisfied", as well as *satisfaction of the individual's interpersonal relationships.*[6] We also considered *participation in clubs or other groups,*[7] *satisfaction with free time*[8] and *satisfaction with leisure activities*[9] for each wave to control for these aspects, which are recognized to have an influence on life satisfaction. Finally, we included a dichotomous variable stating *whether the interviewee lived with a partner* in the model, predicting the impact of the birth of children to consider lone parents in the analysis.

The inclusion of other satisfaction variables as controls can be criticized for theoretical reasons, but similar models were run without these variables with equivalent results.

Analytical Tool

To evaluate the mid-term impact of the events shaping family trajectories with longitudinal data, we estimated a set of multilevel linear models (MLMs) (Hox 2002; Singer and Willett 2003) using the SPSS software (which is notably similar to the SAS Proc Mixed procedure).

These MLMs were designed for longitudinal data (Hox 2002; Singer and Willett 2003) with several observations in a varying number per individual. For these mod-

[4] "How satisfied are you with your state of health, where 0 means 'not at all satisfied' and 10 is 'completely satisfied'?"

[5] "Please tell me to what extent, generally, your health is an impediment in your everyday activities, in your housework and in your work or leisure activities? Note that 0 means 'not at all' and 10 is 'a great deal'."

[6] "How satisfied are you with your personal, social and familial relationships, where 0 means 'not at all satisfied' and 10 is 'completely satisfied'?"

[7] "Do you take part in clubs or other group activities, including religious groups?"

[8] "How satisfied are you with the amount of free time you have, where 0 means 'not at all satisfied' and 10 is 'completely satisfied'?"

[9] "How satisfied are you with your leisure time activities, where 0 means 'not at all satisfied' and 10 is 'completely satisfied'?"

els, repeated observations of the same individual constitute a sub-level[10] of the analysis that takes the form of a composite multilevel model for change (Hox 2002; Singer and Willett 2003). The continuous dependent variables (positive and negative effects) are the linear sum of the structural components (first bracket of Eq. 5.1 below), which have the same effect for all individuals, whereas error terms[11] are randomly distributed among individuals.

$$Y_{ij} = \left[\gamma_{00} + \beta_1 . x_{1ij} + \beta_2 . x_{2ij} + \ldots + \beta_p . x_{pij} \right] + \left[\mu_{0j} + \varepsilon_{ij} \right]$$

$$\text{where } i = \textit{wave index and } j = \textit{individual index} \tag{5.1}$$

$$\text{where } \mu_{0j} \sim N\left(0, \tau_{00}\right); \text{cov}\left(\varepsilon_{ij,}\varepsilon_{i'j}\right) = \sigma^2 \rho^{|i-i'|}$$

The residuals (last bracket of Eq. 5.1) are divided into two parts. In addition to the varying error term for each observation (εij), which is common to every regression equation, we also considered a second error term (μ0j) that remains constant for all observations of the same individual. This approach allowed us to structure the residuals and correlate them across waves.

The chosen model is a first-order autoregressive structural model of the covariance of the residuals (AR1), which is a common choice for repeated measures. It means that, for a given individual, the residuals are correlated from one observation to the next, but in a variable fashion as a function of their proximity. Significant AR1 diagonal (covariance) and AR1 rho (correlation with the preceding observation) coefficients in our analyses demonstrate the pertinence of this choice.

Our models are estimated separately for each sex and are not weighted for two reasons: first, weights distort the gathered data on the basis of sociodemographic parameters, but nothing ensures that representativeness will be reached concerning the variable of interest, namely life-satisfaction; and second, indicators used for weighting are already controlled in our models.

Results

The Family Construction

Table 5.1 presents the first two transitions associated with the construction of the family, namely the *formation of the union* and the transition from *cohabitation to marriage*.

[10] Our models distinguish only two levels (observations and individuals), given the fact that equations are run separately for women and for men. Intra-household correlations within partners living together are thus avoided.

[11] Error terms have a standard normal distribution (a mean of 0), an unknown variance and a structure that can be modeled.

Table 5.1 Impact of the formation of the union and the passage from cohabitation to marriage on life satisfaction – SHP 2001–2014, unweighted

	Formation of the union				Cohabitation to marriage (without children)				Cohabitation to marriage (general model)			
	Women		Men		Women		Men		Women		Men	
	Net impact	Sig.	Net impact	Sig.	Net impact	Sig.	Net impact	Sig.	Net impact	Sig.	Net impact	Sig.
Intercept	2.982	0.000	2.606	0.000	3.508	0.000	3.465	0.000	3.823	0.000	3.551	0.000
Age younger than 30 years	−0.151	0.043	−0.130	0.137	0.210	0.043	0.003	0.980	0.210	0.024	0.067	0.494
30–44 years	−0.318	0.000	−0.355	0.000	0.147	0.157	−0.103	0.331	0.093	0.312	−0.053	0.576
45–64 years	−0.342	0.000	−0.326	0.000	0.064	0.494	−0.189	0.059	0.058	0.508	−0.188	0.036
65 years and older – Reference												
Wave	0.006	0.053	0.013	0.003	0.006	0.225	0.004	0.487	0.002	0.564	0.010	0.013
Level of education – Standardized 0–10	0.015	0.056	0.004	0.630	0.011	0.179	0.024	0.012	0.011	0.101	0.013	0.090
Working time – % of full-time job	0.002	0.000	0.003	0.000	0.001	0.178	0.003	0.001	0.000	0.387	0.003	0.000
Household income – In 10,000 CHF	0.001	0.245	0.005	0.092	0.000	0.994	0.000	0.987	0.002	0.182	0.000	0.754
Satisfaction with health status – 0–10	0.139	0.000	0.158	0.000	0.161	0.000	0.137	0.000	0.153	0.000	0.138	0.000
Health impediment – 0–10	−0.020	0.000	−0.024	0.001	−0.008	0.356	0.000	0.978	−0.017	0.007	−0.008	0.217
Satisfaction with financial situation – 0–10	0.209	0.000	0.209	0.000	0.156	0.000	0.158	0.000	0.145	0.000	0.145	0.000
Satisfaction with personal relationships – 0–10	0.140	0.000	0.164	0.000	0.131	0.000	0.157	0.000	0.132	0.000	0.158	0.000
Satisfaction with free time – 0–10	0.028	0.000	0.028	0.001	0.041	0.000	0.042	0.000	0.036	0.000	0.035	0.000
Satisfaction with leisure activities – 0–10	0.100	0.000	0.080	0.000	0.062	0.000	0.059	0.000	0.055	0.000	0.058	0.000

Participation in a club or group – 0–1	0.064	0.031	0.051	0.157	0.012	0.757	0.013	0.747	−0.014	0.651	0.024	0.443
2 years before transition – t-2	0.070	0.467	−0.072	0.430	−0.057	0.549	0.028	0.763	−0.042	0.569	0.012	0.868
1 year before transition – t-1	0.188	0.021	0.136	0.079	0.095	0.234	0.034	0.665	0.156	0.010	0.054	0.356
Year of transition – t0	0.229	0.004	0.309	0.000	0.201	0.009	0.246	0.001	0.243	0.000	0.222	0.000
1 year after transition – t + 1	0.204	0.025	0.249	0.004	0.204	0.032	0.166	0.069	0.222	0.000	0.151	0.010
2 years after transition – t + 2	−0.049	0.636	0.173	0.089	0.296	0.013	0.050	0.663	0.158	0.015	0.106	0.085
Number of children <18 years									0.006	0.796	−0.004	0.832
Birth of child since last wave									0.251	0.000	0.086	0.086
Year of transition * birth of child since last wave									−0.154	0.283	−0.031	0.829
Number of observations	10,664		6524		3802		3395		6563		5944	
Number of individuals	1903		1338		1064		971		1421		1279	
Number of transitions	251		272		182		183		303		287	
−2 restricted likelihood	34,224		20,499		10,712		9481		18,391		16,138	
AIC	34,230		20,505		10,718		9487		18,397		16,144	
BIC	34,252		20,526		10,737		9505		18,418		16,164	
Individual random effect, AR1 diagonal (cov)	1.188	0.000	1.113	0.000	0.801	0.000	0.773	0.000	0.812	0.000	0.703	0.000
Individual random effect, AR1 rho (corr)	0.072	0.000	0.122	0.000	0.112	0.000	0.139	0.000	0.121	0.000	0.119	0.000
Random effect variance	0.554	0.000	0.499	0.000	0.267	0.000	0.290	0.000	0.279	0.000	0.384	0.000

The formation of the union is characterized by the transition from the single-person household to the couple living together, without any other person (especially children), to control for the influence of other events.

In our sample, 251 women and 272 men experienced this transition during the 14 waves considered. The coefficient indicated that the positive impact of the formation of the union on life satisfaction can be perceived one year before the transition (t-1), especially for women (0.19, $p = 0.021$, compared to 0.14, $p = 0.079$ for men), and reaches a peak just in the year of the transition (t0) (0.23 for women, 0.31 for men). The positive impact generally lasts one more year (t + 1) for both women and men (0.20 and 0.25) and vanishes two years after the transition (no longer significant for both sexes).

In studying the transition from cohabitation to marriage (182 transitions for women and 183 for men in the simple model, and 303 and 287 in the general model, respectively), we found an increase in life satisfaction from both women and men the in the year of transition (t0) (0.20 and 0.24 for women and 0.25 and 0.22 for men, respectively) and one year after (t + 1) (0.20 and 0.22, and 0.17 and 0.15 for men, respectively). In the second year after marriage (t + 2), its positive impact was still perceivable among women (0.30 and 0.16) but was no longer significant among men. Additionally, the positive impact starts before the transition (t-1) in the general model, but only for women (0.16). Even when we control for the number of children in the household and for the birth of a child during the previous 12 months (given that this event is often concomitant with marriage in Switzerland), the results did not change. However, when marriage and the birth of a child happened in the same year, we did not find a supplementary impact on life satisfaction.

The models presented in Table 5.2 were run to predict the impact of the next step in the family construction, the *birth of children*. Therefore, we distinguished the rank of children and separately analysed the birth of the first, the second and the third (and subsequent) child (or children).

The impact of this transition on life satisfaction follows a different pattern according to the rank of children and the sex of the respondents. We first noted a positive impact at the time of each birth among women, even if this positive impact decreased somewhat with the rank of children (0.39 for the 1st child, 0.23 for the 2nd child, 0.21 for the 3rd child and subsequent children). The impact is also positive the year before (t-1) each of those transitions (0.29, 0.14 and 0.21, respectively), revealing a positive effect of pregnancy on life satisfaction. Furthermore, this positive influence generally does not last among women; it can only be marginally noted one year after the birth of the third child (0.20, $p = 0.036$).

Table 5.2 Impact of the birth of children on life satisfaction – SHP 2001–2014, unweighted

	Birth of children			
	Women		Men	
	Net impact	Sig.	Net impact	Sig.
Intercept	3.682	0.000	3.692	0.000
Age younger than 30 years	0.188	0.000	0.168	0.000
30–44 years	−0.095	0.000	−0.128	0.000
45–64 years	−0.121	0.000	−0.146	0.000
65 years and older – Reference				
Wave	−0.004	0.011	−0.001	0.709
Level of education – Standardized 0–10	−0.004	0.208	−0.011	0.000
Working time – % of full-time job	0.000	0.063	0.001	0.000
Household income – In 10,000 CHF	0.002	0.000	0.003	0.000
Satisfaction with health status – 0–10	0.142	0.000	0.149	0.000
Health impediment – 0–10	−0.019	0.000	−0.023	0.000
Satisfaction with financial situation – 0–10	0.165	0.000	0.150	0.000
Satisfaction with personal relationships – 0–10	0.145	0.000	0.141	0.000
Satisfaction with free time – 0–10	0.028	0.000	0.028	0.000
Satisfaction with leisure activities – 0–10	0.066	0.000	0.066	0.000
Participation in a club or group – 0–1	0.042	0.000	0.063	0.000
Living together with a partner	0.247	0.000	0.300	0.000
2 years before birth of 1st child	−0.024	0.724	0.025	0.698
1 year before birth of 1st child	0.285	0.000	0.166	0.006
Year of birth of 1st child	0.390	0.000	0.170	0.005
1 year after birth of 1st child	0.080	0.234	0.151	0.021
2 years after birth of 1st child	0.050	0.495	0.151	0.032
2 years before birth of 2nd child	0.097	0.199	0.078	0.287
1 year before birth of 2nd child	0.138	0.053	0.046	0.497
Year of birth of 2nd child	0.229	0.001	0.053	0.411
1 year after birth of 2nd child	−0.088	0.172	0.127	0.044
2 years after birth of 2nd child	0.048	0.486	0.028	0.677
2 years before birth of 3rd child	0.044	0.669	0.165	0.089
1 year before birth of 3rd child	0.214	0.028	0.013	0.889
Year of birth of 3rd child	0.262	0.004	0.106	0.219
1 year after birth of 3rd child	0.200	0.036	0.134	0.136
2 years after birth of 3rd child	0.127	0.213	0.130	0.181
Number of observations	51,893		42,312	
Number of individuals	8034		6979	
Number of births of 1st child	316		292	
Number of births of 2nd child	289		270	
Number of births of 3rd child	138		137	
−2 restricted likelihood	154,140		120,122	
AIC	154,146		120,128	
BIC	154,173		120,154	
Individual random effect, AR1 diagonal (cov)	0.986	0.000	0.855	0.000
Individual random effect, AR1 rho (corr)	0.127	0.000	0.132	0.000
Random effect variance	0.382	0.000	0.363	0.000

The situation is different for men; only the birth of the first child has a notable impact, but this impact is more constant and persistent on the mid-term (0.17 at t-1 and t0, and 0.15 at t + 1 and t + 2). Apart from a marginal impact one year after the birth of the second child (0.13, $p = 0.044$), other successive births do not convey such a positive feeling of satisfaction.

The Family Dissolution

Table 5.3 shows the impact of the *dissolution of the union*, namely living without a partner after having experienced cohabitation during the previous wave. We distinguished two forms of dissolution: the generic separation, irrespective of the reason (break up, divorce, widowhood, etc.), to which we added a specific effect in case of widowhood, to take into account the very different nature of this event.

The impact of separation on life satisfaction shows a similar pattern for women and men, but with a temporal gap. The negative impact is felt earlier and stronger by women (−0.21, −0.49 and − 0.63 at t-2, t-1 and t0, respectively), but it vanishes sooner (−0.28 at t + 1, no longer significant at t + 2). On the other hand, men tend to perceive a somewhat smoother impact until the time of the event (−0.18, −0.36, −0.61, at t-2, t-1 and t0, respectively), but the influence tends to persist over time (−0.53 at t + 1 and − 0.26 at t + 2).

The total influence of *widowhood* on life satisfaction is composed of the impact of generic separation cumulated[12] to the specific effect of widowhood, given that the latter also comprises a separation. The total effect of widowhood is particularly detrimental to life satisfaction for both women and men at the time of the event (−1.1 and − 0.97, respectively), as well as the year after (−0.49 and − 0.53 at t + 1, respectively). As for generic separation, the effect lasts longer for men and is still perceivable two years after (−0.26), but can be observed sooner among women (−0.49 in t-1).

We also included a specific effect that measured the interaction of the presence of at least a minor child in the household at the time of the separation. Interestingly, its effect is slightly positive for women (0.16, $p = 0.081$) but largely negative for men (−0.44, $p = 0.002$). In case of separation, the presence of a child seems then to represent a resource for women, helping attenuate the negative effect on life satisfaction, but engenders an increased dissatisfaction for men.

The last transition we examined was the *departure of children* from the family nest while the couple remained together. In general, the impact of this transition was not significant in the short term or in the medium term for both women and men. The only exception included the departure of the last (often the youngest) household's child: in this case, the life satisfaction of fathers slightly increases (Table 5.4).

[12] In the calculation, only significant impacts were taken into account.

Table 5.3 Impact of the dissolution of the union on life satisfaction – SHP 2001–2014, unweighted

	Dissolution of the union			
	Women		Men	
	Net impact	Sig.	Net impact	Sig.
Intercept	3.892	0.000	3.886	0.000
Age younger than 30 years	0.162	0.000	0.010	0.815
30–44 years	−0.023	0.449	−0.126	0.000
45–64 years	−0.053	0.035	−0.162	0.000
65 years and older – Reference				
Wave	−0.009	0.000	−0.002	0.163
Level of education – Standardized 0–10	0.009	0.019	0.008	0.055
Working time – % of full-time job	0.000	0.402	0.002	0.000
Household income – In 10,000 CHF	0.003	0.000	0.002	0.022
Satisfaction with health status – 0–10	0.142	0.000	0.144	0.000
Health impediment – 0–10	−0.015	0.000	−0.020	0.000
Satisfaction with financial situation – 0–10	0.176	0.000	0.162	0.000
Satisfaction with personal relationships – 0–10	0.137	0.000	0.130	0.000
Satisfaction with free time – 0–10	0.034	0.000	0.036	0.000
Satisfaction with leisure activities – 0–10	0.056	0.000	0.059	0.000
Participation in a club or group – 0–1	0.027	0.054	0.052	0.000
Presence of children <18 years – 0–1	0.000	0.998	0.017	0.364
2 years before end of union	−0.210	0.001	−0.183	0.004
1 year before end of union	−0.489	0.000	−0.362	0.000
Year of end of union	−0.625	0.000	−0.610	0.000
1 year after end of union	−0.279	0.000	−0.532	0.000
2 years after end of union	−0.054	0.392	−0.258	0.000
2 years before widowhood	0.158	0.153	0.437	0.016
1 year before widowhood	−0.093	0.364	0.354	0.042
Year of widowhood	−0.471	0.000	−0.359	0.037
1 year after widowhood	−0.215	0.043	0.297	0.123
2 years after widowhood	−0.032	0.774	−0.116	0.582
Year of end of union * presence of children <18 years	0.158	0.081	−0.438	0.002
Number of observations	35,345		29,770	
Number of individuals	5155		4587	
Number of ends of union	620		400	
Number of widowhoods	144		34	
−2 restricted likelihood	102,858		82,573	
AIC	102,864		82,579	
BIC	102,890		82,604	
Individual random effect, AR1 diagonal (cov)	0.933	0.000	0.791	0.000
Individual random effect, AR1 rho (corr)	0.130	0.000	0.111	0.000
Random effect variance	0.356	0.000	0.371	0.000

Table 5.4 Impact of the departure of children on life satisfaction – SHP 2001–2014, unweighted

	Departure of children			
	Women		Men	
	Net impact	Sig.	Net impact	Sig.
Intercept	3.934	0.000	3.948	0.000
Age younger than 30 years	0.349	0.000	0.138	0.141
30–44 years	0.018	0.718	−0.116	0.016
45–64 years	−0.040	0.379	−0.196	0.000
65 years and older – Reference				
Wave	−0.006	0.005	0.005	0.035
Level of education – Standardized 0–10	0.008	0.128	0.011	0.037
Working time – % of full-time job	0.000	0.150	0.002	0.000
Household income – In 10,000 CHF	0.002	0.019	0.001	0.296
Satisfaction with health status – 0–10	0.135	0.000	0.142	0.000
Health impediment – 0–10	−0.018	0.000	−0.026	0.000
Satisfaction with financial situation – 0–10	0.167	0.000	0.155	0.000
Satisfaction with personal relationships – 0–10	0.156	0.000	0.133	0.000
Satisfaction with free time – 0–10	0.028	0.000	0.030	0.000
Satisfaction with leisure activities – 0–10	0.048	0.000	0.050	0.000
Participation in a club or group – 0–1	0.027	0.143	0.074	0.000
Number of children <18 years	−0.007	0.571	−0.015	0.223
2 years before departure	0.009	0.791	0.070	0.042
1 year before departure	0.012	0.697	0.015	0.639
Year of departure	0.009	0.824	−0.069	0.079
1 year after departure	−0.024	0.454	0.004	0.900
2 years after departure	−0.033	0.353	−0.022	0.555
Departure of last child	0.037	0.510	0.163	0.005
Number of observations	19,470		16,532	
Number of individuals	2875		2528	
Number of departure of children	1133		919	
Number of departure of last child	485		371	
−2 restricted likelihood	54,772		44,200	
AIC	54,778		44,206	
BIC	54,802		44,229	
Individual random effect, AR1 diagonal (cov)	0.827	0.000	0.711	0.000
Individual random effect, AR1 rho (corr)	0.114	0.000	0.117	0.000
Random effect variance	0.367	0.000	0.351	0.000

Conclusion and Discussion

In this study, we evaluated the relationship between life satisfaction and five family transitions, using a longitudinal approach. Specifically, we studied mid-term individual trajectories, with the aim to understand not only the impact of several events on well-being, but to capture their duration. Focusing on the Swiss context, we used MLMs for their power in studying changes.

Our main findings can be summarised as follows. First, the creation of a couple increases men's and women's well-being, but the positive effect tends to vanish after a couple of years. Our first hypothesis is therefore confirmed and enables us to extend the previous findings on the "honeymoon effect" in the Swiss context. An increase in life satisfaction also appears for the second event (transition from cohabitation to marriage), and it is clearly stronger for women than for men. The birth of children is associated with increased happiness, but this association is differentiated over time and, again, between females and men. Women declare being happier until the time of the birth, whilst men show an effect the year after the birth and only for the first child.

It is not surprising that the break in a relationship causes unhappiness for the individuals involved but, in this case, women and men react differently. Women seem to suffer more at the moment of the disruption and the years before this event. However, they seem to improve their well-being quickly after the event. On the other hand, men show their unhappiness only at the time of the break, but continue to suffer during the subsequent years. Our results also show that the departure of a child does not induce a significant change in the level of satisfaction, as previous literature has underlined. However, when the effect appeared (as in case of men), it was positive. We therefore interpreted it as if Swiss parents were prepared for this event and tended to have an alternative role in which they continued to build their identity.

To the best of our knowledge, our study can be considered the first that takes into consideration both the association of the mentioned five family events with life satisfaction and their duration over time in the Swiss context. We underlined how family events have a crucial impact on the happiness of individuals and how strong the differences between genders are. In focusing on the Swiss context, it is not hazardous to think that at least part of the divergences between men and women are connected with the conservative gender culture, which determines that men invest rather in the labour market and that still associates women with the main roles of wife and mother. The next step would be to confirm these findings in different cultural contexts, as data from the CNEF project could allow.

References

Aassve, A., Goisis, A., & Sironi, M. (2012). Happiness and childbearing across Europe. *Social Indicators Research, 108*(1), 65–86.

Amato, P. R., & Booth, A. (1991). Consequences of parental divorce and marital unhappiness for adult well-being. *Social Forces, 69*(3), 895–914.

Angeles, L. (2010). *Adaptation and anticipation effects to life events in the United Kingdom* (Department of Economics Discussion Paper 08). University of Glasgow. http://repo.sire.ac.uk/bitstream/handle/10943/134/SIRE_DP_2010_01.pdf?sequence=1&isAllowed=y. Accessed 25 June 2016.

Anusic, I., Stevie, C. Y., & Lucas, R. E. (2013). Testing set-point theory in a Swiss National Sample: Reaction and adaptation to major life events. *Social Indicators Research, 119*, 1265–1288.

Beaupré, P., Turcotte, P., & Milan, A. (2006). When is junior moving out? Transitions from the parental home to independence. *Canadian Social Trends, 82*, 9–15.

Billari, F. C. (2009). *The happiness commonality: Fertility decisions in low-fertility settings*. Keynote address at conference on How generations and gender shape demographic change: Toward policies based on better knowledge, UNECE, Geneva, Switzerland. Retrieved from www.unece.org/fileadmin/DAM/pau/_docs/ggp/2008/GGP_2008_GGConf_Publ_1_Chapter-1.pdf

Blanchflower, D. G., & Oswald, A. J. (2004). Money, sex and happiness: An empirical study. *Scandinavian Journal of Economics, 106*(3), 393–415.

Bouchard, G. (2014). How do parents react when their children leave home? An integrative review. *Journal of Adult Development, 21*(2), 69–79.

Clark, A. E., Diener, E., Georgellis, Y., & Lucas, R. E. (2008). Lags and leads in life satisfaction: A test of the baseline hypothesis. *The Economic Journal, 118*(529), F222–F243.

Dare, J. S. (2011). Transitions in midlife women's lives: Contemporary experiences. *Health Care for Women International, 32*, 111–133.

Della Giusta, M., Jewell, S. L., & Kambhampati, U. S. (2011). Gender and life satisfaction in the UK. *Feminist Economics, 17*(3), 1–34.

Dolan, P., Peasgood, T., & White, M. (2008). Do we really know what makes us happy? A review of the economic literature on the factors associated with subjective well-being. *Journal of Economic Psychology, 29*(1), 94–122.

Erickson, J. J., Martinengo, G., & Hill, E. J. (2010). Putting work and family experiences in context: Differences by family life stage. *Human Relations, 63*, 955–979.

Harkins, E. B. (1978). Effects of empty nest transition on self-report of psychological and physical well-being. *Journal of Marriage and the Family, 40*, 549–556.

Hox, J. J. (2002). *Multilevel analysis. Techniques and applications*. Mahwah: Lawrence Erlbaum Associates.

Johnson, D. R., & Wu, J. (2002). An empirical test of crisis, social selection, and role explanations of the relationship between marital disruption and psychological distress: A pooled time-series analysis of four-wave panel data. *Journal of Marriage and Family, 64*(1), 211–224.

Kalmijn, M. (2009). Country differences in the effects of divorce on well-being: The role of norms, support, and selectivity. *European Sociological Review, 32*(5), 475–490.

Kalmijn, M., & Moden, C. W. S. (2009). Are the negative effects of divorce on well-being dependent on marital quality? *Journal of Marriage and Family, 68*(5), 1197–1213.

Kohler, H. P., Behrman, J. R., & Skytthe, J. R. (2005). Partner children = happiness? The effects of partnerships and fertility on well-being. *Population and Development Review, 31*(3), 407–445.

Lavee, Y., Sharlin, S., & Katy, R. (1996). The effect of parenting stress on marital quality an integrated mother-father model. *Journal of Family Issues, 17*(1), 114–135.

Lipps, O. (2010). *Income imputation in the Swiss Household Panel 1999–2007* (FORS Working Paper Series, 1).

Lucas, R. (2005). Time does not heal all wounds. A longitudinal study of reaction and adaptation to divorce. *Psychological Science, 16*(12), 945–950.

Lucas, R., & Clark, A. E. (2006). Do people really adapt to marriage? *Journal of Happiness Studies, 7*, 405–426.

Lucas, R., Clark, A. E., Georgellis, Y., & Diener, E. (2003). Reexamining adaptation and the set point model of happiness: Reactions to changes in marital status. *Journal of Personality and Social Psychology, 84*(3), 527–539.

Myrskylä, M., & Margolis, R. (2014). Happiness: Before and after kids. *Demography, 51*(5), 1843–1866.

Raup, J. L., & Myers, J. E. (1989). The empty nest syndrome: Myth or reality? *Journal of Counseling and Development, 68*, 180–183.

Simon, R. W. (1992). Parental role strains, salience of parental identity and gender differences in psychological distress. *Journal of Health and Social Behavior, 33*(1), 25–35.

Singer, J. D., & Willett, J. B. (2003). *Applied longitudinal data analysis: Modeling change and event occurrence*. Oxford: University Press.

Stutzer, A., & Frey, B. (2006). Does marriage make people happy or do happy people get married? *The Journal of Socio-Economics, 35*, 326–347.

Tillmann, R., Voorpostel, M., Antal, E., Kuhn, U., Lebert, F., Ryser, V.-A., Lipps, O., & Wernli, B. (2016). The Swiss household panel study: Observing social change since 1999. *Longitudinal and Life Course Studies, 7*(1), 64–78.

Umberson, D., Pudrovska, T., & Reczek, C. (2010). Parenthood, childlessness, and well-being: A life course perspective. *Journal of Marriage and Family, 72*, 612–629.

Vignoli, D., Pirani, E., & Salvini, S. (2014). Family constellations and life satisfaction in Europe. *Social Indicators Research, 117*(3), 967–986.

White, L., & Edwards, J. N. (1990). Emptying the nest and parental well-being: An analysis of national panel data. *American Sociological Review, 55*, 235–242.

Williams, K., & Umberson, D. (2004). Marital status, marital transitions, and health: A gendered life course perspective. *Journal of Health and Social Behavior, 45*(1), 81–98.

Zimmermann, A., & Easterlin, R. (2006). Happily ever after? Cohabitation, marriage, divorce, and happiness in Germany. *Population and Development Review, 32*(3), 511–528.

Chapter 6
The (Un)Healthy Migrant Effect. The Role of Legal Status and Naturalization Timing

Gina Potarca and Laura Bernardi

Introduction

All throughout the Western world, immigrants now constitute a sizeable and fast growing segment of the population, making pivotal contributions to the economic and cultural growth of host societies (e.g., Dustmann and Frattini 2014; Eraydin et al. 2010). Despite these benefits, the discourse promoted by the media and right-wing populist parties focuses on the challenges posed by immigration, and little on the challenges faced by immigrants themselves, particularly regarding health. From a utilitarian point of view, low immigrant health has direct costs in terms of health-care expenses. It also produces indirect costs by reducing immigrants' economic input in the host country as well as in their country of origin via decreased international remittances (Kennedy et al. 2006; Neuman 2014; Rechel et al. 2013). From a humanitarian point of view, an advanced and inclusive society ought to make efforts to reduce social inequalities in health, and to ensure that the human needs, primordially good health, of all of its residents are met, irrespective of origin or nativity (Davies et al. 2010).

The literature on origins and health inequalities identified a so-called 'immigrant epidemiological paradox', which refers to the fact that foreign-born migrants report better health compared to both natives and second generation immigrants of the same origin group, and that this difference is reduced with increasing duration of stay in the country of destination (e.g., Antecol and Bedard 2006). The bulk of research examining such paradox is mainly U.S. focused, with recent advances in Europe (for a review, see Domnich et al. 2012). The few studies that examined the immigrant paradox in European contexts found some evidence in support of the healthy immigrant effect (e.g., Borgdorff et al. 1998), but the phenomenon is far

G. Potarca (✉) · L. Bernardi
Swiss National Centre of Competence in Research LIVES, Lausanne & Geneva, Switzerland
e-mail: gina.potarca@unige.ch; laura.bernardi@unil.ch

R. Tillmann et al. (eds.), *Social Dynamics in Swiss Society*, Life Course Research and Social Policies 9, https://doi.org/10.1007/978-3-319-89557-4_6

from being generalized. On the contrary, a fairly substantial amount of studies reveal that immigrants experience worse health compared to natives (e.g., Solé-Auró and Crimmins 2008). The factors behind this reversed health pattern are largely under-researched. While both objective and self-perceived discrimination have been shown to be key factors negatively affecting the physical and mental health of European immigrants (e.g., Schunck et al. 2015), researchers call for further investigations into the role of other more structural aspects, such as socio-economic or legal integration, with potentially deleterious effects on immigrant health (Riosmena et al. 2015). Though legal vulnerability and the stress of acquiring native citizenship are highly likely to perturb immigrants' health (Mehta and Elo 2012), it has so far received insufficient systematic attention.

In this study, we examine whether immigrants are more likely to report worse health than natives in the context of Switzerland, and whether these differences could be explained by means of citizenship status and naturalization timing. By means of rich longitudinal data from the Swiss Household Panel from the years 1999 till 2014, and multilevel logistic regression modeling, we investigate if the detrimental effect of legal disadvantage and restrictive access to citizenship on health occurs over and above the one generated by economic vulnerability. We predominantly focus on second generation migrants, for whom we can differentiate between different life course stages of naturalization, assuming that the earlier migrants receive Swiss nationality, the smaller the health differences with respect to natives are.

The obstacles European immigrants face in gaining legal stability have become even more strenuous in recent years, against a background of austerity measures and adverse immigration policies (Barbero 2015). Switzerland is a country in which, despite economic prosperity and a large intake of highly skilled migrants (Liebig et al. 2012), state anti-immigrant efforts have gained momentum in the last few years, supported by popular votes (e.g., the 2014 anti-mass immigration referendum vote supporting stricter quotas on foreigners) and the rising political influence of the right-wing Swiss People's Party (Abu-Hayyeh et al. 2014). Documenting the link between legal integration and immigrant health in the Swiss context is thus a fruitful research task not only because of the large size of its immigrant group (i.e., more than a quarter of the population), but also because of the exclusionist legal conditions that immigrants settle into (Castles 1995).

Background

The Immigrant Health Paradox

Despite fewer socio-economic resources and a limited access and use of health care (Ku and Matani 2001), recently arrived immigrants enjoy better health than both the native-born and immigrants that have been residing in the host country, and thus acculturated, for a long time (Antecol and Bedard 2006; Newbold 2005). Scientists have been trying to decrypt the puzzle of this immigrant health paradox by advancing several explanations, including: the health selectivity of immigration, meaning that it is mostly individuals with positive health that choose to immigrate (Akresh and Franck 2008) or are allowed entry through immigrant medical screening (Breuss et al. 2002; Zencovich et al. 2006); the 'salmon-bias' hypothesis, suggesting that unhealthy migrants are more likely to emigrate, resulting in a stock of above-average healthy immigrants left in the host country (Palloni and Arias 2004); and the 'cultural buffering' explanation referring to the lifestyle habits of immigrants belonging to less modern cultures, which often exclude or condemn unhealthy behaviors such as smoking, alcohol consumption, heavy diets, etc. (Cho et al. 2004; Hamilton and Hummer 2011). Previous studies examining European contexts found some evidence of an epidemiological paradox, but most often used difficult-to-compare methodologies and focused on one origin group or a single geographical region. Immigrants were linked to better health than natives across a series of outcomes, ranging from perinatal health in Spain (Restrepo-Mesa et al. 2010), nutrition-related non-communicable diseases in France (Méjean et al. 2007), or disability levels in Germany (Giuntella and Mazzonna 2015). Recent research that looks at multiple health metrics at once and across various immigrant groups reveals that immigrant-native health differentials are highly dependent on origin group (Cebolla-Boado and Salazar 2016; Juárez and Revuelta-Eugercios 2014, 2016; Pacelli et al. 2016), with certain groups experiencing more negative health with reference to natives than others.

There are also studies that unequivocally find that immigrants have worse health than natives. For instance, examining differences in functional ability, disability, disease presence and behavioral risk factors among individuals aged 50 years and older in 11 European countries, Solé-Auró and Crimmins (2008) discovered that immigrants aged 50 years and older report worse health than natives, even after adjusting for socio-economic status. Other cross-national studies also point out immigrants' health disadvantage when looking at self-rated health (Malmusi 2015) or mental health outcomes (Safi 2010; Sieberer et al. 2012). The authors often explain the poor health of migrants by invoking the exposure to health hazards in their country of origin, the precarious residential and employment conditions in the host country, but also the stress of the migration process itself (Rechel et al. 2013). While integrating into a new society, immigrants commonly face a complex and strenuous set of social, cultural, economic and institutional hurdles, increasing their vulnerability to physical and mental illness (Davies et al. 2010).

Legal Status

One factor that might contribute to the emergence of health inequalities between immigrants and natives is the legal trajectory that immigrants go through in the process of assimilation. First, access to permanent resident status or citizenship is a direct determinant of health disparities (Riosmena et al. 2015). Health insurance coverage of U.S. immigrants was shown to differ by citizenship status, with non-citizens being much less likely to receive employer-sponsored health insurance or government coverage, as well as being less likely to sign private health insurance contracts given low wage (Carrasquillo et al. 2000; Derose et al. 2009). The recently implemented Patient Protection and Affordable Care Act in the U.S. continues to exclude undocumented migrants, student and employment visa holders, and short-term legal residents (Joseph 2016). Given restricted access to conventional sources of care, one would expect immigrants to more frequently make use of complementary and alternative medicine (CAM) treatments, but research shows that non-citizens are less likely to use CAM compared to naturalized citizens, and even less so compared to natives (Elewonibi and BeLue 2015). Second, restriction to naturalization and legal long-term residence hampers health indirectly because of processes of spillover across life domains and accumulation of disadvantages by which "exclusion in one sector can influence inequalities in another, producing a synergistic matrix of social conditions that drive health inequities" (WHO Regional Office for Europe 2010, p. 8).

Denial of citizenship rights produces vulnerability in terms of social status, well-being and ultimately health (ib.). Legal status is for instance a large source of disparities in housing cost burden, with unauthorized immigrants being the most affected by housing affordability problems (McConnell 2013). The economic recession in recent years has also accelerated the restriction of universal rights for immigrants, particularly those who cannot comply with strict work and resident permit requirements, leading to a climate of anxiety among non-citizens and non-natives (Barbero 2015). Immigrants with an uncertain legal status may also be more likely to accept atypical, precarious and demanding jobs with non-standard work schedules through their life course, more so than natives (Halpin 2015), leading to a higher prevalence of work-related illnesses. Furthermore, legal status insecurity and holding a transitory residence status could erode health through the simple effect of uncertainty causing psychological distress (Howell and Sweeny 2016).

In Switzerland, some studies encountered a mortality advantage among immigrants (Degrate et al. 1999; Zufferey 2016). Other health-based research though shows that immigrants have worse self-rated health and daily functioning than natives, a disparity that is often larger than in other European countries (Solé-Auró and Crimmins 2008). Also employing a cross-national comparative perspective, Malmusi (2015) discovers a substantial health gap between immigrants and natives in Switzerland (even after controlling for variation in socio-economic status and living conditions), in opposition to the better health experienced by immigrants in multicultural and assimilationist countries. The author indicates that health disparities are particularly apparent in national contexts characterized by exclusionist immigration policies, with strict requirements for long-term residence, naturalization, and family reunification, and where immigrants usually hold a temporary guest worker position and have no political rights. For instance, to currently apply for naturalization in Switzerland, in addition to the procedure's high costs, the residency requirement is of 12 years,[1] with a minimum cantonal residency prerequisite varying between 2 and 5 years (State Secretariat for Migration 2016). According to the Migrant Integration Policy Index (Huddleston et al. 2015), when compared to other Western European countries, Switzerland scores fairly low when it comes to access to citizenship as well as anti-discrimination laws. Despite the fact that international comparisons rate Switzerland favorably in terms of access and responsiveness of health care services (Huddleston et al. 2015), other evaluations point out that the Swiss medical system fosters a high share of out-of-pocket costs, mainly due to high user chargers and the non-coverage of certain services (i.e., dental care), which places a large financial burden on lower- and middle-income households (De Pietro et al. 2015). Furthermore, the compulsory health insurance system in Switzerland run by competing private insurers is subject to much public debate and criticism given issues such as poor transparency, high costs, or competition driven by risk-selection instead of quality services (De Pietro and Crivelli 2015). The challenges of navigating a fragmented health insurance system are even higher for immigrants, who are new to it, with the consequence being a further depreciation of their health.

Based on this argumentation and the current evidence, we expect *residents with immigrant background to display worse health than the native Swiss*, above and beyond differences in socio-economic conditions. We anticipate that these disparities will be especially strong for *immigrants that have not acquired Swiss citizenship* or *those that have been naturalized in adulthood*. For the latter, in line with Riosmena et al. (2015) we imply that the health disadvantage of having had a vulnerable legal status in the early phases of the life course cannot be compensated by later-age naturalization. Therefore, we assume that the difference *in health status between immigrants having Swiss nationality at birth and natives will be the smallest*.

Data and Methods

Data Source

The data for this study come from the Swiss Household Panel (SHP). The SHP is running since 1999, with further refreshment samples (meant to ensure the continuing representativeness of the population in Switzerland) added in 2004 and recently in 2013. For this study, we select a sample of 10,010 native and immigrant respondents with at least one measurement point between 1999 and 2014 (i.e., 16 waves). The average number of participations is 10.4 (min 1, max 16), with 5.2% of respondents having participated only once and 23.5% having participated all 16 times. For the purpose of avoiding post-retirement changes in health and the onset of chronic

[1]As of January 2018 the minimum residency duration is lowered to 10 years, but conditions are stricter (e.g., no naturalization for residents with temporary residence permit, a written language test).

health conditions with the advent of old age, we restrict the analysis to individuals who were between 18 and 60 years old at entry into the panel, in a strategy similar to Mazzonna and Peracchi (2012).

Measurement of Variables

The dependent variable is general self-rated health, assessed through the question: 'We are now going to talk about various aspects of your health. How do you feel right now?' and the following 5-item scale: (1) very well, (2) well, (3) so, so (average), (4) not very well, and (5) not well at all. Self-assessed health is a common way of measuring health in previous studies of health in general, as well as for comparisons between native and immigrant groups (Neuman 2014). Given the skewed distribution of the variable, the scale is dichotomized so that 0 signifies good health, and 1 signifies poor health, describing respondents that report 'so, so (average)', 'not very well', and 'not well at all' health.

We distinguish between six *origin* groups: (1) natives, (2) ex-Yugoslavs and Turks,[2] (3) Southern Europeans (originating from Italy, Spain, or Portugal), (4) Western Europeans (from Germany, France or Austria), (5) other European countries, and (6) other non-European countries. Respondent's origin and generation type (for immigrants) were computed based on extensive information on both parents' nationality, respondent's current nationality, whether having had Swiss nationality at birth, and whether born in Switzerland. If the individual has current Swiss nationality, was born Swiss and both parents have Swiss nationality, the respondent was coded as 'native'. If either one or both of the parents have foreign nationality and the respondents migrated to Switzerland after the age of 16, he or she was coded as 'first generation' and assigned the specific nationality group of the foreign parent (or of the mother, if both are foreigners) as origin. If either one or both parents are non-Swiss nationals and respondents came to reside in Switzerland between the ages of 6 and 16, they are coded as 'middle generation' and are given the foreign parent's or mother's nationality group as origin. If however they migrated to Switzerland before the age of 6 (or were born in Switzerland), they are coded as 'second generation' and are given the foreign parent's or mother's nationality group as origin.

Legal Status is measured by using information on the year of birth and the year that the immigrant respondent acquired Swiss nationality. Four distinct categories are created, as follows: (1) Swiss since birth, (2) naturalized in early life (i.e., before the age of 18), (3) naturalized as adult (i.e., after 18), and (4) non-Swiss. *Socio-economic*

[2] We acknowledge that grouping respondents from Ex-Yugoslavia and Turkey into a single category does not account for their heterogeneous background; yet, these immigrant groups are often treated as one group both in research and in the public discourse (e.g., Liebig et al. 2012). For the sake of comparability with previous studies, and to avoid small issues related with small sample sizes we comply with this practice for this paper.

status is captured via three distinct variables: educational level reached (with categories: (1) low, (2) medium, (3) high), employment status (with options: (1) active occupied; (2) unemployed; (3) not in labour force), and the natural logarithm of household income.

Control Variables include gender, respondent's age (in years), squared age, survey period (with options: 1999–2003, 2004–2008, and 2009–2014[3]), and marital status (with categories: (1) single, never married; (2) married; (3) separated, divorced; (4) widow(er); and (5) registered partnership).

Analytical Plan

First, we generate descriptive statistics on the distribution of both dependent and independent variables by nativity. Second, we use multilevel logistic regression with random individual-level intercepts to estimate poor self-rated health. The nested approach accounts for the non-independence of observations within individuals (Snijders and Bosker 2012), in addition to allowing for unbalanced panel structure or missing within-subject observations (Singer and Willett 2003).

Results

Descriptive Results

The baseline (i.e., corresponding to the year of entry into the panel) characteristics of the native and immigrant respondents are shown in Table 6.1. We first notice that the percentage of poor self-rated health for immigrants is higher than for natives. The difference is small, but being statistically significant, already pointing out to the health disadvantage of the former. In terms of citizenship status among immigrants, almost half (48.9%) do not have Swiss nationality, 26.2% were born Swiss, 19.5% were naturalized in adulthood,[4] and 5.5% became Swiss in early life. The immigrant sample is also comprised of 34.9% Southern Europeans, 33.8% Western Europeans, 10.2% immigrants from Former Yugoslavia and Turkey, 10.4% from other European countries, and 10.7% from outside of Europe. In terms of distribution of citizenship status by origin, further cross-tabulations (not shown here) reveal that whereas Southern and Western Europeans are over-represented among immigrants who are

[3] The cut-offs reflect equal intervals of four (or five) years. Survey period is categorized to avoid collinearity issues with age.

[4] Only a small number of observations (i.e., $n = 125$) in our sample were recorded before the respondent received Swiss nationality. Supplementary analyses removing such observations and thus only including information on self-rated health post-naturalization, showed identical results.

Table 6.1 Descriptive statistics for sample of native and immigrant respondents ($N = 10{,}010$)

	Natives	Immigrants
	%/ M (SD)	*%/ M (SD)*
Dependent variable		
Poor self-rated health	11.6	14.5
Independent variables		
Citizenship status		
Swiss since birth		26.2
Naturalized in early life		5.5
Naturalized as adult		19.5
Non-Swiss		48.9
Origin group		
Former Yugoslavia & Turkey		10.2
Southern Europe		34.9
Western Europe		33.8
Other European		10.4
Others		10.7
Generation type		
First generation		51.9
Middle generation		6.1
Second generation		42.0
Gender		
Male	46.7	46.6
Female	53.3	53.4
Educational level		
Low	11.1	18.5
Medium	73.9	58.0
High	15.0	23.5
Employment status		
Active occupied	86.3	82.1
Unemployed	1.4	3.1
Not in labour force	12.4	14.8
Marital status		
Single, never married	21.8	16.4
Married	72.4	77.3
Separated, divorced	5.1	5.8
Widow(er)	0.6	0.4
Registered partnership	0.1	0.1
Age (range 18–60)	41.28 (10.53)	39.99 (9.60)
Household income, ln (range 7.31–72,884.54)	10.96 (0.50)	10.89 (0.53)
N	*7123*	*2886*

Source: SHP, 1999–2014.
Note: M = mean, SD = standard deviation. All figures related to both dependent and independent time-varying factors correspond to the values measured at year of entry.

born Swiss or became Swiss early in life, Turks and ex-Yugoslavs are over-represented among those who are naturalized as adults or not at all.

Overall, there are slightly more women in the sample than men. In terms of qualifications, immigrants are much more represented among the highly educated than the natives (23.5% versus 15%), with a large fraction of the Swiss natives (73.9%) having medium level education. Immigrants however are marginally less likely to be actively employed compared to natives. They are also less likely to be single (never married), and are on average slightly younger at entry. Finally, there are no particular differences between the native and the immigrant sample in terms of household income.

Multivariate Analysis: Multilevel Models

Table 6.2 presents the results of three multilevel models of self-rated health. Model 1 estimates the origin group differences in health while including several confounders. Model 2 adds variables gauging respondents' socio-economic conditions, namely educational level, employment status, and household income. To test our main hypothesis, Model 3 includes a measure of citizenship status for a sub-sample that excludes first generation immigrant respondents, since the distinction between holding Swiss nationality since birth, being naturalized in early life, or later in adulthood is only possible to make for the second generation. Finally, given multicollinearity when having both origin group and citizenship status in the same model (recall the origin by citizenship status cross-tabulation results mentioned earlier), the former is excluded from Model 3. All models are estimated on unweighted data. We prefer not using weighted data however given its smaller sample size, as longitudinal weights are only constructed for original sample members, leaving aside so-called 'cohabitants'. Additional analyses including weights that correct for non-response reveal similar results.

Findings corresponding to Model 1 show that, as expected, immigrant respondents belonging to almost all origin groups are significantly more likely to be in poor self-rated health than Swiss native respondents, with immigrants from Former Yugoslavia and Turkey being predominantly worse off. We initially posited that these differences would hold even after adjusting for variation in socio-economic profile. Results in Model 2 indicate that controlling for education, employment status and household income slightly attenuate some of the differences, but immigrants are still linked to lower self-rated health than natives, irrespective of origin. Our central hypothesis proposed that immigrants' health would be particularly disadvantaged in terms of health if they are not naturalized or acquired Swiss citizenship later in life, as opposed to at birth or earlier. Findings resulting from Model 3 entirely confirm our expectation.

While the differences between native Swiss, on the one side, and immigrants born with Swiss nationality of who received it early in life, on the other side, are non-significant, second generation immigrants who got naturalized in adult age or,

Table 6.2 Multilevel logistic models of poor self-rated health among native and immigrant respondents

	Model 1		Model 2		Model 3	
	Coef.	SE	Coef.	SE	Coef.	SE
Fixed effects						
Origin group (ref. native)						
Former Yugoslavia & Turkey	1.251***	(0.171)	1.041***	(0.170)		
Southern Europe	0.676***	(0.092)	0.502***	(0.093)		
Western Europe	0.288**	(0.092)	0.321***	(0.092)		
Other European	0.280†	(0.161)	0.418**	(0.160)		
Others	0.702***	(0.164)	0.606***	(0.165)		
Citizenship status (ref. native)						
Swiss since birth					0.130	(0.105)
Naturalized in early life					0.143	(0.247)
Naturalized as adult					0.377†	(0.224)
Non-Swiss					0.658***	(0.195)
Educational level (ref. low)						
Medium			−0.517***	(0.083)	−0.446***	(0.098)
High			−0.729***	(0.106)	−0.609***	(0.123)
Employment status (ref. active occupied)						
Unemployed			0.503***	(0.128)	0.468**	(0.157)
Not in labour force			0.419***	(0.055)	0.408***	(0.061)
Household income, ln			−0.343***	(0.047)	−0.322***	(0.052)
Gender (ref. male)						
Female	0.531***	(0.058)	0.379***	(0.059)	0.383***	(0.065)
Age	0.049***	(0.015)	0.096***	(0.015)	0.106***	(0.017)
Age squared	−0.00006	(0.000)	−0.001***	(0.000)	−0.001***	(0.000)
Marital status (ref. single, never married)						
Married	−0.225**	(0.086)	−0.411***	(0.088)	−0.475***	(0.094)
Separated, divorced	0.198	(0.133)	0.084	(0.134)	0.047	(0.144)
Widow(er)	−0.419	(0.370)	−0.581	(0.382)	−0.842*	(0.419)
Registered partnership	−1.007	(0.620)	−0.984	(0.615)	−0.716	(0.638)
Survey period (ref. 1999–2003)						
2004–2008	−0.138**	(0.044)	−0.086†	(0.046)	−0.097†	(0.051)
2009–2014	−0.069	(0.047)	0.035	(0.049)	0.017	(0.054)
Intercept	−5.210***	(0.332)	−1.717**	(0.603)	−2.124**	(0.666)
Random effects						
Variance (level-two)	3.593***	(0.142)	3.320***	(0.137)	3.229***	(0.148)
N (individuals)	10,010		10,010		8316	
N (observations)	60,064		56,101		47,796	
− 2 log likelihood	−19534.363		−18149.83		−14852.078	

Source: SHP, 1999–2014.

Note: Coef = coefficient; SE = standard error; ref. = reference category. † $p < 0.10$; *$p < 0.05$; **$p < 0.01$; ***$p < 0.001$.

even more so, those who are still without Swiss nationality are significantly more likely to be in poor health than natives.

Supplementary analyses (available from authors) that estimate Model 3 by immigrant group show that the largest effects are noticed for Western and Southern European immigrants. For the Turks and former Yugoslav group, the differences are non-significant. Another set of auxiliary analyses looking at the comparison between natives and first generation immigrants only, illustrates a negative gradient of health along legal status, with non-naturalized first generation reporting worse health than native. To address health-driven attition, other analyses either looked at respondents in their first year of panel participation, or included a measure of participation gaps to specifically account for potential health-related temporary exits from the panel, but did not reveal dissimilar results. Finally, we re-ran the analysis using several other health-related outcome variables (e.g., satisfaction with health, health impediment in everyday activities, frequency of depression) and encountered similar findings and hierarchies.

Conclusions

Immigrants' health is shaped by specific vulnerabilities, including diminished empowerment and autonomy over life choices (Davies et al. 2010), exposure to anti-migrant attitudes, difficulties in the labour and housing markets, in the educational and welfare systems, or in terms of political and social participation. Given the position of disadvantage experienced by this large and expanding demographic segment of the population, it is essential to assess and understand how immigrants fare in terms of health when compared to natives.

Long-term health risk factors have occasionally been linked to the legal status of migrants, as this determines access to health and social services (Riosmena et al. 2015). While some attention had been given to monitor the health profile of undocumented migrants (e.g., Wendland et al. 2016), much less has been done to assess the health of immigrants with respect to holding native citizenship (or not) and the life course stage in which it was granted. In this study we set out to disentangle the link between legal status and immigrant health in Switzerland, a context with exclusionist immigration policies and a recent rise in nativism (Abu-Hayyeh et al. 2014). In line with most European studies (e.g., Solé-Auró and Crimmins 2008), we found no evidence of a Swiss epidemiological paradox. On the contrary, immigrants display worse health than natives. We also saw that later naturalization produces negative spill-over effects on health. Migrants who did not receive Swiss nationality or who acquired it more recently fare even worse in health than natives, illustrating that being naturalized later in life does not compensate for early-life legal vulnerability (Riosmena et al. 2015).

The study is not without drawbacks. One such limitation is that we were unable to examine the effect of other forms of legal statuses, given the limited variation in terms of types of residence permit held by immigrant respondents with non-Swiss citizenship in the sample (the majority of them declare having a permanent residence permit, while a panoply of non-permanent permits are also possible and held by many immigrants, ranging from refugee permits to limited working permits). In addition, we do not have data on undocumented migrants, for whom the stress and urgency of legal integration would be presumably higher. Further research should address the potential hardship faced by this subgroup of migrants, as well as those with temporary residence permit, to apply for and obtain appropriate health coverage. For instance, undocumented migrants in Switzerland face a number of difficulties in realising their formal right to subscribe to health insurance, depending on their economic situation, place of residence, administrative status, and the actual practices of different insurance companies to accept undocumented migrants (Bilger et al. 2011). Among other limitations we encountered by using SHP data we note the selective panel attrition and the underrepresentation of highly vulnerable segments of the population, including migrant groups, the lower educated, the unemployed or those with a poor health status (Rothenbühler and Voorpostel 2016). As a consequence, we most likely underestimate the potentially larger health differences between immigrants and natives in the general population. Furthermore, we could not trace risk factors, patterns of disease, and living conditions in the immigrants' countries of origin, nor could we account for lifestyle factors (smoking, diet, etc.). Nevertheless, previous research indicates that immigrants tend to have better (not worse) diet quality than natives (Méjean et al. 2007), meaning that adjusting for lifestyle factors would not tone down the health differences identified in this study.

Taken these limitations into account, our results are certainly a conservative test of the influence of legal status on immigrants' health and the epidemiological disadvantage associated with the delayed or denied acquisition of political rights in Switzerland. Insights into the effects of citizenship on wage rise (Steinhardt 2012), employment opportunities (Fougere and Safi 2009) and remittances (Piracha and Zhu 2012) show that legal status is an important condition for economic and labour integration and the reduction of social inequalities between migrants and natives. We add to this literature by showing the negative effects of a non-permanent or non-timely achieved legal status on immigrants' health. Further research is needed to exactly calculate the societal costs of the immigrants' health disadvantage due to the current naturalization policy. Our findings though already cast sufficient doubts on a naturalization policy that considers the acquisition of the Swiss nationality more as a privilege to be deserved than as a tool to promote integration.

References

Abu-Hayyeh, R., Murray, G., & Fekete, L. (2014). Swiss referendum: Flying the flag for nativism. *Race & Class, 56*(1), 89–94.

Akresh, I. R., & Frank, R. (2008). Health selection among new immigrants. *American Journal of Public Health, 98*(11), 2058–2064.

Antecol, H., & Bedard, K. (2006). Unhealthy assimilation: Why do immigrants converge to American health status levels? *Demography, 43*(2), 337–360.

Barbero, I. (2015). Scapegoat citizens in times of austerity: The impact of the crisis on the immigrant population in Spain. *Social Identities, 21*(3), 244–256.
Bilger, V., Hollomey, C., Wyssmüller, C., & Efionayi-Mäder, D. (2011). *Health care for undocumented migrants in Switzerland. Policies – People – Practices.* Vienna: Federal Office of Public Health, International Center for Migration Policy Development, Swiss Forum for Migration and Population Studies – University of Neuchâtel.
Borgdorff, M. W., Veen, J., Kalisvaart, N. A., & Nagelkerke, N. (1998). Mortality among tuberculosis patients in the Netherlands in the period 1993-1995. *European Respiratory Journal, 11*(4), 816–820.
Breuss, E., Helbling, P., Altpeter, E., & Zellweger, J. P. (2002). Screening and treatment for latent tuberculosis infection among asylum seekers entering Switzerland. *Swiss Medical Weekly, 132*(15–16), 197–200.
Carrasquillo, O., Carrasquillo, A. I., & Shea, S. (2000). Health insurance coverage of immigrants living in the United States: Differences by citizenship status and country of origin. *American Journal of Public Health, 90*(6), 917–923.
Castles, S. (1995). How nation-states respond to immigration and ethnic diversity. *Journal of Ethnic and Migration Studies, 21*(3), 293–308.
Cebolla-Boado, H., & Salazar, L. (2016). Differences in perinatal health between immigrant and native-origin children: Evidence from differentials in birth weight in Spain. *Demographic Research, 35*, 167–200.
Cho, Y., Frisbie, W. P., Hummer, R. A., & Rogers, R. G. (2004). Nativity, duration of residence, and the health of Hispanic adults in the United States. *International Migration Review, 38*(1), 184–211.
Davies, A. A., Basten, A., & Frattini, C. (2010). Migration: A social determinant of migrants' health. *Eurohealth, 16*(1), 10–12.
Degrate, A., Testa-Mader, A., & Clerici, N. (1999). Mortality in the Swiss and foreign immigrants in the Canton of Ticino. *Epidemiologia e Prevenzione, 23*(2), 84–89.
De Pietro, C., & Crivelli, L. (2015). Swiss popular initiative for a single health insurer… once again! *Health Policy, 119*(7), 851–855.
Derose, K. P., Bahney, B. W., Lurie, N., & Escarce, J. J. (2009). Review: Immigrants and health care access, quality, and cost. *Medical Care Research and Review, 66*(4), 355–408.
Domnich, A., Panatto, D., Gasparini, R., & Amicizia, D. (2012). The "healthy immigrant" effect-does it exist in Europe today? *Italian Journal of Public Health, 9*(3), 1–7.
Dustmann, C., & Frattini, T. (2014). The fiscal effects of immigration to the UK. *The Economic Journal, 124*(580), F593–F643.
Elewonibi, B. R., & BeLue, R. (2015). Prevalence of complementary and alternative medicine in immigrants. *Journal of Immigrant and Minority Health, 18*(3), 600–607.
Eraydin, A., Tasan-Kok, T., & Vranken, J. (2010). Diversity matters: Immigrant entrepreneurship and contribution of different forms of social integration in economic performance of cities. *European Planning Studies, 18*(4), 521–543.
Fougere, D., & Safi, M. (2009). The effects of naturalization on immigrants' employment probability (France, 1968–1999). *International Journal of Manpower, 30*(1–2), 83–96.
Giuntella, O., & Mazzonna, F. (2015). Do immigrants improve the health of natives? *Journal of Health Economics, 43*, 140–153.
Halpin, B. W. (2015). Subject to change without notice: Mock schedules and flexible employment in the United States. *Social Problems, 62*(3), 419–438.
Hamilton, T. G., & Hummer, R. A. (2011). Immigration and the health of U.S. black adults: Does country of origin matter? *Social Science and Medicine, 73*(10), 1551–1560.
Huddleston, T., Bilgili, Ö., Joki, A.-L., & Vankova, Z. (2015). *Migrant integration policy Index 2015*. Barcelona/Brussels: CIDOB and MPG.
Howell, J. L., & Sweeny, K. (2016). Is waiting bad for subjective health? *Journal of Behavioral Medicine, 39*(4), 652–664.

Joseph, T. D. (2016). What health care reform means for immigrants: Comparing the affordable care act and Massachusetts health reforms. *Journal of Health Politics, Policy and Law, 41*(1), 101–116.

Juárez, S. P., & Revuelta-Eugercios, B. A. (2014). Too heavy, too late: Investigating perinatal health outcomes in immigrants residing in Spain. A cross-sectional study (2009–2011). *Journal of Epidemiology and Community Health, 68*(9), 863–868.

Juárez, S. P., & Revuelta-Eugercios, B. A. (2016). Exploring the 'Healthy migrant Paradox' in Sweden. A cross sectional study focused on perinatal outcomes. *Journal of Immigrant and Minority Health, 18*(1), 42–50.

Kennedy, S., McDonald, J. T., Biddle, N. (2006). *The healthy immigrant effect and immigrant selection: Evidence from four countries.* Social and Economic Dimensions of an Aging Population (SEDAP) Research papers no. 164.

Ku, L., & Matani, S. (2001). Left out: Immigrants' access to health care and insurance. *Health Affairs (Project Hope), 20*(1), 247–256.

Liebig, T., Kohls, S., & Krause, K. (2012). *The labour market integration of immigrants and their children in Switzerland.* OECD Social, Employment and Migration Working Papers, No. 128, OECD Publishing.

Malmusi, D. (2015). Immigrants' health and health inequality by type of integration policies in European countries. *The European Journal of Public Health, 25*(2), 293–299.

Mazzonna, F., & Peracchi, F. (2012). Ageing, cognitive abilities and retirement. *European Economic Review, 56*(4), 691–710.

McConnell, E. D. (2013). Who has housing affordability problems? Disparities in housing cost burden by race, nativity, and legal status in Los Angeles. *Race and Social Problems, 5*(3), 173–190.

Mehta, N. K., & Elo, I. T. (2012). Migrant selection and the health of U.S. immigrants from the former Soviet Union. *Demography, 49*(2), 425–447.

Méjean, C., Traissac, P., Eymard-Duvernay, S., El Ati, J., Delpeuch, F., & Maire, B. (2007). Diet quality of North African migrants in France partly explains their lower prevalence of diet-related chronic conditions relative to their native French peers. *The Journal of Nutrition, 137*(9), 2106–2113.

Neuman, S. (2014). *Are immigrants healthier than native residents?* IZA World of Labor no. 208.

Newbold, K. B. (2005). Self-rated health within the Canadian immigrant population: Risk and the healthy immigrant effect. *Social Science and Medicine, 60*(6), 1359–1370.

Niessen, J., Huddleston, T., & Citron, L. (2015). *Migrant integration policy index.* Brussels: British Council and Migration Policy Group.

Pacelli, B., et al. (2016). Differences in mortality by immigrant status in Italy. Results of the Italian network of longitudinal metropolitan studies. *European Journal of Epidemiology, 31*(7), 691–701.

Palloni, A., & Arias, E. (2004). Paradox lost: Explaining the Hispanic adult mortality advantage. *Demography, 41*(3), 385–415.

De Pietro, C., Camenzind, P., Sturny, I., Crivelli, L., Edwards-Garavoglia, S., Spranger, A., Wittenbecher, F., & Quentin, W. (2015). Switzerland: Health system review. *Health Systems in Transition, 17*(4), 1–288.

Piracha, M., & Zhu, Y. (2012). Precautionary savings by natives and immigrants in Germany. *Applied Economics, 44*(21), 2767–2776.

Rechel, B., Mladovsky, P., Ingleby, D., Mackenbach, J. P., & McKee, M. (2013). Migration and health in an increasingly diverse Europe. *The Lancet, 381*(9873), 1235–1245.

Restrepo-Mesa, S. L., Estrada-Restrepo, A., González-Zapata, L. I., Agudelo-Suárez, A. A., & Ronda-Pérez, E. (2010). Factors related to birth weight: A comparison of related factors between newborns of Spanish and Colombian immigrant women in Spain. *Archivos Latinoamericanos de Nutrición, 60*(1), 15–22.

Riosmena, F., Everett, B. G., Rogers, R. G., & Dennis, J. A. (2015). Negative acculturation and nothing more? Cumulative disadvantage and mortality during the immigrant adaptation process among Latinos in the United States. *International Migration Review, 49*(2), 443–478.

Rothenbühler, M., & Voorpostel, M. (2016). Attrition in the Swiss household panel: Are vulnerable groups more affected than others? In M. Oris, C. Roberts, D. Joye, & M. E. Stähli (Eds.), *Surveying human vulnerabilities across the life course* (pp. 221–242). Springer International Publishing.

Safi, M. (2010). Immigrants' life satisfaction in Europe: Between assimilation and discrimination. *European Sociological Review, 26*(2), 159–176.

Schunck, R., Reiss, K., & Razum, O. (2015). Pathways between perceived discrimination and health among immigrants: Evidence from a large national panel survey in Germany. *Ethnicity & Health, 20*(5), 493–510.

Sieberer, M., Maksimovic, S., Ersoez, B., Machleidt, W., Ziegenbein, M., & Calliess, I. T. (2012). Depressive symptoms in first-and second-generation migrants: A cross-sectional study of a multi-ethnic working population. *International Journal of Social Psychiatry, 58*(6), 605–613.

Singer, J. D., & Willett, J. B. (2003). *Applied longitudinal data analysis: Modeling change and event occurrence*. New York: Oxford University Press.

Snijders, T., & Bosker, R. (2012). *Multilevel analysis: An introduction to basic and applied multilevel analysis* (2nd ed.). London: Sage Publishing House.

Solé-Auró, A., & Crimmins, E. M. (2008). Health of immigrants in European countries. *International Migration Review, 42*(4), 861–876.

State Secretariat for Migration. (2016). Available at https://www.sem.admin.ch/sem/en/home/themen/buergerrecht/faq.html

Steinhardt, M. F. (2012). Does citizenship matter? The economic impact of naturalizations in Germany. *Labour Economics, 19*(6), 813–823.

Wendland, A., Ehmsen, B. K., Lenskjold, V., Astrup, B. S., Mohr, M., Williams, C. J., & Cowan, S. A. (2016). Undocumented migrant women in Denmark have inadequate access to pregnancy screening and have a higher prevalence hepatitis B virus infection compared to documented migrants in Denmark: A prevalence study. *BMC Public Health, 16*, 426.

WHO Regional Office for Europe. (2010). *How health systems can address health inequities linked to migration and ethnicity*. Available at http://www.euro.who.int

Zencovich, M., Kennedy, K., MacPherson, D. W., & Gushulak, B. D. (2006). Immigration medical screening and HIV infection in Canada. *International Journal of STD & AIDS, 17*(12), 813–816.

Zufferey, J. (2016). Investigating the migrant mortality advantage at the intersections of social stratification in Switzerland: The role of vulnerability. *Demographic Research, 34*(32), 899–926.

Part II
Resources, Work & Living Conditions

Chapter 7
The Association Between Self-Reported Health Problems and Household Prosperity

Maurizia Masia, Monica Budowski, and Robin Tillmann

Introduction

This chapter focuses on the relationship between individual health and its financial effects on the household in Switzerland in terms of its welfare, a topic which to date has been rarely explored scientifically. Given the widely documented national and international research findings on the association between social inequality and health, this topic warrants attention. Two major explanatory models have emerged in the social science debates about health inequalities on the individual level: the causality hypothesis and the selection hypothesis. The causality hypothesis has a long tradition of research, revealing that higher socioeconomic status leads to better health and, conversely, lower socioeconomic status to worse health. It has repeatedly been confirmed that socioeconomic factors such as income, education, and social status affect health (e.g. Allanson et al. 2010). International findings have also made clear that the effect of socioeconomic factors on health is not country-dependent. In Europe, in Australia, Canada, and the US, mortality rates are highest for people with lower occupational status, lower educational levels, and lower incomes (Mackenbach 2006). Longitudinal analyses have provided information about the long-term effects of socioeconomic factors on health and studied the selection effect of health (Dragano and Siegrist 2009; Rueda et al. 2012). Selection in this context refers to the process of social mobility: as the likelihood of upward

M. Masia (✉) · M. Budowski
Division of Sociology, Social Policy and Social Work, Department of Social Sciences, University of Fribourg, Fribourg, Switzerland
e-mail: maurizia.masia@unifr.ch; monica.budowski@unifr.ch

R. Tillmann
FORS-Swiss Centre of Expertise in the Social Sciences, Lausanne, Switzerland
e-mail: robin.tillmann@fors.unil.ch

R. Tillmann et al. (eds.), *Social Dynamics in Swiss Society*, Life Course Research and Social Policies 9, https://doi.org/10.1007/978-3-319-89557-4_7

social mobility is greater for healthy people, there is a higher risk of social decline for those who are sick (Connolly et al. 2007).

From a life course perspective and focusing on individuals, the existence of health-related selection processes is undisputed. Epidemiological and health inequality research has explored and discussed both causal and selective health mechanisms, which are not thought to be mutually exclusive. Nevertheless, the causal hypothesis with its focus on individuals has continued to receive more attention in research and thus overshadowed research both on health selection mechanisms and the consequences of ill health beyond individual circumstances. Research in countries of the Global North has neither paid sufficient attention to the consequences of a household member's ill health for the household's welfare and social mobility nor for other household members.[1]

In this contribution, we ask whether the household's welfare, i.e., material well-being, is affected when a household member's health deteriorates. Deterioration in health is a complex phenomenon that cannot be defined solely according to the dichotomy of "healthy" vs. "sick" (Erhart et al. 2009). From an individual and subjective perspective, the experience of being healthy or sick is certainly important. Therefore, the subjective perception of well-being reflects whether a person feels ill or healthy; this perception may change between points in time on a temporal continuum over the life course. Ill health may be interpreted as a phase of imbalance between risks and protective factors occurring when an individual lacks the physical and/or mental resources to cope with the various requirements of everyday life (Hurrelmann 2006). The onset of ill health may also be understood as a critical life event that disrupts individuals' normal contexts of activity requiring adaptions for everyday activities (Filipp and Aymanns 2009).

With this in mind, we ask whether and to what extent the onset of a member's ill-health affects his or her household's welfare, when this member's function is that of a breadwinner. The "breadwinner" refers to the "sole-earner" in a household or to a "co-earner" contributing a substantial proportion to household income. Household members with no substantial contribution to the household income ("secondary earners") are not considered breadwinners. Analytically, we focus on sole-earner households. In sole-earner households one member takes over the breadwinner role and secures household income, whereas in multiple-earner households various household members as co-earners each contribute substantially and share the function of the breadwinner to secure household income together. When combining the resource and the deprivation approach, welfare, i.e., material well-being, may be understood as the result of different living standards and income situations (Townsend 1979). For our analysis, we concentrate on the changes over time in three "welfare positions" ("prosperity", "precariousness", and "poverty"). The dynamic relationship between the deterioration of breadwinner's health for the household and the household's welfare may be considered a function of the demographic, resource-specific, and psy-

[1]There is, however, an ongoing debate and research in countries of the Global South for example with regards to "catastrophic health expenditures" and the economic burden of illnesses for household and their strategies.

chosocial characteristics of households when comparing the situation before and after the deterioration of the breadwinner's health. The Swiss Household Panel (SHP) provides the data for our empirical analysis.

Health and Welfare in the Household: A Theoretical Framework

A private household may, in general, be classified as belonging to an individual's everyday experience. Private households as units of analysis may include one or many individuals. Multi-person households may be differentiated into couple households with or without children, households with single parents and children, and others. A functional household's constitutive characteristics are that to provide material and immaterial services to meet the household members' welfare-relevant needs and goals, and that some activities and expenditures are shared (Casimir and Tobi 2011; Egner 1976).

The resource approach emphasizes economic aspects and the extent to which individual household members take on a provider status. The relative amount of income that each person contributes to the household determines the provider status (Blood and Wolfe 1960). The breadwinning function of household members may be distinguished according to the following categories: "sole-earner", "co-earner", or a member who contributes no (substantial) income, a "secondary earner". If the breadwinner function relies on one person, households are considered to be "sole-earner households"; if this function is shared by more co-earning household members substantially contributing to household income, they constitute "multiple-earner households". It may be argued that the household's welfare goes beyond economic terms and also depends on the emotional and symbolic tasks that household members take over (albeit generally unequally distributed) on the basis of solidarity amongst the household members (Galler and Ott 1993). Household organization, thus, depends the distribution of income generation, unpaid housekeeping and caregiving. The latter are, when necessary, still performed in the majority of cases by women in the household (Daly 2011; Budowski et al. 2016). Moreover, to better understand how households allocate income generation for the household and its usage, it is relevant to consider not only tangible but also intangible resources, such as education, health, and social support (Thébaud 2010). Household members mobilize their personal, social, and economic potential and organize their work in order to ensure the provision of welfare-relevant contributions to the household (e.g., prosperity, health, or prestige).

Adopting the life course perspective as a "status biography" (Levy 1996), the individual life courses of household members may be considered both as products of employment and income-specific configurations, and as contingent on the household's standard of living and welfare. The position and role structures within the household shape its welfare over time and, depending on social conditions, are associated with different capacities and limitations for the members to achieve desired objectives. As we focus on the function of the breadwinner within the household, we conceptualize the onset of his or her health deterioration as a critical event that may interfere with routine activities and affect the household's welfare (Filipp and Aymanns 2009). Such an event may influence the way the household is organized, for example, the household members' division of labor. Daily activities are expected to change both for the person with ill-health and for the other household members and to be contingent on the household situation. Coping strategies may be required, for example, to deal with the consequences of the breadwinner's ill-health-related inability to work (and particularly income-loss) that may lead to material burdens.

Hypotheses

From a life course perspective, a deterioration in a breadwinner's health may be conceptualized as a critical event that causes an interruption of familiar and everyday household procedures (Filipp and Aymanns 2009). Following this line of argument, it is reasonable to expect that the effects of a breadwinner's deterioration in health depends both on the severity of his or her health conditions and on his or her provisioning function, i.e., the positions and role structure within the household. These elements should contribute to explaining an enhanced risk of decline in household welfare. The first hypothesis therefore makes explicit the relationship between the deterioration of the breadwinner's health (sole-earner or co-earner), use of healthcare services, and the risk of change to a less favorable welfare position:

H_1: As a result of a breadwinner's chronic, mental and physical illness and his or her increased use of healthcare services, the risk of descent in household welfare position is likely to augment.

The impact of a breadwinner's health deterioration on household welfare position needs to be understood in light of household-dependent factors. Research into poverty and inequality has shown that sociodemographic factors play a key role in explaining deprivation and income in the household (Callens and Croux 2009; Halleröd and Gustafsson 2011). Whereas a greater number of children living in the household is associated with an increased risk of poverty, a greater number of adults is associated with additional income potential in the household (Jenkins 2000). Thus, apart from the breadwinner's deterioration in health, sociodemographic factors influence the household's welfare leading to hypotheses H_2 and H_3:

H_2: If more adults live in the household prior to the deterioration of the breadwinner's health, the risk of descent in household welfare position is likely to diminish.

H_3: If more children live in the household prior to the deterioration of the breadwinner's health, the risk of descent in household welfare position is likely to augment.

The household is a dynamic unit over time. From the perspective of different points in time and at the household level, some studies have provided evidence that demographic processes (e.g., the birth of a baby, the departure of a household member) or critical events (e.g., divorce, death) impact on household income (Chen and Korinek 2010; Jenkins 2000; Sauerborn et al. 1996). Thus, hypothesis (H_4) is:

H_4: An increase in the number of adults in a household (when compared to before the deterioration of the breadwinner's health) reduces the risk of descent in household welfare position as a result of the deterioration of the breadwinner's health.

Considering the importance of cumulative disadvantages, it is probable that an accumulation of psychosocial strain affects the behavior of household members after the deterioration of a breadwinner's health (Jungbauer-Gans and Gross 2009; Steinkamp 1999). These stressful events may reflect in behavior-specific risk factors affecting the household members' coping strategies, thereby making it more difficult to achieve material security. Therefore, we put forth the following hypotheses (H_5 and H_6):

H_5: The higher the level of psychosocial strain in the household before the deterioration of the breadwinner's health, the more likely will be a descent in household welfare position.

H_6: The greater the number of chronically ill people living in the household prior to the deterioration of the breadwinner's health, the greater the risk of a descent in household welfare position.

Considering cumulative disadvantages and advantages, we assume that the household may reorganize itself after the deterioration of the breadwinner's health. This reorganization need not be interpreted in terms of risk only, but may also be done in terms of favorable or risk-reducing resources (Keck and Sakdapolrak 2013). Household members' individual characteristics and their social relationships may work as protective factors. Therefore, the resource-specific configuration of the household (e.g., education, health, and social support) may buffer the risks of descent in household welfare after the deterioration of the breadwinner's health. Hypothesis 7 states this relationship:

H_7: Higher intangible resources (highest level of education, average health, average social support) within the household prior to the deterioration of the breadwinner's health are likely to protect against a descent of the household's welfare position.

Based on the accumulation model, and adopting a dynamic perspective on the household, we expect that a deterioration of the breadwinner's health will lead to an accumulation of psychosocial strain in the household. The risks to household welfare may therefore intensify, so that a decline of the household's welfare position becomes more likely. In contrast, the event may also lead to a change in employment status of other household members. If there is a potential for additional income, the risk that the household welfare position declines may be reduced. The compensatory possibilities offered by other members in the household become more important. This results in the following two hypotheses (H_8, H_9):

H_8: Greater psychosocial strain in the household as a result of the deterioration of the breadwinner's health increases the risk of descent in household welfare position.

H_9: An increase in the workload of all adults in the household as a result of the deterioration of the breadwinner's health reduces the risk of descent in household welfare position.

Methodological Issues and Operationalization

The empirical test of our hypotheses is based on data from the first 16 waves of the Swiss Household Panel (SHP, 1999–2014). The SHP contains a large range of variables related to the household, such as living conditions, standard of living, and certain activities. It also contains a large array of information about individual household members (e.g., health status, life events, occupation, education, employment level, occupational prestige, health, etc.).

In order to analyze how the household's welfare position is affected by a household's breadwinner's deterioration of health, we employ data from the entire panel for all household members who had suffered a deterioration in (self-reported) health. All households were included in the analyses, in which one household member aged 18 to 64 years had suffered a deterioration of health within a time frame of four years (single person households were excluded). A deterioration of health was defined to have occurred when a household member experienced a (subjective) deterioration of health (i.e., when interviewees answered with point 4 or less on an 11-point scale regarding the question: "In the last 12 months, has your health improved or worsened, if 0 means "greatly worsened" and 10 "greatly improved") and when his or her health status remained unchanged for two further years thereafter. The longitudinal data were pooled at the time point at which (subjective) health deteriorated. Hence, the results are not interpreted per calendar year, but in relation to the onset of the household member's deterioration in health. Data were available one year before the point in time health deteriorated (t_{-1}), in the year in which health deteriorated (t_0), and for the two following years. A before/after comparison (from t_{-1} to t_0) was conducted in order to perform an inferential statistical analysis of the change in household welfare position. In the SHP data (1999–2014), 859 persons experienced a deterioration of health within a four-year time frame as described above.

As is commonly known, poverty rates fluctuate considerably according to how income poverty thresholds are defined. In the Swiss case, previous research has shown that poverty rates fluctuate from about 6 to 23% for the years 1999 to 2003, depending on the selected income level (50, 60, or 70% of the median) (Tillmann and Budowski 2006). This kind of poverty threshold represents an indirect poverty measure because it is based on income. Direct measures of poverty include household expenditures or fulfilling certain criteria that correspond to an "acceptable standard of living" in a given context (Townsend 1979). According to Gordon and Spicker (1999), the direct measure of an "acceptable standard of living" is considered superior to the expenditure approach. Following Townsend's studies, we conceptualize poverty with a measure that integrates income, and possession of goods and opportunities for activities and services. The monetary poverty threshold is set at 60% of the median equivalized household income. Deprivation consists of the lack of goods (e.g., a car, a washing machine, a dishwasher, or a computer) or activities or services (e.g., eat at a restaurant at least once a month, take a week's holiday away from home each year, save money in a private pension fund, or invite friends to the household at least once a month) due to financial reasons that a majority of households in Switzerland does not lack.

We combined these two aspects (income and deprivation) to construct three welfare positions. The first household welfare position is defined by non-poverty; for reasons of comprehensibility we refer to it as "prosperity". The second household welfare position is defined as "precarious": the household is deprived in two or more items yet avails an income level above the poverty threshold or, alternatively, the household with an income level below the poverty threshold yet is deprived at most in one item. The third welfare position is defined as consistently "poor" (an income level below the poverty threshold and deprived in two or more items).

The effects of the deterioration of the breadwinner's health are considered in terms of his or her household's movements across these different welfare positions (prosperity, precariousness, and poverty). To compare the welfare position before and after the deterioration of the breadwinner's health (i.e., from t_{-1} to t_0), we created a dependent variable capturing the household's movement. Households remaining at the same welfare position before the deterioration of the breadwinner's health (t_{-1}) and after it (t_0) are considered "stable". Households changing their welfare position (from t_{-1} to t_0) are considered either to ascend (i.e. be "upwardly mobile") or to descend in welfare position (i.e. be "downwardly mobile"). The operationalized independent variables included in the analysis model are shown in Table 7.1.

Results

The Development of Health-Related Factors

To empirically ground the perceived deterioration of health as a critical life event, we examined how various health-related variables, for example, physical and psychological health problems and the use of healthcare services changed in the course of the defined time period (four subsequent years). To compare the changes in different health-related variables we present the percentage change in health over time (see Fig. 7.1).

Figure 7.1 shows a clear pattern of change emerging regarding (physical and psychological) health problems and the use of healthcare services accompanying the subjectively perceived deterioration in health. The rates increase for all three indicators by more than 5%. Although the health care system is utilized more intensively after the onset of ill-health (t_0), the level of use a year later (t_1) is practi-

Table 7.1 Operationalization of the independent variables

Health factors	These factors capture three different aspects of the breadwinner's health: physical and psychological health and use of healthcare services. The three health indicators were extracted by means of an exploratory factor analysis from nine items available in the SHP. The ranges of values (min/max) of these three factors are: −4.74/6.56 (psychological strain), −7.06/6.88 (physical problems), −3.58/4.95 (use of health care services).
Number of adults	Number of adults in the household
Number of children	Number of children (up to age 17) in the household
Psychosocial strain	For each adult member of the household the summative index "number of psychosocial strain" calculates the number of strains and captures the amount of strains that all adult household members reported on the household level (e.g., problems with their own children, conflicts with a close relationship, the break, illness or the death of a close relationship). Alongside the mean number of psychosocial strains within a household, the mean intensity of the strain for the household is calculated as the arithmetic mean of all scores as a household characteristic. The survey collects the information on the subjective rating of each strain on a Likert scale ranging from 0 "not at all burdened by strain" to 10 "completely burdened by strain".
Number of chronic illnesses	Number of people with chronic illnesses in the household
Highest education level	Highest education level represented in the household (adults only), converted into the number of years of education; values range from 0 (no schooling) to 21 (PhD-degree)
Health	The mean health of all adult household members; subjective ratings on a Likert scale ranging from 1 "very poor" to 5 "very good"
Mean social support	For each adult member of the household the summative index "social support" describes the practical and emotional support received from partners, relatives, neighbors and friends. The mean social support is the arithmetic mean of all scores as a household characteristic (scale: 0–10 points).
Total employment load	Accumulated work load of all adult household members. In our dataset, the total employment load after a deterioration of breadwinner's health varied from −200 to +200 (this corresponds to +/−2 fulltime jobs in the household).

cally the same again as it was before the onset (t_{-1}). Physical health problems show a similar pattern of change, whereby the increase in physical health problems after the initial deterioration of health is not significant. In contrast, psychological strain increases more strongly and then decreases gradually over time. Thus, subjectively perceived deterioration of health shows different effects over time, whereby it may be assumed that the effect of this life event is health-specific. Based on these considerations, we now focus on the household and, more specifically, address the topic of how a breadwinner's deterioration of health particularly affects the household's welfare. The regression analysis allows for generating more detailed information about the relevance of the breadwinner's deterioration of health with respect to a change in the household's welfare position.

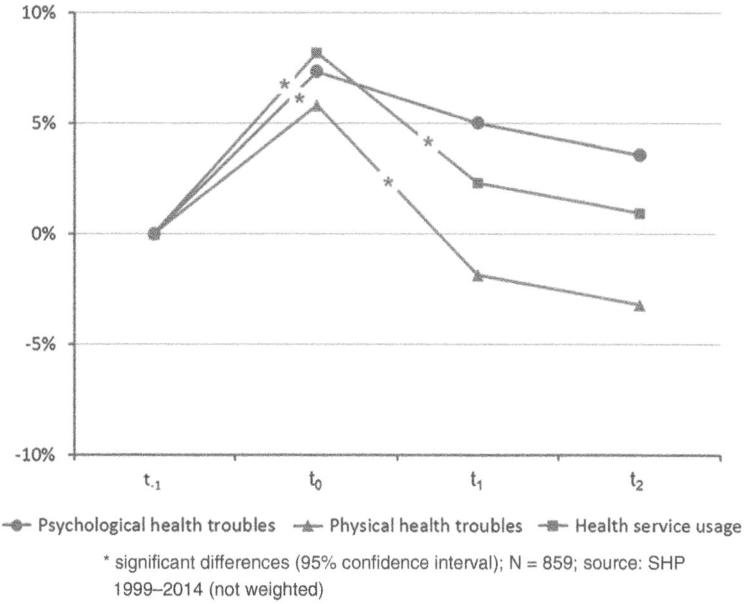

Fig. 7.1 Changes in health problems and the use of health-care services over four years (in percentages of levels before the subjectively perceived deterioration of health)

Factors Influencing the Household's Welfare Position

The multinomial logistic regression modeling procedure analyzes the effects of a breadwinner's deterioration of health on the household's welfare position. To empirically substantiate the relevance of the breadwinner function in sole-earner households by means of an exploratory group comparison between two types of households, we estimate two logistic models: one for "sole-earner households" (i.e., households with a breadwinner who contributes 80% or more to the household's income) and another for the "multiple-earner households" (i.e., households where co-earning members contribute between 40 and 80% to the household's income). The multivariate analysis serves to test the postulated effects of the independent variables (H_1 to H_9) on the probability of the dependent categorical variable "household welfare position" (i.e., the three categories: remaining stable, ascent or descent in welfare position) following the breadwinner's deterioration in health. A stable welfare position was the reference category; the estimated coefficients of the households in the other two positions (ascent or descent in welfare position) are interpreted on the basis of this reference category.

Table 7.2 provides the estimated results of the multinomial regression with respect to ascent and descent of household welfare position as the result of a deterioration of health in the household. The first model (sole-earner household) tests the extent to which a change in the breadwinner's psychological and physical health

Table 7.2 Effects on the probability of ascent and decline in household welfare position after the deterioration of the breadwinner's health differentiated according to "sole-earner household" (model 1) and "multiple-earner household" (model 2): multinomial logistic regression coefficients (dependent variable: change in household welfare position)

	Model 1: Sole-earner household				Model 2: Multiple-earner household			
	Descent in position[a]		Ascent in position[a]		Descent in position[a]		Ascent in position[a]	
Independent variables	B	Exp(B)	B	Exp(B)	B	Exp(B)	B	Exp(B)
Constant	−2.465		7.806*		9.276		8.822	
Variables at point in time t_{-1}:								
Number of adults (household)	−3.949*	0.019*	−0.518	0.596	0.762	2.143	0.893	2.442
Number of children (household)	1.384*	3.992*	0.348	1.416	−0.120	0.887	0.519	1.681
Extent of psychosocial strain (household)	−0.237	0.789	0.190	1.209	0.889	2.432	−0.966	0.381
Number of chronically ill (household)	0.749	2.115	0.102	1.107	1.544*	4.682*	−0.423	0.655
Highest level of education (in years)	−0.017	0.983	−0.364*	0.695*	−0.760*	0.468*	−0.296	0.744
Mean health (household)	0.122	1.130	−1.473*	0.229*	−2.270	0.103	−0.733	0.481
Mean social support (household)	0.515	1.674	−0.082	0.921	−0.193	0.824	−0.341	0.711
Change in variables (Δ) from t_{-1} to t_0:								
Δ Psychological health troubles (breadwinner)	0.704*	2.022*	−0.116	0.890	−0.011	0.989	−0.467	0.627

Δ Physical health troubles (breadwinner)	0.242	1.273	0.161	1.174	0.014	1.014	−0.285	0.752
Δ Use of health care services (breadwinner)	−0.344	0.709	0.291	1.337	−0.053	0.949	0.037	1.038
Δ Number of adults (household)	−0.146	0.864	1.716*	5.562*	1.852	6.372	0.231	1.260
Δ Extent of psychosocial strain (household)	−0.018	0.982	−0.200	0.819	1.277	3.587	0.505	1.658
Δ Total employment load (household)	−0.047*	0.954*	0.003	1.003	−0.025*	0.976*	0.001	1.001
Model-fit	Pseudo R^2		−2 log-likelihood	Chi^2 (df)	Pseudo R^2		−2 log-likelihood	Chi^2 (df)
	Cox-Snell	Nagelkerke			Cox-Snell	Nagelkerke		
	0.309	0.458	167.964	74.792* (26)	0.306	0.513	92.802	56.804* (26)

*$p < 0.05$
[a]reference group: no change in welfare position (“stable”); number of households: n1 = 216 (“descent in position” = 39; “ascent in position” = 47), n2 = 165 (“descent in position” = 23; “ascent in position” = 23); source: SHP 1999–2014 (not weighted)

as well as the use of health-care services after deterioration of health affect the probability of descent in household welfare position. An important finding is contrary to the postulated effects: only the increase of psychological strain augments the risk of descent in household welfare position. The changes in the health-related variables following the deterioration of a co-earner's health, however, are not able to explain a change in the household's welfare position. Thus, the first hypothesis (H_1) can only be partly confirmed.

The relationship between the demographic- and resource-specific household characteristics before the breadwinner's health deteriorated and the likelihood of a change in the household's welfare position is revealed in Table 7.2. In sole-earner households a larger number of adults in the household considerably reduces the risk of descent, whereas a greater number of children in the household increases the risk of descent. These results confirm the second and the third hypotheses. In addition, the increase in the number of adults in a household supports an ascent in household welfare position. The risk of descent, however, is not significantly reduced. Therefore, hypothesis 4 must be rejected. In multiple-earner households, none of the demographic variables (number of adults in the household, number of children in the household, and change of number of adults in the household) exerts an influence on the probability of change in household welfare.

Hypotheses 5 and 6 must be rejected, because neither the number of chronically ill household members nor the extent of psychosocial strain in the household are found to exert an influence on the probability of change in household welfare. For multiple-earner households, the risk of descent in welfare position increases significantly with a growing number of chronically ill members in the household. When the effect of resource-specific factors is integrated into the analysis, households with members with higher educational levels tend to show greater stability in welfare position than those with lower educational levels. Both the likelihood of sole-earner households ascending in welfare position and the risk of multiple-earner households descending in welfare position decreases. A higher average health status in the household seems to support stability and also lower the risk of ascent in welfare position. Contrary to our expectations, however, the average social support on the household level has no effect on the probability of a change in household welfare position. The seventh hypothesis may thus be rejected.

A change in psychosocial strain in the household has no significant effect on a change in household welfare position. An increase in the household's total employment load reduces the risk of descent in welfare position for both types of households. Hypothesis 8 may thus be rejected; whilst hypothesis 9 may be accepted.

Discussion and Conclusion

This contribution dealt with the relationship between a household breadwinner's health deterioration and the change in the household's welfare (operationalized by three welfare positions). From a life course perspective, there is, overall, empirical evidence that a deterioration in health not only affects individual modes of dealing with everyday activities but also the household's complex structure of roles and positions. In this regard, there is a clear association between the deterioration of the breadwinner's psychological health troubles in sole-earner households and the risk of a decline in household welfare. In contrast, the deterioration of a breadwinner's physical health troubles has no effect on the household's welfare in both household types.

In agreement with previous research (see Chen and Korinek 2010; Jenkins 2000), our findings show that while a greater number of adults in a household lowers the risk of a household of experiencing a decline in welfare, a greater number of children considerably increases this risk. Moreover, our analysis shows that the average health status in a sole-earner household tends to exert a stabilizing effect on the household's welfare following the deterioration of the breadwinner's health. Not only risk but also protective factors come into play and contribute to explaining the change of a household's welfare: both demographic factors and an increase in the overall employment load clearly lower the risk of the household to experience a decline in welfare. As such, the results suggest that in order to compensate for anticipated losses in employment or income due to the deterioration of a breadwinner's health, other household members activate their potential income generation capabilities by taking employment or increasing their employment loads.

Our findings support the thesis that the increase in psychological health troubles of the breadwinner (in sole-earner households) and the demographic and resource-specific factors of the household are relevant for explaining the change of the household's welfare position as a result of a deterioration of the breadwinner's health. The analysis further substantiates empirically that demographic and resource-specific household factors (e.g., psychosocial strain) vary in relevance, depending on the organization of the provider status amongst the household members. In this regard, the comparison of the sole-earner and multiple-earner households reveals striking differences: in multiple-earner households, neither the type of illness nor demographic factors (e.g., number of adults or children in the household) are relevant regarding its change in welfare position. Moreover, other household-related factors are more important, such as the number of chronically ill household members.

The results further suggest that not all of the household-related characteristics studied here are associated with change in household welfare position. Rather, it is the interaction of the provider status amongst the household members (e.g., sole-earner or multiple-earner household) and household composition that contribute to explaining to some extent the change in household welfare position. Further research that explores the effects of changes in a household member's health more deeply would be highly desirable: at the household level, it would be important to study the effects of health deterioration of members with different roles regarding income contribution in households ranging from the traditional sole-earner household to the modern dual-earner household. Therewith, more knowledge about the influence of position and role constellations of the household members on health-specific mechanisms and their effects on household welfare could be generated.

References

Allanson, P., Gerdtham, U.-G., & Petrie, D. (2010). Longitudinal analysis of income-related health inequality. *Journal of Health Economics, 29*(1), 78–86.

Blood, R. O., & Wolfe, D. M. (1960). *Husbands and wives: The dynamics of married living*. New York: Free Press.

Budowski, M., Knobloch, U., & Nollert, M. (Eds.). (2016). *Unbezahlt und dennoch Arbeit*. Zürich: Seismo.

Callens, M., & Croux, C. (2009). Poverty dynamics in Europe: A multilevel recurrent discrete-time hazard analysis. *International Sociology, 24*(3), 368–396.

Casimir, G. J., & Tobi, H. (2011). Defining and using the concept of household: A systematic review. *International Journal of Consumer Studies, 35*, 498–506.

Chen, F., & Korinek, K. (2010). Family life course transitions and rural household economy during China's market reform. *Demography, 47*(4), 963–987.

Connolly, S., O'Reilly, D., & Rosato, M. (2007). Increasing inequalities in health: Is it an artefact caused by the selective movement of people? *Social Science & Medicine, 64*(10), 2008–2015.

Daly, M. (2011). What adult worker model? A critical look at recent social policy reform in Europe from a gender and family perspective. *Social Politics, 18*(1), 1–23.

Dragano, N., & Siegrist, J. (2009). Die Lebenslaufperspektive gesundheitlicher Ungleichheit: Konzepte und Forschungsergebnisse. In M. Richter & K. Hurrelmann (Eds.), *Gesundheitliche Ungleichheit. Grundlagen, Probleme, Perspektiven* (2nd ed., pp. 181–194). Wiesbaden: VS Verlag für Sozialwissenschaften.

Egner, E. (1976). *Der Haushalt. Eine Darstellung seiner volkswirtschaftlichen Gestalt*. Berlin: Duncker und Humblot.

Erhart, M., Wille, N., & Ravens-Sieberer, U. (2009). Die Messung der subjektiven Gesundheit: Stand der Forschung und Herausforderungen. In M. Richter & K. Hurrelmann (Eds.), *Gesundheitliche Ungleichheit. Grundlagen, Probleme, Perspektiven* (2nd ed., pp. 335–352). Wiebaden: VS Verlag für Sozialwissenschaften.

Filipp, S.-H., & Aymanns, P. (2009). *Kritische Lebensereignisse und Lebenskrisen. Vom Umgang mit den Schattenseiten des Lebens*. Stuttgart: Kohlhammer.

Galler, H. P., & Ott, N. (1993). *Empirische Haushaltsforschung. Erhebungskonzepte und Analyseansätze angesichts neuer Lebensformen*. Frankfurt/New York: Campus Verlag.

Gordon, D., & Spicker, P. (1999). *The international glossary on poverty*. London/New York: Zed Books.

Halleröd, B., & Gustafsson, J.-E. (2011). A longitudinal analysis of the relationship between changes in socio-economic status and changes in health. *Social Science & Medicine, 72*(1), 116–123.

Hurrelmann, K. (2006). *Gesundheitssoziologie. Eine Einführung in sozialwissenschaftliche Theorien von Krankheitsprävention und Gesundheitsförderung* (6th ed.). Weinheim: Juventa.

Jenkins, S. P. (2000). Modelling household income dynamics. *Journal of Population Economics, 13*(4), 529–567.

Jungbauer-Gans, M., & Gross, C. (2009). Erklärungsansätze sozial differenzierter Gesundheitschancen. In M. Richter & K. Hurrelmann (Eds.), *Gesundheitliche Ungleichheit. Grundlagen, Probleme, Perspektiven* (2nd ed., pp. 77–98). Wiesbaden: VS Verlag für Sozialwissenschaften.

Keck, M., & Sakdapolrak, P. (2013). What is social resilience? Lessons learned and ways forward. *Erdkunde, 67*(1), 5–19.

Levy, R. (1996). Zur Institutionalisierung von Lebensläufen. Ein theoretischer Bezugsrahmen. In J. Behrens & W. Voges (Eds.), *Kritische Übergänge. Statuspassagen und sozialpolitische Institutionalisierung* (pp. 73–113). Frankfurt am Main: Campus.

Mackenbach, J. P. (2006). *Health inequalities: Europe in profile*. London: Departement of Health.
Rueda, S., Chambers, L., Wilson, M., Mustard, C., Rourke, S. B., Bayoumi, A., et al. (2012). Association of returning to work with better health in working-aged adults: A systematic review. *American Journal of Public Health, 102*(3), 541–556.
Sauerborn, R., Adams, A. T., & Hien, M. (1996). Household strategies to cope with the economic costs of illness. *Social Science & Medicine, 43*(3), 291–301.
Steinkamp, G. (1999). Soziale Ungleichheit in Mortalität und Morbidität. In W. Schlicht & H. H. Dickhuth (Eds.), *Gesundheit für alle: Fiktion oder Realität?* (pp. 101–154). Stuttgart/New York: Schattauer.
Thébaud, S. (2010). Masculinity, bargaining, and breadwinning: Understanding men's housework in the cultural context of paid work. *Gender and Society, 24*(3), 330–354.
Tillmann, R., & Budowski, M. (2006). La pauvreté persistante: un phénomène de classe, de cumul de désavantages ou d'individualisation? *Revue suisse de sociologie, 32*(1), 329–348.
Townsend, P. (1979). *Poverty in the United Kingdom*. London: Penguin.

Chapter 8
Between Social Structure Inertia and Changing Biographies: Trajectories of Material Deprivation in Switzerland

Pascale Gazareth, Katia Iglesias, Eric Crettaz, and Christian Suter

Introduction

In contemporary societies, attaining a decent standard of living which allows people to lead a socially integrated life is a key issue for human rights and social policy. However, social inequalities reduce the chances of reaching this standard of living. Social structure is actually still a strong determinant of poverty risks, which impacts durably the lower classes and are transmitted from generation to generation, whether we consider material or immaterial poverty. Despite decades of social and educational policy, structural determinants like social origin, education, or occupational position still play a major role in explaining poverty or prosperity. Social structure is, then, a powerful factor of inertia for what concerns the persistence of poverty in contemporary societies (*class hypothesis*).[1]

[1] The theoretical framework we present in this introductory section was commonly used in previous researches on the same topic (see Section 2). Due to place restriction, we concentrate on the most important aspects for our purpose and renounce to cite the large literature related to this framework. For a more detailed presentation including corresponding literature, see Section 1.1 of Heeb and Gutjahr about the dynamics of poverty (Heeb and Gutjahr 2012).

P. Gazareth (✉) · C. Suter
Department of sociology, University of Neuchâtel (CH), Neuchâtel, Switzerland
e-mail: pascale.gazareth@unine.ch; christian.suter@unine.ch

K. Iglesias
School of Health, University of Applied Sciences of Western Switzerland, Fribourg, Switzerland
e-mail: katia.iglesias@hefr.ch

E. Crettaz
School of Social Work, University of Applied Sciences of Western Switzerland, Geneva, Switzerland
e-mail: eric.crettaz@hesge.ch

R. Tillmann et al. (eds.), *Social Dynamics in Swiss Society*, Life Course Research and Social Policies 9, https://doi.org/10.1007/978-3-319-89557-4_8

Yet, social structure is more porous today than it was until the end of the Second World War. According to the *individualization hypothesis* (Beck 1992), uncertain life events such as a job loss, matrimonial and other family changes, or health issues, surpass the effect of the social structure; hence, poverty is less predictable, or more precisely, democratized (middle and upper classes are also concerned) and without predetermined temporal structure (poverty occurs in various short-term or long-term episodes in discontinuous and heterogeneous biographies). Moreover, social positions are not as fixed as they were. Job opportunities and successes, as well as marriage, are well-known factors of social elevation; symmetrically, economic set-backs or divorce are factors of social downgrading.

The literature on this topic reveals that both hypotheses (class vs. individualization) are valid in Switzerland, though to a varying degree (class having a larger impact than individualization). Other hypotheses also emerged, like the cumulating (dis)advantages or the life course perspectives. They suppose a sequential view of poverty: rather than a permanent (class) position or unstructured patterns (individualization), poverty evolves in time following trajectories of reinforcement of the original social position (increasing poverty over the life course) or specific patterns related to successive life course phases (e.g.: poverty is higher at the entry into independent adulthood when young people have unstable and low paid jobs, then reduces in middle-age when they gain stable occupational and social positions, reduces again after the departure of grown-up children and with the accumulation of goods and savings, then increases after retirement when pensions replace wages, and finally when old-age dependence impacts the financial situation with high costs for care).

We are interested in changes and inertia at the bottom of the social structure during the last decades.[2] Based on poverty trajectories, we examine which part of the population experienced the inertia of the social structure and remained durably in low economic strata – and which part moved from its initial position or faced individualized biography patterns. We also consider the main drivers of the various observed trajectories. In other words: What characteristics or events are related to inertia or, on the contrary, to changing socio-economic trajectories, and what do they reveal of the respective forces of change and inertia in contemporary Switzerland?

[2]This contribution is part of the research project 'Income and wealth inequality, deprivation and wellbeing in Switzerland, 1990–2013', supported by the Swiss National Science Foundation (SNF; request 100017_143320 / 1). We use data collected by the Swiss Household Panel (SHP; www.swisspanel.ch), which is based at the Swiss Centre of Expertise in the Social Sciences FORS. SHP is financed by the SNF. We express our most grateful thank you to Ursina Kuhn who helped preparing the data and the deprivation trajectories.

What Do We Know About Poverty Trajectories in Switzerland?

Poverty is mostly defined in material terms and indirectly measured through income. In a longitudinal perspective, income is affected by yearly variations (e.g. irregular secondary incomes, compensation for inflation) which do not necessarily reflect real changes in the socio-economic positions (Lollivier and Verger 2005), and render the analysis of poverty trajectories more complex. In addition, income is known to be affected by measurement errors which are cumulating in longitudinal analyses (Whelan and Maître 2006). Even if these difficulties can be overcome, some scholars developed an alternative approach to poverty measurement, with a focus on 'material deprivation', which is more directly connected with the standard of living of the population and less affected by measurement errors in longitudinal analyses.[3]

Material deprivation as defined by Townsend in the 1970s is a direct measure of poverty based on the difficulty of households to face expenses in order to have a decent living and to be able to participate to social life. In Townsend's words material deprivation is defined as: 'the absence or inadequacy of those diets, amenities, standards, services and activities which are common or customary in society' (Townsend 1979, p. 915). This measure is considered as a complementary measure to income poverty because the correlation between both is only partial: Households facing material deprivation without income poverty or income poverty without material deprivation are many. This can be explained by non-income resources or by special needs of the households that blur the relation between income and the real socio-economic situation of the population. Thus, we focus on longitudinal analyses of material deprivation in Switzerland, and leave aside the literature devoted to the dynamics of income poverty.

Three research teams were active on this topic during the last decade in Switzerland, all using data from the Swiss Household Panel. Based on data from 1999 to 2003 and analyzing episodes of consistent poverty (combination of income poverty and material deprivation), Tillmann and Budowski (2006) highlighted that a large part of the Swiss population was durably preserved from poverty (85%), when 5% faced persistent poverty and 10% occasional poverty. They confirmed the strength of inertia forces measured by the relation between persistent poverty and determinants associated with the social class (socioprofessional position, education).

Later, Gazareth and Suter compared transitions between two five-year periods at the beginning and at the end of the interval from 1999 to 2007 (Gazareth and Suter 2010). Using a deprivation measure with three positions (no deprivation, low, high), they found smaller proportions of stability patterns in the population with 46% durably non-deprived, 20% in long-lasting low deprivation, and 5% in persistent

[3] They are, however, affected by adaptative preferences (Halleröd 2006; Crettaz and Suter 2013). This topic will be further discussed below.

high deprivation. Changing patterns mostly concerned transitions from or to the intermediate position (30%), while transitions between both extreme positions were seldom observed. These findings confirm the strength of social structures' inertia but also that change is more frequent when considering deprivation in more detail; yet, it is restricted to transitions to a close position. In addition, Gazareth and Suter revealed that SHP data on deprivation are affected by selective attrition: households facing deprivation are more likely to drop out of the survey.[4] This necessarily affects the proportion of households measured in the various transitions, and potentially also their characteristics.

Furthermore, Crettaz and Suter (2013) highlighted that people facing long-lasting deprivation tend to adapt their aspirations to their objective possibilities. They are, then, more likely to mention personal preferences rather than financial constraints when lacking items (*adaptative preferences*). The phenomenon also affects the proportion of the population measured in the various transitions.

Finally, based on a continuous index of material deprivation and latent growth analyses, Heeb and Gutjahr concluded that four main types of trajectories appear when analyzing material deprivation from 1999 to 2008 (Heeb and Gutjahr 2012). They found that 80% of the population was durably preserved from material deprivation and 5% durably exposed to that form of poverty. This is comparable to Tillmann and Budowski and confirms the large impact of the inertia forces of the social structure. A contrario, 10% experienced a progressive reduction of the material deprivation they endured at the beginning of the period and 5% faced a progressive increase. For these 15%, poverty is a changing reality, potentially affected by singular individual events or cumulative processes. As panel data suppose a progressive aging of the sample, a part of these 'trajectories of change' could also reflect life course effects, like the improvement of the material situation of young people who entered independent adulthood at the beginning of the data collection.

Among people durably affected by material deprivation, Heeb and Gutjahr found more people with low education, more women, more individuals in lone parent households (and less in couple households), and more unemployed persons. A contrario, living in a couple, having a higher educational level, and being in employment characterize those durably preserved from poverty. Regarding an increase in material deprivation, low education, separation or divorce, and unemployment were found to be associated to a higher risk, and age (40 to 64 in comparison to 65 and more) and living in a couple with children were found to be related to a lower risk. Finally, among people experiencing a decrease in material deprivation, the following groups were over-represented:

- Unemployed, lowly educated persons, younger people (<24 and 25–39), individuals living alone, and married persons in the first wave.
- Employed persons (as opposed to students or homemakers) and widows (vs married people) in the last wave.

[4] Further tests confirm that attrition impacts the data durably, not only in first waves (Gazareth and Iglesias 2017).

The researchers conclude that trajectories of poverty are clearly connected with social stratification and with life course transitions. Traditional drivers of vertical inequality like education and (un)employment distinguish the destiny of the various social groups, as gender or age do. Only divorce, and mainly lone parenthood, could be related to the deregulation theses.

Building on those previous results on Switzerland, we address these questions in new ways. First, we considered a longer period (15 years) which allows us to draw conclusions about the long-term evolution of the social structure. Second, as poverty depends on the needs and resources of households (considered as communities of people sharing goods and resources), we focused our analysis at the household level instead of at the usually considered individual level. Third, as we deal with time and change, we introduced this dimension by constructing dynamic measures of the main drivers we analyzed; this is probably our most original contribution.

Methods

Data

We used Swiss Household Panel (SHP) data from 1999 to 2013 including the first two samples (SHP I starting in 1999 and SHP II starting in 2004). Material deprivation data are collected in SHP in the household questionnaire and are measured through questions about goods or activities ('items') that the household cannot afford. Nine[5] items are available in every wave and can be used for longitudinal analyses: one week vacation away from home once a year, invite friends at least once a month, meal at a restaurant minimum once a month, car for private use, color TV, washing machine for exclusive use, dishwasher, computer at home, and going to the dentist if needed (knowing that dental care is not included in the obligatory health insurance in Switzerland).

Trajectories of Deprivation

Trajectories shall be understood as the successive statuses a household occupies within a given period with regard to the dimension under observation (material deprivation). The number of trajectories we can theoretically observe corresponds

[5] A tenth item is available on all waves but was removed from our analyses: the third pillar (private pension plan). Gazareth and Iglesias (2017) explain that this item is submitted to measurement problems, like the confusion about which saving plans should be included or not. In addition, the existence of a compulsory second pillar for employees makes that item less relevant for Switzerland.

to the number of statuses (2 – not deprived or deprived)[6] raised to the power n (n being the number of observations: 15 waves), or 32,768 trajectories (without taking into account possible missing informations within waves). An important matter is, then, to reduce the number of trajectories in order to have an overview of the main types of trajectories present in the data. This can be attained mostly by gathering similar sequences together.

Gathering similar sequences together is complicated. Basically, three main trajectories can be defined: the 'never deprived' (households never reporting any enforced lack for any item), the 'always deprived' (with households reporting every year at least one enforced lack), and the 'crossing the line', which can be separated in several subgroups based on the number of observations (waves) in deprivation (mainly deprived or mainly not deprived), and/or the direction of changes (moving into poverty or out of poverty) the successive observations underline. Manual or statistical methods can be used to gather the trajectories together. We present results based on the manual construction of seven trajectories: (1) Non-deprived (no deprivation or max. once), (2) Mainly non-deprived (2 or 3 deprivation episodes, or 3 deprivation episodes and at least 7 non-deprivation episodes), (3) Mainly deprived (analogous to mainly non-deprived), (4) Durably deprived (always deprived or max. once non-deprived), (5) Moving into deprivation (several non-deprivations episodes followed by several deprivation episodes[7]), and (6) Moving out of deprivation (analogous to Moving into deprivation), (7) Fluctuating (without any clear direction). Trajectories 1 to 4 refer to stable positions, and 5 to 7 to changing positions. We decided to include households facing one exception to their main status into the 'non-deprived' or the 'durably deprived' categories. Indeed, such exceptions are not relevant for defining the socio-economic position of the household on a large period.

The treatment of missing values is a critical issue for sequence analysis: missings can occur within a sequence, at the beginning or at the end of the sequence. From 1999 to 2013, the maximum length of sequences is 15 observations for SHP I, and 10 for SHP II. We had, then, to choose a compromise between few highly comparable cases (long trajectories with same length) and more but less comparable cases (use of much of the available information). We present results based on households

[6] The choice of a binary index is coherent with our purpose, as we are mostly interested in changes in socio-economic positions defined as out-of-poverty versus in-poverty, and not in changes taking into account the severity of poverty. Many theoretical considerations are in favor of a more complex measurement. However, due to the very asymmetrical distribution of deprivation (the large majority of households are non-deprived), the results do not vary much if we deal with more than one deprivation status, and the possibilities to analyze a continuous measure are reduced (problems with the statistical assumptions). Yet, using a binary measure brings some limitations, like emphasizing transitions from positions around the poverty threshold.

[7] More precisely: One change from non-deprived to deprived with the first two observations not deprived and the last two deprived; two changes from non-deprived to deprived, with the last three observations deprived, max. Once deprived in the first three waves, and at least three time non-deprived in total; two changes from non-deprived to deprived with two episodes non-deprived within the first three observations, rest deprived; one change from deprived to non-deprived and return to deprived, with the first observation deprived, at least three episodes non-deprived, and at least the last three observations deprived.

with at least 9 observations from 1999 to 2013 (N = 4319). This includes 53% of the initial sample and 39% of the refreshment sample.[8]

Determinants

A rich literature provides theoretical inputs and empirical results about the determinants of poverty, and material deprivation more specifically (for details see e.g. Layte et al. 2001; Suter and Paris 2002; Figari 2012). We first present the determinants associated with our framework at the individual level as analyzed traditionally.

Determinants of material deprivation can be divided in four groups. First, determinants associated with vertical inequality (social origin, education, income, occupational position), referring to the class conception of poverty, have to be considered. They should be associated with unchanging deprivation trajectories, because poverty is seen as a permanent and transgenerational phenomenon. Second, ascriptive characteristics referring to horizontal inequality, like gender, age or ethnicity/nationality, are also essential. They shall be related to stable trajectories, as they remain unchanged over the life course for most individuals, except for age.

Third, critical life events (disruptions in the occupational trajectory, divorce, sickness) are taken into account as determinants related to the individualization hypothesis. Their influence should result in unstructured trajectories with short periods of poverty following such events. Fourth, as standard of living is related to the composition of the household and the sharing of resources and expenses between members, these attributes also have to be part of the analysis. Changes in the household structure (arrival of new members or departure of others, like grown-up children) are associated with durably changing trajectories, especially when the changes affect the main earners in the household. This last group of determinants coincides to some extent with the third one (e.g. divorce) but is also strongly connected to life-course transitions, as age can be. This consideration is important for the interpretation: the influence of some determinants is possibly multiple, which pleads for various hypotheses depending on how these factors affect deprivation trajectories.

As mentioned earlier, material deprivation refers essentially to the economic situation of the household, as most of the resources and durables are shared by all members even if they belong to one member specifically. Due to heterogeneous individual characteristics like higher and compulsory education within the same household, the relation with the deprivation status of the household is confused when analyzed at the individual level (mostly when all members, except young

[8] Hence, sequences of various lengths (9 to 15 observations) are considered: observations are missing in 26% of the households at the beginning of the sequence and in 14% at the end (non-participation); 32% present gaps inside the sequence (whole or partial non-response). All in all, 62% of the sequences with at least 9 observations are incomplete. This is an important issue for the validity of the inference on the global population.

children, are interviewed like in SHP). In order to avoid this confusion, individual characteristics must be transposed at the household level. In doing so, the respective influence of the various members has to be taken into account. We assume that material deprivation is mostly related to the situation of the adult or couple who contributes mainly to the household's income (usually the parents in family households).

Consequently, for most individual attributes, we considered the situation of the 'head' of the household defined as the main earner (ME) and his or her partner, if any (whatever the marital status or sex). For some characteristics such as health-related impediment in everyday activities, we considered whether any household member was affected (because impediment of any member leads to particular expenses that affect the standard of living of the whole household).

In a similar way, we used dynamic determinants based on variables dealing with changes or events that occurred during the period. Education of the household head for example was constructed as the highest degree achieved by the head in all waves, but also as movement (no change, increase, decrease,[9] varying). In other instances, we used the mode value within the period, or the percentage of years in which a specific characteristic, situation or event was observed, or the occurrence of some events at least once. For every determinant, we defined a construction and thresholds that take into account theoretical considerations (expected impact of the determinant) as well as the size and distribution of the created subgroups in the sample. The resulting variables are presented in Table 8.1.

The analysis of the determinants was performed using multinomial logistic regressions. We first ran univariate models in order to test the potential influence of our determinants one-by-one. Then, we ran multivariate models to assess each determinant's strength. We used a stepwise procedure to select a model with the higher explicative capacity (pseudo R2). Further models were tested for explorative purposes.

Results

Trajectories of Deprivation

A large majority of the households (82.4%) stayed durably in the same status from 1999 to 2013 (see Table 8.2). Among those with changing trajectories, the larger groups are those who experienced fluctuating changes of status (9.7%), or who moved out of deprivation (5.6%). Only a small group faced a durable entry into poverty (2.3%). These percentages at the household level are globally consistent with those found at the individual level (Tillmann and Budowski 2006; Heeb and Gutjahr 2012). The strength of inertia forces appears clearly, as well as the good

[9] As head can change, a decrease in level of education is possible, for example after divorce.

Table 8.1 Variable construction for the main determinants of trajectories

Variable	Categories: Reference category vs. other	Level
Education of head: highest level over the whole observation period (hereafter 'over obs.')	Upper secondary vs. compulsory; tertiary	HEAD
Education of head: change over obs.	Unchanged vs. increase; decrease; variation	HEAD
Log of net HH income (mean value over obs. + value at first obs.); Variation of net HH income: last 3 obs. divided by first 3 obs.; Reported change in income since previous interview: mean value over obs.[a]	Continuous	HH
Unbalanced HH budget (i.e. HH gets into debts or eats assets) (% of obs.)	Never vs. <25%, 25–100%	HH
Homeowner (% of obs.)	Never vs. <2/3, 2/3+	HH
Retirement of HH head	Never vs. event (retirement occurred after 1st obs.); always (retired since 1st obs.)	Head
Death of a close person since previous interview; Illness or accident since previous interview (if still affecting)	Never vs. min. once	ALL
Health-related impediment in daily activities (any member) (% of obs.)	Never vs. <25%; 25–50%; >50%	ALL
Head reporting: bad health[b]; deterioration of health since previous interview; chronic health condition (% of obs.)	Never vs. <25%; 25–50%; >50%	Head
HH composition: New partner of head; Separation of head; Lone parent HH	Never vs. min. once	HH
Dependent child(ren) in HH (share of obs.)	Never vs. <2/3, 2/3+	HH

Notes: Level: ME = Main Earner; Head = ME + partner if any; All = all members 15+; HH = Household characteristic (identical for all members).

[a]For each observation: Income improved since previous interview = 1; decreased = (−1); no change = 0.

[b]'How do you feel right now?': 'so, so' (average), 'not very well', or 'not well at all'.

Table 8.2 Trajectories of material deprivation, 1999–2013: min. 9 observations

Stable trajectories		Moving trajectories	
Non-deprived	61.6%	Moving into deprivation	2.3%
Mainly non-deprived	12.5%	Moving out of deprivation	5.6%
Mainly deprived	4.1%	Fluctuating	9.7%
Durably deprived	4.3%		

Source: Swiss Household Panel (SHP I and SHP II, unweighted), own calculation.

situation of the Swiss population over the period; deprivation remains low, and entries into poverty are scarce.

However, two methodological issues challenge the representativeness of our results, especially the relative size of our trajectories: non-randomized attrition and panel conditioning. Attrition is characterized by deprived households being more likely to drop out of the survey, especially during the first waves (Gazareth and

Iglesias 2017). Trajectories that deal with deprivation should, thus, be underestimated. Further analyses would be necessary to know which ones exactly, and to what extent. Conversely, the households participating in at least 9 waves are clearly more stable (and wealthy) than households in the whole Swiss population. More generally, how random the many missing observations are is a crucial issue. The effects of panel conditioning, that is, the transformation in the cognitive process when answering several times the same questions, are more difficult to anticipate (answers about the reason for lacking items are possibly concerned), but tests based on measures of subjective wellbeing confirm that SHP data are affected (Iglesias et al. 2017).

Adaptative preferences also challenge the results by affecting mainly the stated reason for lacking an item (Crettaz and Suter 2013). Some households could seem to move out of deprivation, yet are actually durably affected by deprivation and have gotten used to it. As a consequence of these limitations, the real comparative strengths of change and inertia in Swiss society are probably somewhat different. If the comparative strengths are not fully representative, it is reasonable to say that the general patterns are not affected.

Determinants

Three groups of determinants, classified by the strength of their relation to deprivation trajectories, emerged from the initial one-by-one regressions.

The first group includes the three determinants with the strongest predictive power for the trajectories (pseudo R2 between 0.030 and 0.082). They are all related to the financial situation of the household: household income, unbalanced budget, and reported change in income since previous interview.

The second group (pseudo R2 between 0.011 and 0.020) is more diverse. The economic situation is still present (home ownership), but also determinants related to vertical or horizontal inequalities (HH head's highest education, main earner's sex), as well as health (any member with health-related impediment in everyday activities and head reporting bad health) and two determinants related to the structure of the household (depending child(ren) in household, lone parent household).

The last group includes determinants with a weak predictive power for trajectories (pseudo R2 between 0.05 and 0.01): Age of the main earner, all members being less than 25 at first participation, region where the household mainly lived, change in the household head's education, social origin (education of the father, financial problems during childhood), household being jobless (all non-retired members are unemployed or out-of-employment). In addition, many life events we tested show a marginal relationship (pseudo R2 < 0.05) to the trajectories: separation or (re)partnering of household head, retirement, accident or illness since previous interview, or death of a closely related person since previous interview (connected with possible inheritance). Nationality, usually influent in socio-economic phenomenons, also presents a very weak relation to the deprivation trajectories.

Table 8.3 Main determinants of trajectories of material deprivation 1999–2013: beta coefficients of multinomial logistic regression with non-deprived trajectory as reference

	Mostly non-deprived	Mostly deprived	Durably deprived	Moving out of deprivation	Fluctuating
	β	β	β	β	β
Income (mean of log net)	−1.66***	−3.34***	−3.94***	−1.65***	−2.52***
Unbalanced budget (ref. never)					
<25% of observations	0.74***	0.92***	1.33***	0.80***	1.00***
25% and more	0.40*	1.63***	1.74***	0.77**	1.35***
Evolution of income since previous interview (mean)	−0.01***	−0.02***	−0.04***	n.s.	−0.02***
Homeowner (ref. never)					
<2/3 of observations	n.s.	−0.94***	−0.94***	n.s.	−0.36*
2/3 and more	−0.51***	−1.33***	−1.68***	−0.87***	−0.80***
Health-related impediment (ref. never)					
<25% of observations	n.s.	n.s.	n.s.	n.s.	0.45*
25–50%	n.s.	0.57*	n.s.	0.50*	0.90***
More than 50%	0.54**	1.09***	1.39***	0.75**	0.89***
Retirement (ref. never)					
occurred within period	−0.62***	−1.13***	−1.01**	−0.60*	−1.02***
yes since 1st obs.	−0.99***	−2.05***	−1.89***	−0.93**	−1.77***
Dependent child(ren) (ref. never)					
<2/3 of observations	0.61***	n.s.	1.09***	1.12***	n.s.
2/3 and more	0.54***	0.75**	1.19***	0.90***	0.73***
Constant	16.25***	33.06***	38.78***	14.98***	24.85***

Notes: P value: * <0.05, ** <0.01, *** <0.001, n.s. = not significant. Households with min. 9 observations. N = 4319.
Source: Swiss Household Panel (SHP I and SHP II, unweighted), own calculation.

Table 8.3 presents our best multivariate model (pseudo R2 of 0.171), which deals with seven determinants. The trajectory 'moving into deprivation' was excluded in this model.[10]

The determinants related to the economic situation of the household strongly impact on deprivation trajectories, what was expected and confirms previous results (Heeb and Gutjahr 2012). In particular, compared to remaining non-deprived all over the period, the chance of being in deprived trajectories decreases when the mean household's income increases over the period, with larger beta coefficients for more unfavorable trajectories (from β= −1.7 for the 'mostly non-deprived' trajectory to β= −3.9 for the 'durably deprived'). This pattern is similar

10 Too many estimates in regard to the small number of households available in the sample; similar results.

for unbalanced budget: Having an unbalanced budget at least once compared to never (budget always balanced) increases the chance to be in deprived trajectories compared to remaining non-deprived all over the period. The more often the budget was unbalanced over the period, the greater the β coefficient – except for the 'mostly non-deprived' and 'moving out of deprivation' trajectories. In other words, and not surprisingly: deprived households have less money and have problems balancing their budget. Coherently, being a homeowner at least two third of the time compared to never, decreases the chance to be in 'mostly non-deprived' and 'moving out of deprivation' trajectories compared to remaining non-deprived all over the period; and being a homeowner at least once compared to never decreases the chance of being in 'mostly', 'durably' or 'fluctuating' deprived trajectories compared to remaining non-deprived all over the period. Regarding the mean reported change in income since previous interview, the chance of being in deprived trajectories compared to remaining non-deprived all over the period decreases when the mean change in income increases, except for the 'moving out' trajectory.

The other determinants of our final model are more interesting: Durable impairment due to a health condition, retirement, and many years with dependent child(ren). They are all related to life course and life events. Having health-related impediment more than 50% of the time compared to not having any impediment increases the chance of being in deprived trajectories compared to remaining non-deprived all over the period.[11] Impediment in 25 to 50% of the time compared to not having any impediment increases the chance of being in the 'mostly deprived', 'fluctuating' or 'moving out' trajectories compared to remaining non-deprived. However, the causality in the relation between deprivation and health cannot be observed from our analyses.

In relation to the life course hypothesis, retirement has a 'protective' effect: the fact that the household head or his/her parnter has retired (since the beginning of the period or during the period) compared to 'no one ever retired' decreases the chance of being in a deprived trajectory compared to remaining non-deprived, with β coefficients larger when retirement lasts longer (retired at first observation).[12] Finally, having dependent children compared to never having dependent children increases the chance of being in a deprived trajectory compared to remaining non-deprived, especially 'durably deprived'.

Results in Table 8.3 globally show that the chosen determinants are impacting the chance of being in deprived trajectories compared to remaining non-deprived, and that the β coefficient usually increases when the trajectory implies more deprivation phases. Furthermore, the impact of a factor depends on the number of years

---

[11] The stepwise procedure confirms that the impact of impairment is not related to age.

[12] In the literature, retirement is usually seen as a risk of deprivation. However, in Switzerland, the retired own a large part of the wealth. Attrition and adaptative preferences could also explain this, as both contribute to hide poverty in old age.

during which it affects the household. All in all, these factors have a larger impact on trajectories with long-lasting deprivation; and the impact is larger when the unfavorable situation of the determinant lasts.

Conclusion

'Les faits sont têtus' ('facts are stubborn', literally) is a French saying meaning that, when reality is strong enough (homogenous and stable), it always appears as it is, whatever the way you look at it. The alternative and innovating methodology we used to measure trajectories of deprivation and their determinants delivers relatively similar results to previous researches. Using trajectories dealing with a longer period of observation, based on a binary measure of deprivation, and constructed at the household level rather than at the individual level (as is usually done in mainstream research), reveals similar patterns of stable and moving trajectories to those found in previous studies. Like Tillmann and Budowski (2006), as well as Heeb and Gutjahr (2012), we found that about 80 percent of households remained in a (mostly) stable position (which was expected following the class hypothesis), with a large majority of survey participants never reporting any deprivation or only once over the 9 to 15 waves they participated in. Among those who experience change, most households display fluctuating patterns without any clear structure (which was expected following the individualization hypothesis). Trajectories related to durable transition into or out of deprivation are scarce.

This chapter therefore fills a gap, because results that rely on similar concepts and definitions always raise the same question: are their findings robust? Our clearly different approach – based on the use of household-level variables and on a different treatment of time-varying factors – leads to similar conclusions; therefore, we can be reassured that these results are quite robust.

Indeed, our results show the strength of inertia forces over the last decade. Yet, some elements mitigate this conclusion. First, we classified the mostly (non-) deprived trajectories as stable. These trajectories, representing 17 percent of the households, could also be associated to moving patterns and related to the individualization or life course hypothesis: they potentially correspond to non-definitive transitions following unpredictable life events or life course transitions, rather than to temporary deviations from a durably stable position. When keeping these 17 percent out of the stable households, the proportion of stability becomes even smaller than in Gazareth and Suter (2010), which is coherent (the longer the period, the higher the probability of change).

In addition, methodological issues affect the representativeness of panel data (which are the only data allowing such analyses of trajectories). Non-randomized attrition is the most problematic issue. It reinforces the strength of inertia because households facing deprivation are more likely to drop out (Gazareth and Iglesias

2017), including households in transitional life course phases that drop out before any change can be measured (e.g. a household headed by a young adult entering stable occupational position but dropping out before moving out of deprivation). By and large, the many missing observations challenge the results. Furthermore, adaptative preferences improve the probability of false identification of 'moving-out-of-poverty' trajectories. In conclusion, although we think that our results convincingly show that structural factors still represent powerful determinants of the poverty risk, they should not be taken as an exact quantification of this phenomenon, because of the methodological challenges mentioned above.

The analysis of the determinants of trajectories confirms the influence of factors related to unchanging vertical or horizontal inequality. The longer the households face unfavorable social conditions, the higher the risk they follow trajectories with many deprivation phases, like the mostly or durably deprived ones. This conclusion is coherent with the class hypothesis, but also with the cumulative (dis)advantages hypothesis. It pleads in favor of pursuing efforts engaged to reduce social inequalities, such as redistributive and social policy, educational support for children of the lower class, or the prevention of discrimination.

Life course transitions are clearly another driver of deprivation trajectories. Dependent children and retirement appear as the life events with the strongest impact in our analyses. Most interestingly, the'moving out of deprivation' trajectory is more likely if a household had dependent children for only a part of the period (less than 2/3 of observations), what can be partly related to grown-up children. This emphasizes the importance of family policy and support.

Health issues, and in particular the resulting impediments in everyday activities, is the last determinant with a clear impact on deprivation trajectories. This impact, however, is related to the duration of the (bad) health condition: when occurring occasionally (in less than 25 percent of the observations), impediment has no significant impact, except for the risk of fluctuating trajectory that increases slightly, what is coherent with the individualization hypothesis. If it occurs more frequently (25–50 percent), the 'mostly deprived' and 'moving out of deprivation' trajectories are also concerned. The last result is interesting: it indicates that overcoming an impediment contributes to moving out of deprivation. Finally, if impediment characterizes most of the experience of a household (that is, it affects one/several household member/s in at least half of the observations), all trajectories containing deprivation phases are more likely, especially the 'durably deprived' one. Without further analyses, it is hard to determine the direction of the causality; it is probably circular in some cases.

In summary, our contribution confirms the importance of inertia forces in Switzerland (class and cumulative hypotheses) and the limited or mostly temporary effect of life events (individualization hypothesis). In addition, life course transitions are found to have a clear impact on changes in social positions (but probably not much on changes in the social structure). Finally, it is noteworthy that the way in which we measure deprivation, the household composition and the changes in the situation of the household, has only a limited impact on the results, and so has the length of the observed period.

Our findings suggest that some of the claims that have been made regarding the individualization of social inequalities and the decline of social class (e.g. Beck 1992; Bauman 2000), are not confirmed empirically, and that the classical determinants of social inequalities remain powerful predictors. Sure enough, critical life events can have an impact; however, the scale of this impact is nowhere near as great as the effect of 'classical' poverty factors. This discrepancy between the assumed individualization of risks and what has been observed in recent years is attributable to the fact that these 'grand theories' of the new modernity (Goldthorpe 2002; Atkinson 2007) are not based on rigorous empirical work. Facts are, indeed, quite stubborn.

References

Atkinson, W. (2007). Beck, individualization and the death of class: A critique. *British Journal of Sociology, 58*(3), 349–366.

Bauman, Z. (2000). *Liquid modernity*. Cambridge: Polity.

Beck, U. (1992). *Risk society: Towards a new modernity*. New Delhi: Sage.

Crettaz, E., & Suter, C. (2013). The impact of adaptive preferences on subjective indicators: An analysis of poverty indicators. *Social Indicators Research, 114*, 139–152.

Figari, F. (2012). Cross-national differences in determinants of multiple deprivation in Europe. *The Journal of Economic Inequality, 10*, 397–418.

Gazareth, P., & Iglesias, K. (2017). *Material deprivation from 1999 to 2013 in Switzerland: How index construction impacts on measured patterns of evolution*. FORS Working Papers Series.

Gazareth, P., & Suter, C. (2010). Privation et risque d'appauvrissement en Suisse, 1999–2007. *Swiss Journal of Sociology, 36*(2), 213–234.

Goldthorpe, J. (2002). Globalisation and social class. *West European Politics, 25*(3), 1–28.

Halleröd, B. (2006). Sour grapes: Relative deprivation, adaptative preferences and the measurement of poverty. *Journal of Social Policy, 35*, 371–390.

Heeb, J.-L., & Gutjahr, E. (2012). Are there patterns of poverty trajectories? The dynamics of deprivation between classes, individualism, and cumulative disadvantage. *Swiss Journal of Sociology, 38*(2), 267–290.

Iglesias, K., Gazareth, P., & Suter, C. (2017). Explaining the decline in subjective well-being over time in panel data. In G. Brulé & F. Maggino (Eds.), *Metrics of subjective well-being*. Cham: Springer.

Layte, R., Whelan, C. T., Maître, B., & Nolan, B. (2001). Explaining levels of deprivation in the European Union. *Acta Sociologica, 44*(2), 105–121.

Lollivier, S., & Verger, D. (2005). Trois apports des données longitudinales à l'analyse de la pauvreté. *Economie et statistique, 383–385*, 245–282.

Suter, C., & Paris, D. (2002). Ungleichheit und Deprivation: Die Schweiz im Drei-Länder-Vergleich. *Swiss Journal of Sociology, 28*(2), 217–240.

Tillmann, R., & Budowski, M. (2006). La pauvreté persistante: un phénomène de classe, de cumul de désavantage ou d'individualisation? *Swiss Journal of Sociology, 32*(2), 329–348.

Townsend, P. (1979). *Poverty in the United Kingdom: A survey of household resources and standards of living*. London: Penguin.

Whelan, C., & Maître, B. (2006). Comparing poverty and deprivation dynamics: Issues of reliability and validity. *The Journal of Economic Inequality, 4*, 202–323.

Chapter 9
Trajectories of Vulnerability: A Sequence-Analytical Approach

Felix Bühlmann

Dynamics of Vulnerability

A growing proportion of the European population faces situations of vulnerability. Stable employees feel more and more at risk of losing their job or of experiencing a deterioration of their employment situation (Gallie et al. 1998). The share of standard employment relationships are declining, whereas atypical and precarious employment is on the rise (Rodgers & Rodgers, 1989; Hipp et al. 2015). In addition, joblessness in different forms—invalidity insurance, social assistance, early retirement—has also grown in recent decades (Paugam 2005). One of the unresolved issues is the relative scope of these phenomena. First, the advocates of what we could call exclusion thesis contend that only a small and marginal group is touched by material poverty and that this deprivation is inherently accompanied by isolation and segregation (Paugam 2005). A second approach, most famously brought forward by Robert Castel (2002), contends that not only the margins but also the larger zones of the labour market are characterised by precariousness. In a third perspective, it is asserted that work, even in formerly prestigious and well-paid occupations, is less and less socially recognised (Bourdieu 1999; Paugam 2000).

We argue that none of these three perspectives alone appropriately describes the current situation. They ought not to be conceived as alternative conceptual framings, but as facets of the same phenomenon. Life course sociology seems to be a particularly promising approach to link these facets of vulnerability together. In this contribution, we relate the different expressions of vulnerability to each other through the use of sequence analysis and investigate the development of the share of

F. Bühlmann (✉)
LINES/LIVES, University of Lausanne, Lausanne, Switzerland
e-mail: felix.buhlmann@unil.ch

R. Tillmann et al. (eds.), *Social Dynamics in Swiss Society*, Life Course Research and Social Policies 9, https://doi.org/10.1007/978-3-319-89557-4_9

individuals in precarious jobs, unemployment, and situations of exclusion during the period from 2000–2010 in Switzerland. Event mining techniques are used to investigate the odds of transition between crucial states of vulnerability and precariousness. Finally, we examine how the membership to different trajectories of vulnerability is influenced by cohort, gender, educational level or ethnic origin.

This chapter begins with a discussion of the three mentioned facets of vulnerability and an explanation of how they can fruitfully be linked together by a biographical approach. Then, we present the data and the Swiss case and discuss the results at greater length. In the concluding section, the findings and the heuristic value of the employed research strategy are discussed.

A Biographical Approach to Vulnerability

Subjective insecurity, precariousness, and exclusion are phenomena that emerge as the result of the interplay between the dynamics of the labour market and welfare policies. In this article, we seek to bring together the literatures addressing each of the issues and then discuss how they can be blended into a biographical approach.

The first step towards vulnerability is often a certain feeling of insecurity in an otherwise stable job. This subjective impression of job insecurity can be approached, for example, by the premonition that one will lose one's job within the next 12 months. According to Gallie et al. (1998), insecurity has become, in recent years, an increasingly relevant dimension of the well-being *at* and the satisfaction *with* work. It can be hypothesised that the feeling of job insecurity depends on the subjective impression of being in danger of becoming unemployed, previous spells of unemployment or the salience of unemployment as an issue in the media or personal entourage. Regardless of whether the threat behind this feeling is real, it can have psychological consequences and lead to a generalised hunch that one's work performance is not adequately rewarded (Paugam 2000).

When insecurity ceases to be a feeling but becomes linked to precarious employment conditions, we can speak of precariousness. Precarious employment embraces a large number of situations that differ from the male standard employment situation: part time employment fixed-term and otherwise temporary contracts, work at home, work in pseudo self-employment, on-call work (and all other forms of forced flexibility), night and weekend work, several employments, poorly paid jobs, or underemployment (Kalleberg 2000; 2009; Hipp et al. 2015). Night, weekend, or on-call work may prevent people from enjoying their social lives, meeting friends, and participating in clubs and associations. Others, such as temporary and fixed-term contracts, make it difficult for people to plan ahead and schedule important events, such as having children or buying a house.

Exclusion became a major analytical category at the beginning of the 1990s, first in France, later also in the German context (Kronauer 1996). In France, it developed jointly with concepts such as "precariousness" and "new poverty" (Paugam 2005). When, in the early 1990s, the unemployment rate and the number of those dependent on social assistance rose dramatically in almost all European countries, a growing group of "excluded" or "dispensables" people emerged. As a consequence of the enduring absence from the labour market, these people were unable to provide for the living cost of their households and depended on social assistance or invalidity insurance (Kronauer 1996). Not surprisingly, exclusion renders it difficult to live according to socially and culturally recognised norms and therefore often leads to social stigmatisation.

According to Castel (2002), different degrees or zones of precariousness are related to each other. The reserve army of the excluded put pressure on both groups in the zones of vulnerability and security. Those who are in the zone of vulnerability may want to move to the zone of security because they are afraid of falling back into the zone of exclusion. From a biographical angle, the fears that are typical for each zone, may be based on personal experiences and biographical mobility between one or several of these zones. A biographical approach, focused on how people pass through different forms of vulnerability, is, therefore, a simple but effective strategy to get a comprehensive glance at all these phenomena. We can reasonably assume that during their life courses, the same people go through situations of subjective insecurity, precariousness, and exclusion. As in theories of labour market segmentation, these zones may be defined by an absence of mobility between them and a large amount of mobility within them. Biographical mobility between groups is an important aspect of the activation, maintenance and reinforcement of boundaries between different welfare categories at the margins of the labour market (Lamont and Molnàr 2002; Scherschel et al. 2012). By studying the individual boundary crossing through entry into (or exit from) different situations of vulnerability, it is possible to understand the meaning of these boundaries as well as the categories of people who are labelled as "precarious" or "excluded." Situations of vulnerability, which are easily and regularly crossed by biographical movements, might lose their symbolic power of distinction, demarcation, and discrimination. They will be considered permeable and biographically reversible.

It has insistently been argued that precariousness or exclusions should be considered dynamically, not statically (Bane and Ellwood 1983; Leisering and Leibfried 1999). However, despite the progress made in dynamic poverty research, we believe the dynamic character of vulnerability can still be explored further. The studies of poverty spells tell little about the order and the velocity of the processes with which a person passes through a situation of vulnerability. Hence, it is different to be excluded all of a sudden to go through a long and slow process of precariousness. What is more, we can assume that a short precarious situation may remain ephemeral, whereas a longer spell in the same situation can lead to psychological and social repercussions. A biographical approach is, therefore, a promising strategy to gain a comprehensive and relational perspective on these three forms of vulnerability. Our inquiry will be guided by three research questions: (a) What is the overall and comparative proportion of individuals feeling insecure, employed in precarious jobs, or finding themselves in situations of exclusion during the period from 2000–2010? (b) What transition and mobility patterns can we observe between different situations of vulnerability? (c) Which typical trajectories of vulnerability can we distinguish, and how can these types be explained by cohort, gender, educational level, or ethnic origin?

Data and Method

Analysis of trajectories of vulnerability must rely on longitudinal data. Therefore, this article is based on data from the Swiss Household Panel (SHP) (Voorpostel et al. 2011). As the same respondents are interviewed every year, it is possible with these data to construct trajectories of a certain length. In the present case, we have used the waves 2 to 11, covering the years 2000–2010 in yearly intervals.[1] This period covers both the relatively prosperous early 2000s and the years of crisis from 2008 to 2010. The analysis has been limited to the population aged between 20 and 65 years in all waves. This means that the sample is constrained to those who, in 2010, were between 30 and 65 years old. In general, we must assume that those in vulnerable situations are underrepresented in the SHP and more concerned by attrition (Voorpostel et al. 2011). In addition, we have excluded all trajectories with more than three missing years.[2] This leaves us with 1332 individuals. The following table compares our subsample to the entire sample concerning a series of key socio-demographic variables (Table 9.1).

Groups, which according to the literature are threatened by vulnerability, are slightly underrepresented in the sequential sub-sample (immigrants, people with only compulsory education, younger cohorts)—very likely as a consequence of a higher attrition rate of these groups. However, other potentially vulnerable groups

Table 9.1 Comparison of Sub-sample and SHP Sample

	Sub-sample 2010 (30–65 years)		SHP Sample 2010 (30–65 years)	
	%	n	%	n
Women	58.3	777	52.8	2938
Foreigners	8.9	119	12.6	4862
Compulsory education	5.0	66	8.2	452
30–39 years	12.9	172	19.5	1086
40–49 years	38.7	515	35.1	1953
50–64 years	48.4	645	45.4	2527
Total	100	1332	100	5566

[1] The first wave in 1999 features not all variables on social assistance and invalidity and was thus not taken into account.

[2] An alternative would have been to use techniques of multiple imputation (see Halpin 2016). Because of the relative large number of missing values we have to be aware of possible selection effects and interpret the results cautiously.

are overrepresented (women) or fairly well represented (50–65 year old people). In general, the differences between the sub-sample and the whole SHP sample are not very large. It is also noteworthy that for the year 2006, we must deal with a filter error for one of the central variables (time limited contracts) and have about 5% more missing values compared to the other years.

The construction of the variables draws on the gradual conceptualisation of precariousness proposed by Paugam (2000), but differs on important point from it. As opposed to France, Switzerland has a relatively liberal labour law and lacks, in particular, a strong legal protection of categories considered as the stable core of the labour market. Therefore, less stable labour contracts, such as fixed-term contracts or temporary contracts are not as strongly opposed to permanent contracts. As a consequence, certain categorical adjustments were made. Categories were constructed based on the question on the risk of becoming unemployed in the next 12 months, the temporal limitation of the employment contract, and questions about unemployment, social assistance, invalidity insurance, and pre-retirement schemes. We present them here in an order of decreasing security:

- Stable and secure employment (31%)[3]: People in this situation possess a formally stable contract (no temporary or fixed-term employment) and they indicate also that they feel subjectively sure (risk of becoming unemployed estimated at 0 on an 11-item scale from 0 to 10).
- Stable and insecure employment (36%): This group enjoys a formally stable employment, but is considered to be at risk of becoming unemployed in the next 12 months (risk estimated at 1 to 5 on a scale from 0 to 10).
- Stable and very insecure employment (6%): Identical to the second group, except that the risk of becoming unemployed is estimated rather high (6 to 10 on a scale from 0 to 10).
- Unstable but secure employment (2%): Despite experiencing a situation of formal employment precariousness, this group feels subjectively secure.
- Unstable and insecure employment (4%): More consistent, these individuals are both formally and subjectively insecure. Not only is their employment contract non-permanent, but they are considered at risk of becoming unemployed in the next 12 months (1 to 10 on a scale from 0 to 10).
- Registered as unemployed (2%): These people report not being employed at the moment and are officially registered at a Swiss unemployment office. In other words, they are ready and willing to work if they find a job.
- Social assistance, invalidity insurance, pre-retirement (6%): This group is defined as people under 65 who are out of the workforce and simultaneously receive an old-age pension, a payment from the invalidity insurance, or a payment from social assistance.
- Out of workforce (13%): This group is not employed, but, at the same time, declares itself neither unemployed, nor dependent on contributions from one of the aforementioned insurances. Even though the status of this group is probably

[3] These percentages are average values over the period 2000–2010.

heterogeneous, we can assume that its members have left (or never entered) the labour market voluntarily.

In addition, we will test the composition of the trajectories with respect to some basic socio-demographic factors. Therefore, we have defined the following variables: sex (male and female), birth cohort (30–39 years; 40–49 years; 50–65 years), highest educational level (compulsory education; apprenticeship/high school; higher educational education; university/applied university) and nationality (rich countries, southern countries, Swiss).[4]

To respond to our research questions, we used transition mining, sequence analyses, and a multinomial regression model. To examine the transition between different forms of vulnerability, we searched for and counted all transitions and compared their frequency to an expected frequency, based on the proportion of a single state among all the possible states. To study the trajectories of vulnerability, we carried out a sequence analysis conducted with the R-libraries TraMineR (Gabadinho et al. 2009) and WeigthedCluster (Studer 2013). This method, popularised by Abbott, allows the researcher to display trajectories graphically, group them into types according to similarity, and link them to explanatory factors by the means of multinomial logistic regression models or discrepancy analysis (Abbott and Hrycak 1990; Aisenbrey and Fasang 2010; Studer et al. 2011). We used an optimal matching algorithm by calculating the substitution costs empirically and setting the insertion-delition costs at 1.5. Further, we used weighted Ward clustering and decided on the number of solutions on the basis of an extensive evaluation of cluster quality (Studer 2013). The six clusters are represented by a distribution plot, which gives an aggregate overview of the trajectories. Finally, we applied a multinomial regression analysis on the six clusters in order to understand which social categories trajectories are typical.

The Historical Dynamic of Vulnerability (2000–2010)

In a first step, we seek to trace the overall evolution of the above defined forms of vulnerabilities for the period from 2000–2010. Compared to most of the European countries, Switzerland's labour market remained for a long time spared from major crisis in the form of mass unemployment. Even when, in the early 1990s, the unemployment rate rose, its increase was gentler than in many other Western countries. This has specific reasons: unemployment was, for a long time, buffered by the periodic pushing out of the labour market of the foreign workforce and women

[4]In Switzerland the traditional working-class migration from southern countries between 1960-1980s has recently been completed by a group of better educated immigrants from northern European countries. We defined Italy, Portugal, Spain Ex-Yugoslavia as "southern countries" and Germany, France, USA and the UK as "rich countries".

(Streckeisen 2012).[5] In the early 1990s, as women would increasingly crowd into the labour market and the yearly regulation of labour immigration was abandoned, the economic crisis caused a rise in the unemployment rate from about 1% to 4%. Long-term unemployment rose from 20% of the unemployed to over 30% in 1995 and 40% in 1999 (Bühlmann et al. 2012). In addition and as a consequence of the increasing long-term character of unemployment rates, recipients of invalidity insurance and social assistance rose in the 1990s and then particularly in the early 2000s. These two insurance systems, structurally conceived as support of the last order, became the collecting tank of those who were no longer supported by the regular unemployment insurance.

Beyond the increase of those durably excluded from the labour market, we can also trace the rise of precarious jobs through the same period. An increasing proportion of the workforce labours in fixed-term contracts, with temporary agencies, on call or in part-time arrangements. Whereas, for instance, only about 4500 people were working for a temporary agency in 1993, this number rose to 46,000 in 1997, 201,000 in 2003 and even 236,000 in 2009. Also the proportion of employees in fixed-term contracts and employment on call increased about 35%, respectively 38% between 2001 and 2009. This contrasts rather strongly with the stagnation or slight decrease of both full-time jobs and permanent employment during the period of 2001–2009.[6] The parallel rise of exclusion and precarious employment is no coincidence. It has strong institutional links. Beyond new recruitment and personnel administration policies of firms, it was also novel social policies that contributed to the rise of precarious employment. Modification of the unemployment law in the spirit of the "activation policies" reduced the period of unemployment support (especially for younger people), enlarged the definition of jobs that must be accepted, and created a series of re-integration courses and programs, some of which corresponded to precarious forms of employment (Bonvin 2008; Tabin 2000; Streckeisen 2008). How are these official data from the Swiss Labour Force Survey now reflected in the data used for this study? (Fig. 9.1).

The period between 2000 and 2010 was characterised by a massive growth of subjective employment insecurity. This sharp rise, which is not documented in official data as discussed above, has much larger amplitude than the increase of precarious employment conditions. We may speak of a creeping general vulnerability, a growing destabilisation of otherwise stable jobs. This surge in employment insecurity means the proportion of people with a stable and secure job, a situation that is supposed to represent the male norm of the post-war period, became a minority. For the years 2009 and 2010, it amounts to less than 30% of the age group between 20 and 65. More generally, we can observe a rather consistent overall trend towards

[5]The so called « Saisonnierstatut », which allowed Switzerland to limit the number of foreign workers per year at will, and which gave virtually no labour rights to this important foreign part of the workforce, was abandoned in 1991 for non-EU citizens and 2002 also for citizens of the European Union.

[6]These numbers draw on the Swiss Labour Force Survey. See also Pelizzari (2009) for the period 2001–2006.

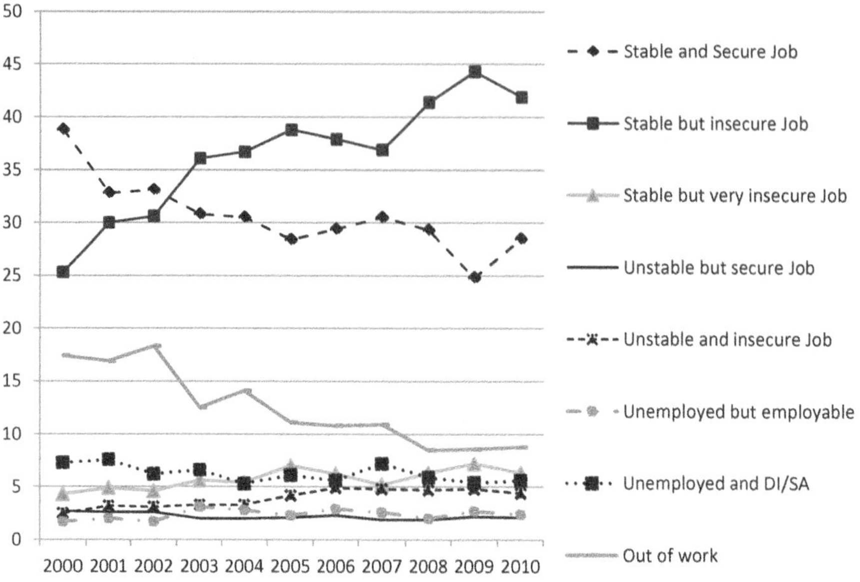

Fig. 9.1 Development of situations of vulnerability in Switzerland, 2000–2010

less security and stability in employment. Most categories of unstable and insecure jobs are on the rise. It is important not to over-interpret this trend though; the most significant rise concerns those who feel *slightly* instable in their job. Very insecure jobs and combinations of insecure and instable jobs do not increase as strongly. In other words, there is a widespread uncertainty in the Swiss society, but this uncertainty is comparatively superficial. To understand how biographical dynamics contribute to this rise of vulnerability in Swiss society, we examine the transition between different states of vulnerability and then carry out a sequence analysis to identify typical trajectories of vulnerability.

Mobility Between Different Forms of Vulnerability

By studying the relative chances of transition between the eight states of vulnerability we have defined, we will first examine whether the pathways into and out of insecurity (respectively, precariousness or exclusion) are abrupt or rather gradual. Second, we ask whether we can identify certain segments of vulnerability *within* which mobility is common, while at the same time mobility *between* these segments is rare. This will shed light on the social boundaries that potentially enclose different situations of vulnerability.

We mine for transition between the states and calculate the relative chances to accede to each of the states from each other state (odds ratios). These odds ratios result from a calculation of the relative chances to move to a state (measured by the share of this state among all states) and the real share of people within the specific state who moved to this state. A value of 1 means that the comparative chances to move to this state equal the chances under a uniform distribution. A value of 0.5 means that the chances are only half what they should be under conditions of a uniform distribution. A value of 2 means that the chances are two times higher than with a uniform distribution (Table 9.2).

In the light grey upper part of the table, the odds of transitions are displayed from relatively stable and secure situations on the left to more and more insecure and excluded situations on the right. The results confirm the trend found on the individual level: generally, people move away from "stable and secure jobs" towards less stable or secure types of employment. Second, we find it more likely to move to a neighbouring state than to "jump" to states that are farther away on the scale of vulnerability. This means the trajectories of vulnerability are rather regular and gradual. It is conspicuous, that there is no specific threshold between unstable jobs and registered unemployment. Moves in and out of unemployment are, thus, relatively common.[7] Third, we can identify a certain caesura between the states "invalidity and social assistance" and "out of workforce" versus all other states. Direct moves to these states of exclusions are relatively rare.

The lower part of the matrix displays the odds to move from marginal and unstable states to more stable forms of employment. Mirror-inverted to the findings above, shifts to secure and stable forms of employment were generally rare in the period of 2000 to 2010. Also in the inverse direction, gradual moves to neighbouring state are more likely than jumps from total exclusion to total stability. It is very unlikely to shift from registered unemployment or social assistance directly to a stable and secure job. The chances to move to a better situation along the scale diminish the better the conditions are in comparison. Third, the only situations that offer relatively good chances to move to stable and secure jobs is from stable but insecure jobs. When it comes to upwards mobility, these two states at the stable pole of the scale seem to constitute a homogenous zone.

Biographical Dynamics of Vulnerability

As a further step, a sequence analysis was carried out to identify and represent seven typical trajectories graphically. The following distribution plots represent the years between 2000 and 2010 as pillars on the x-axis. For each year, the proportional distribution of the states is displayed (Fig. 9.2).

The first type, *stable but insecure jobs* (n = 458), corresponds to a continuous trajectory of employment in formally permanent but subjectively insecure jobs. Even if these jobs are not contractually limited in time, this group feels there is a certain risk that they will become unemployed in the next 12 months. This type is by far the largest group in contemporary Switzerland. Even when there are no formal reasons to feel vulnerable in a job, the very low legal obstacles to lay off people

[7] This is among other things a consequence of the liberal Swiss labour law and is unlikely to happen in other countries which have a stronger protection of permanent labour status.

Table 9.2 Odds ratios of transitions between different states of vulnerability

	Stable and secure job	Stable but insecure job	Stable but very insecure job	Unstable but secure job	Unstable and insecure job	Unemployed registred	Unemployed DI/SA	Out of work force
Stable and secure job	0.00	1.73	3.82	3.30	2.22	1.74	1.29	0.66
Stable but insecure job	2.03	0.00	5.57	3.30	2.56	2.35	0.96	0.66
Stable but very insecure job	0.69	1.16	0.00	3.30	2.91	2.35	0.63	0.57
Unstable but secure job	0.73	0.50	3.29	0.00	6.91	1.74	0.63	0.85
Unstable and insecure job	0.58	0.64	2.79	10.20	0.00	4.24	1.29	0.75
Unemployed registred	0.33	0.56	2.79	2.61	6.03	0.00	1.98	1.79
Unemployed and DI/SA	0.42	0.22	0.78	2.61	2.91	1.63	0.00	6.76
Out of work force	0.45	0.30	0.98	3.30	3.64	3.60	18.24	0.00

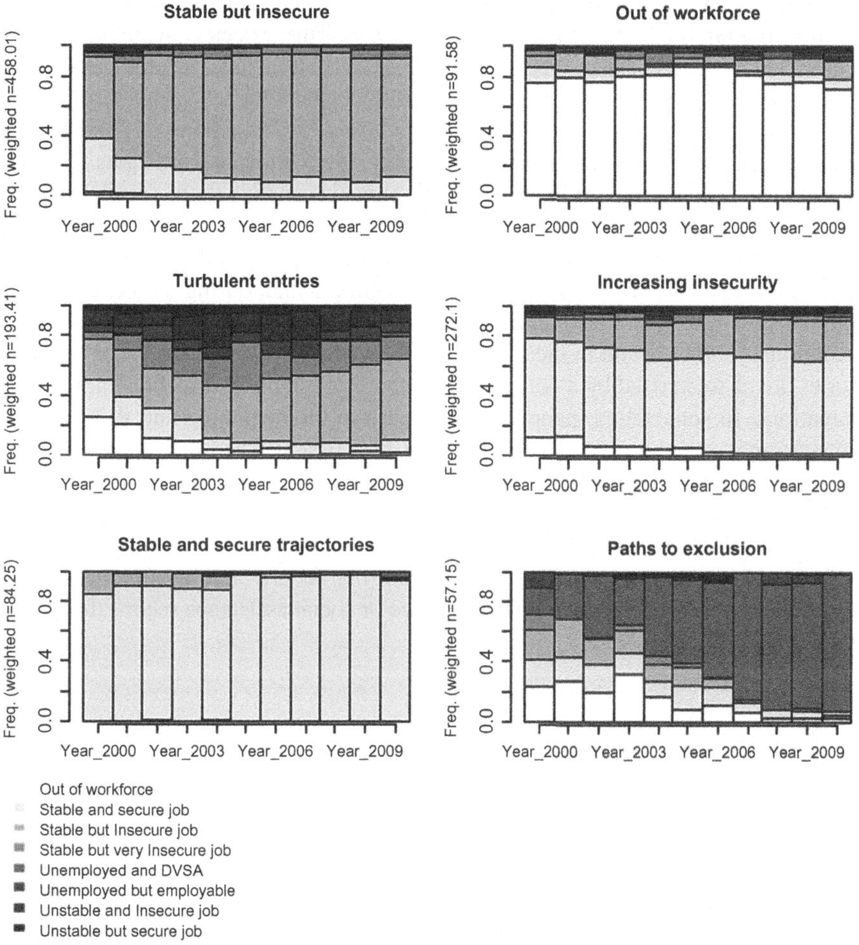

Fig. 9.2 Typology of trajectories of vulnerability 2000–2010

in Switzerland seems to create a widespread fear of losing one's job. Also the individuals in the second cluster, *out of workforce* (n = 92), remain essentially stable over the whole period of 2000 to 2010. This group refrains from participating in the labour market. At the same time, it does not declare itself as unemployed or dependent on social assistance. We can assume that the member of this cluster remain voluntarily out of the labour market. It is probably mainly composed of women who, permanently or for a child rearing period, decide (or are forced) to live a life as a homemaker. *Turbulent entries* (n = 193) include pathways that change between different forms of unsteady employment. Typically, short periods of insecure or unstable employment alternate with spells of unemployment, as well as with stable but insecure jobs. What is conspicuous is the high volatility between different states and the permanence of vulnerability; the members of this type never really reach a secure shore in the form of stable and secure jobs. This trajectory seems to be typical for labour market entries between 2000 and 2010. It includes a certain share that, in the beginning, is out of the workforce and then enters the labour market.

The fourth trajectory (labelled *increasing insecurity*) assembles 272 individuals who are first in stable and secure job and then slowly move towards jobs that they deem exposed to the risk of becoming unemployed even though the formal status of these employments is not changing. These people went through a kind of subjective vulnerabilisation of their employment situation between 2000 and 2010. The trajectory-type, which was supposedly the norm for men during the economically golden post-war years, has survived, but concerns only a rather small group. 84 individuals can be found in the *stable and secure trajectories cluster*. These trajectories are characterised by a continuous sequence of stable and secure employment situations. In some cases, people feel insecure in the beginning and then become increasingly sure towards the end of the ten-year period. The last type is best characterised as *paths of exclusion* (n = 57). Its members were employed or out of work in the early 2000s and then successively fell out of the labour market and are taken care of by the either invalidity insurance, social assistance, or early retirement schemes. Returns from this state to the labour market are rare, even in the form of insecure or instable jobs. Invalidity insurance or social assistance seems, thus, to be an irreversible state.

Explaining Trajectories of Vulnerability

In order to characterise these six trajectory-types socially, we carried out a multinomial regression analysis. This method allows us to characterise the cluster membership by a series of simple socio-demographic variables, such as gender, age group, ethnic origin, and educational level.[8] Stable and secure trajectories were chosen as the reference group. Table 9.3 displays the results of these analyses. Because of the relatively large number of missing values in our analytical sample, the results of this regression analysis have to be interpreted with caution.

Stable but insecure trajectories are common among younger men aged 30–40 and 40–50. Surprisingly, those with a basic education or migrants do not feel particularly threatened. Trajectories out of workforce are above all female trajectories. Virtually no men move voluntarily out of the employment system. This is confirmed by other longitudinal studies on male work trajectories (Widmer et al. 2003) Second,

[8] We deliberately refrained from using variables which do not apply to all types (such as occupation, which makes no sense for people out of the workforce) or which are ambivalent according to their temporal-causal relationship with reference to the trajectories.

Table 9.3 Multinomial regression – factors explaining the trajectory of vulnerability (odds ratios)

		Stable but insecure	Out of Workforce	Turbulent entries	Increasing insecurity	Paths to exclusion
Sex	Men	1.55°	0.07**	1.03	1.15	0.94
	Women	–	–	–	–	–
Cohort	30–40	2.30*	1.21	2.11*	2.33*	0.20°
	41–50	3.01**	1.98°	2.89**	3.17**	0.78
	51–65	–	–	–	–	–
Education	Compulsory	2.94	10.28*	1.50	9.12*	20.10**
	Apprenticeship	1.10	2.85*	0.90	1.40	3.28*
	Higher vocational	1.63	0.56	0.78	1.59	0.92
	University	–	–	–	–	–
Ethnic origin	Swiss	0.52	0.72	0.27*	0.56	0.40
	Rich countries	0.94	1.54	0.40	0.42	0.52
	Poor countries	–	–	–	–	–

° < 0.1; * < 0.05; ** < 0.01.

we see that those with only a compulsory education or an apprenticeship stay for long periods out of the labour market. We can make the hypothesis that rather than women in general, it is women with a small amount of educational capital, who refrain from labour market participation. Women who invested more into education may want to "capitalise" that investment.

When it comes to turbulent entries, we see that these concern above all younger people who make their entry into the labour market. However, with our data it is not possible to compare the labour market entry of different cohorts. Therefore we are not able to say if the labour market entry is more turbulent for the younger cohorts. It seems also that turbulent entries are less prevalent among Swiss citizens than among foreigners from poor countries. However, they are not particularly bound to any educational level: they occur to a broad range of young adults. This is surprising. We would have to dig deeper in order to examine whether this form of vulnerable trajectories may are typical for project-oriented and voluntarily flexible occupations (such as graphic designer, architects or journalists). Paths to exclusion threatens those who only possess a compulsory school degree, those with an apprenticeship, and, much less, those holding a higher vocational degree or a university degree. In addition, similarly to what has been found in other studies, it touches particularly the older cohorts (Oesch and Baumann 2014): it is particularly widespread among poorly trained older workers.

Conclusions

The fear of losing one's job, precarious employment, or long-term exclusion from the labour market have become more urgent over the last decades. However, the real scope of the phenomenon and the angle from which to approach it remain controversial. While certain scholars consider the economic and social exclusion of a minority as the main problem, others frame the issue in terms of precarious employment situations. Still, others deem the declining subjective employment security as the main problem. In this contribution, we sought to relate these three forms of vulnerability with a biographical approach.

A comparative examination of different forms of vulnerability shows that in Switzerland only a minority held a secure and stable job in 2010. Even within a sample such as the SHP, in which marginalised actors tend to be under-represented, less than 30% enjoy stable and secure employment conditions. More severe forms of vulnerability, unstable and insecure jobs, for instance, have also risen, but on a lower initial level and in a much less spectacular way. Subjective insecurity touches a wide range of the Swiss population and increases steeply between 2000 and 2010. It is particularly widespread among young (men). Possibly, the "objectively" turbulent entries into the labour market of those aged between 30–40 years one reason for this subjective feeling of insecurity.

Through an analysis of the transitions between the different forms of vulnerability, we can observe certain social boundaries beyond which circulation is rare (Lamont and Molnár 2002). The findings show that the pathways to precariousness or exclusion are rather incremental. This also means that in countries such as Switzerland, there is no specific protection threshold against unemployment. The only boundaries between zones are constructed by social policies that actually direct mobility. Movements to situations of social assistance or invalidity often make it necessary to pass first through a longer period of unemployment. On the other hand, once somebody finds him- or herself in a situation of unemployment or precarious employment, the way back to stable and secure employment is boarded-up.

A biographical analysis reveals that the younger generation seems to be particularly concerned by vulnerability. Increasing insecurities and turbulent entries, spells of unemployment, and late access to secure jobs are common among the younger generation. When we examine the older age class, it seems that, on one hand, its poorly trained fraction is clearly more in danger of becoming irreversibly excluded. On the other hand, older people are also well represented among the cluster of stable and secure trajectories. Either because they are towards the end of a long career and have achieved positions that are more secure or because they have never gone in their younger years through turbulent phases they seem to feel more confidence about the security of their job.

References

Abbott, A., & Hrycak, A. (1990). Measuring resemblance in sequence analysis: An optimal matching analysis of musicians careers. *American Journal of Sociology, 96*(1), 144–185.

Aisenbrey, S., & Fasang, A. E. (2010). New life for old ideas: The 'second Wave' of sequence analysis bringing the "course" back into the life course. *Sociological Methods and Research, 38*(3), 430–462.

Bane, M. J., & Ellwood, D. T. (1983). *Slipping into and out of poverty: The dynamics of spells*. Cambridge, MA: National Bureau of Economic Research.

Bonvin, J.-M. (2008). Activation policies, new modes of governance and the issue of responsibility. *Social Policy and Society, 7*(3), 367–377.

Bourdieu, P. (1999). *Weight of the world: Social suffering in contemporary society*. Cambridge: Polity Press.

Bühlmann, F., Schmid Botkine, C., Farago, P., Höpflinger, F., Joye, D., Levy, R., Perrig-Chiello, P., & Suter, C. (2012). *Swiss social report 2012: Generations in perspective*. Zürich: Seismo.

Castel, R. (2002). *From manual workers to wage laborers: Transformation of the social question*. New Brunswick: Transaction.

Gabadinho, A., Ritschard, G., Studer, M., & Müller, N. S. (2009). *Mining sequence data in R with the TraMineR package: A user's guide*. Geneva: University of Geneva.

Gallie, D., White, M., Cheng, Y., & Tomlinson, M. (1998). *Restructuring the employment relationship*. Oxford: Oxford University Press.

Halpin, B. (2016). Multiple imputation for categorical time series. *Stata Journal, 16*(3), 590–612.

Hipp, L., Bernhardt, J., & Allmendinger, J. (2015). Institutions and the prevalence of nonstandard employment. *Socio-Economic Review, 13*(2), 351–377.

Kalleberg, A. L. (2000). Nonstandard employment relations: Part-time, temporary and contract work. *Annual Review of Sociology, 26*, 341–365.

Kalleberg, A. L. (2009). Precarious work, insecure workers: Employment relations in transition. *American Sociological Review, 74*(1), 1–22.

Kronauer, M. (1996). Soziale Ausgrenzung" und „Underclass": Über neue Formen der gesellschaftlichen Spaltung. *Sofi-Mitteilungen, 24*, 53–69.

Lamont, M., & Molnár, V. (2002). The study of boundaries in the social sciences. *Annual Review of Sociology, 28*, 167–195.

Leisering, L., & Leibfried, S. (1999). *Time and poverty in western Germany: United Germany in perspective*. Cambridge: Cambridge University Press.

Oesch, D., & Baumann, I. (2014). Smooth transition or permanent exit? Evidence on job prospects of displaced industrial workers. *Socio-Economic Review, 13*(1), 101–123.

Paugam, S. (2000). *Le salarié de la précarité. Les nouvelles formes de l'intégration professionnelle*. Paris: PUF.

Paugam, S. (2005). *Les formes élémentaires de la pauvreté*. Paris: PUF.

Pelizzari, A. (2009). *Dynamiken der Prekarisierung. Atypische Erwerbsverhältnisse und milieusspezifische Unsicherheitsbewältigung*. Konstanz: UVK.

Rodgers, G., & Rodgers, J. (1989). *Precarious jobs in labour market regulation: The growth of atypical employment in Western Europe*. Geneva: International Institute for labour studies.

Scherschel, K., Streckeisen, P., & Krenn, M. (Eds.). (2012). *Neue Prekarität. Die Folgen aktivierender Arbeitsmarktpolitik – europäische Länder im Vergleich*. Frankfurt: Campus.

Streckeisen, P. (2008). *Die zwei Gesichter der Qualifikation. Eine Fallstudie zum Wandel von Industriearbeit*. Konstanz: UVK Verlag.

Streckeisen, P. (2012). Steigende Erwerbslosigkeit und Prekarität in der Schweiz: Das Ende eines „Sonderfalls". In K. Scherschel, P. Streckeisen, & M. Krenn (Eds.), *Neue Prekarität. Die Folgen aktivierender Arbeitsmarktpolitik – europäische Länder im Vergleich* (pp. 47–73). Frankfurt: Campus.

Studer, M., Ritschard, G., Gabadinho, A., & Müller, N. S. (2011). Discrepancy analysis of state sequences. *Sociological Methods & Research, 40*(3), 471–510.

Studer, M. (2013). *WeightedCluster library manual: A practical guide to creating typologies of trajectories in the social sciences with R* (Vol. 24). Lausanne: LIVES Working Papers.

Tabin, J. P. (2000). Les politiques actives du marché du travail. *Les Politiques sociales / Collège international pour l'étude du changement dans les politiques sociales, 3–4*, 38–54.

Voorpostel, M., Tillmann, R., Lebert, F., Weaver, B., Kuhn, U., Lipps, O., Ryser, V. A., Schmid, F., Rothenbühler, M., & Wernli, B. (2011). *Swiss household panel userguide (1999–2010), Wave 12*. Lausanne: FORS.

Widmer, E., Levy, R., Pollien, A., Hammer, R., & Gauthier, J. A. (2003). Entre standardisation, individualisation et sexuation: une analyse des trajectoires personnelles en Suisse. *Schweizerische Zeitschrift für Soziologie, 29*(1), 35–68.

Chapter 10
The Impact of Modernization and Labor Market Conditions on the School-to-Work Transition in Switzerland: A Dynamic Analysis of the Period from 1946 to 2002

Christoph Zangger, David Glauser, and Rolf Becker

Introduction

The transition from the education system into the labor market is a significant and sensitive phase in the life course of young generations given the long-term consequences of work history and impact on future opportunities (Blossfeld 1985, 1987; DiPrete et al. 2001). It is undisputed that the school-to-work transition depends on individual resources, such as social background and attained educational qualification (Buchmann and Sacchi 1998; Jann and Combet 2012; R. Becker and Zangger 2013) and on the structure and organization of the education and the employment system as well as their institutional linkage (Allmendinger 1989; Kerckhoff 1995; Shavit and Müller 2000; Wolbers 2007). In addition, opportunities to attain specific educational credentials and returns to investments in education at the beginning of the occupational career vary over time (e.g., Blau and Duncan 1967). They affect the patterns of labor market entry and the status attainment in the course of people's occupational career, and indicate the openness of the class structure across birth cohorts (Blossfeld 1987; Sørensen 1986; Shavit and Müller 1998). However, this time dependency of these trajectories has often been neglected in previous empirical research. Therefore, there is limited information on the probability and process through which individuals accept profitable employment and the social status they achieve when they enter the labor market. In addition, it is important to understand how these factors are related to (1) the long-term social changes with respect to modernization (e.g., educational expansion, tertiarization of professions and

C. Zangger (✉) · D. Glauser · R. Becker
Department of Sociology of Education, University of Bern, Institute of Educational Science, Bern, Switzerland
e-mail: christoph.zangger@edu.unibe.ch; david.glauser@edu.unibe.ch; rolf.becker@edu.unibe.ch

R. Tillmann et al. (eds.), *Social Dynamics in Swiss Society*, Life Course Research and Social Policies 9, https://doi.org/10.1007/978-3-319-89557-4_10

industries, and increasing social welfare), (2) the economic business cycles in the post-war period (e.g., boom periods, recessions resulting from oil price shocks, dot-com and real estate bubbles, financial and bank crises), and (3) the fluctuating state of the labor market (e.g., decrease in full time employment, increasing youth unemployment).

In this chapter, the transition of different birth cohorts into the labor market is reconstructed as a dynamic process that is time-dependent on the (*a*) transition duration from the education system to the first job (age or life-cycle effect), (*b*) period-specific changes of labor market conditions, the level of modernity in the economy, and the social structure after completing education (period effect), and (*c*) the economic and social conditions at the time of achieving educational qualifications (cohort effect). The age-period-cohort (APC) analysis aims to answer the following questions with respect to Switzerland in the period from 1946 to 2002: (*1*) What is the role of the modernization trend and economic business cycles in determining the speed of transition and the likelihood of attaining a prestigious job? (*2*) Are there still direct effects of social background and educational qualification across cohorts on the likelihood of graduates starting their career and achieving status in their first jobs if the modernization trend and economic business cycle are taken into account? (*3*) Despite the increasing uncertainty due to globalization and labor market competition, are the institutional arrangements of the education system and its linkage to the labor markets effective in providing "safety roads" for young professionals to start their career?

The remainder of this contribution is organized as follows. In the next section, the theoretical background is briefly outlined. Subsequently, the data, operationalization of the variables, methodological design, and statistical procedure are presented. The empirical results are discussed in the fourth section and the findings are summarized in the final concluding section.

Theoretical Background and Hypotheses

Following Shavit and Müller (2000), the organizational structure of the education system and labor markets as well as their institutional linkages affect the extent to which a "safety net" for socially disadvantaged adolescents and a "safety road" for graduates to their first job is provided (Imdorf and Hupka-Brunner 2015; Buchs et al. 2015). Additionally, the attained educational qualification (in terms of credentials) and social background of adolescents (in terms of socio-economic status of parental home) are important factors in the transition from school to work (Müller and Kogan 2010). According to the human capital approach (G. S. Becker 1964), investment in education is a necessary precondition for access to privileged positions in the labor market. Furthermore, the signal theory emphasizes that labor market access depends on attained certificates that signal the productivity of young professionals. Both these theoretical approaches are consistent with the assumptions of the labor queue model (Thurow 1975): the better people are educated, the better their position in front of the entry ports of firms and therefore the higher their chances to get hired in favorable positions.

In the course of the educational expansion, the tertiarization of professions and industries, and the upgrading of successive birth cohorts (Oesch and Rodríguez Menés 2010; Oesch 2013), the attained (vocationally or academically oriented) education has become increasingly important in securing the first job. This is because the supply of well-trained graduates has increased. In this respect, social background and familial social networks might have also become increasingly important for occupational beginners (Franzen and Hangartner 2005; Kramarz and Skans 2014). However, it has to be kept in mind that the institutional interpretation by employers of graduates' credentials, productivity, and desirable qualities depends on macro processes, such as modernization and economic business cycles (Gangl 2002). Crowding-out processes in the school-to-work transition might intensify because of tertiarization and increase in qualification requirements of jobs in the service and administrative areas. Consequently, younger school-leaver cohorts, who benefited from the educational expansion (R. Becker and Zangger 2013; Zangger and Becker 2016), are in a more advantageous position at the start of their career compared to older school-leaver cohorts. The percentage of persons who have completed at most compulsory education level has declined across birth cohorts and is remarkably low for the youngest cohorts. In addition, the Swiss case is characterized by a rather smooth school-to-work transition (OECD 2015): The majority of adolescents who have completed upper secondary education gain access to permanent, secure, and suitable jobs within a short timeframe (Buchs et al. 2015; de Lange et al. 2013).

If the dynamics of the entry process in the labor market are considered in context of the timing and speed of transition and the macro-level situation during this time period, then the process of modernization and the fluctuations of economic cycles will affect labor markets and therefore the school-to-work transition and returns to education in the early phase of employment (Raaum and Røed 2006; Gangl 2002). Presumably, under better economic conditions, the opportunities to enter the labor market immediately after graduation and attain employment in a high-level position will improve (cohort effect). In addition, better economic conditions will lead to a smooth transition into the labor market after leaving the education system (period effect). However, the insider-outsider approach (Lindbeck et al. 1988) provides an additional perspective: If there is a decline in the economy, the situation of recent graduates will become more challenging as they will have to compete against groups that are already employed. Under these conditions, the competition between school-leavers will intensify. Graduates with vocational and academic training increasingly displace the less educated people in the labor market. Furthermore, if the economic recession lasts longer, then the competition among school-leavers that have attained vocational education and training will increase. In contrast, people who have attained a higher education may continue their education, thus, gaining a foothold in the labor market for the future.

Finally, the linear trend of modernization in Switzerland – the combination of educational expansion, size of the labor force, changes in the occupational structures during tertiarization, and increases in qualification requirements – is associated with substantial differences in the patterns of the school-to-work transition between cohorts. On one hand, it is assumed that higher levels of modernity at the time of graduation and training increases the graduates' chances of being hired in a high-level position (cohort effect). On the other hand, continuous modernization during the job search will result in more favorable outcomes (period effect).

In sum, we expect that the school-to-work transition is influenced by age, period, and cohort effects. The age effect will be observed when a long-lasting job search worsens the labor market outcomes of school-leavers in terms of lower employment opportunities and lower chances of being hired in a high-status position (Gebel 2009). Period effects will be observed with the increasing level of modernity and favorable labor market conditions during the job search that will smoothen the transition into the labor market and provide access to prestigious jobs. In addition, and due to the higher level of modernity, we assume that younger school-leaver cohorts are in a more advantageous position at the start of their career (cohort effect).

Data, Variables, and Statistical Procedure

In the following section, we present the data, the operationalization of variables, and the statistical procedure used to test our research hypotheses.

Data and Variables

This study uses data from the retrospective biographical calendar collected in 2002 as part of the Swiss Household Panel (SHP). It allows the identification of respondents' stages across the life course in terms of education, employment, civil status, and housing. Thus, the data are suitable for this study since they allow a time-dependent modeling of the transition from education into employment. The participants include those who left education prior to entering the labor market between 1946 and 2002, which corresponds to birth cohorts born between 1912 and 1986. After excluding missing values, the total sample size consists of 2344 individuals. Education is defined as a categorical variable comprising the following educational levels: "compulsory schooling," "vocational education," "general education," "higher vocational education," and "university (of applied sciences)." The dependent variable is the respondents' status in the labor market after leaving education and is based on the International Socio-Economic Index (ISEI) scores of the first job. However, since not all subjects entered the labor market, this variable was divided into categories in order to include those who were not part of the labor market and those who were unemployed. This resulted in a categorical variable with six values: those not in the labor market, the unemployed, those in the first (lowest),

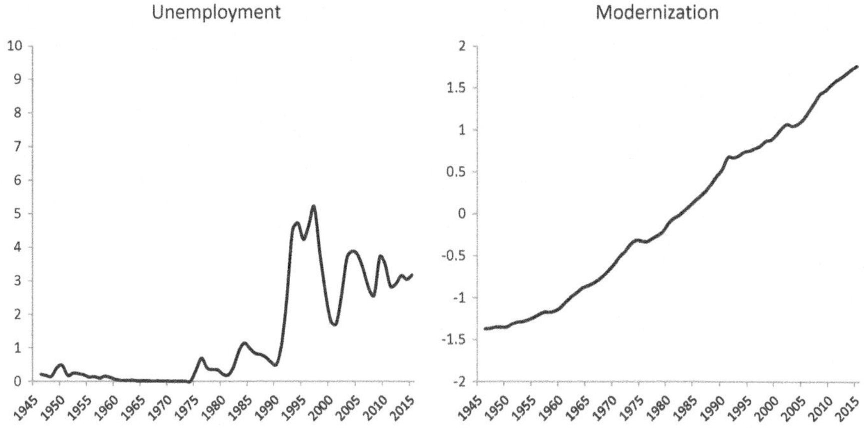

Fig. 10.1 Labor market conditions (unemployment rate in %) and modernization (factor scores) in Switzerland (*Source*: Federal Office of Statistics; Historical statistics of Switzerland online)

second, third, and fourth (highest) quartile in the status distribution. Since the unemployed category was marginal, it was merged with those who are not in the labor market.

Other variables include the respondents' gender, citizenship as a substitute for migration background, and a measure of social background (the highest education of the primary income earner at the age of fifteen years, operationalized the same way as respondents' education). Descriptive statistics for all the variables are listed in the Appendix. Of main interest, however, are the measures for cohort and period effects. In the theoretical section, it was outlined that the changing labor market conditions might have an impact on the successful transition of entrants to their first job. Therefore, the trend of changes in labor market conditions is an important indicator, and is measured in terms of the unemployment rates (left side in Fig. 10.1). Based on the analysis using the historical observation window from 1946 until 2002, it was observed that the most remarkable changes of labor market conditions occurred in the 1970s, 1980s, and 1990s. The unemployment rate at the time of graduation is considered as the first cohort effect and the changing unemployment rates between graduation and entry into the labor market indicate period effects.

It is suggested that the process of modernization is an additional secular development affecting labor market outcomes of graduates. Since modernization is a complex process with different interrelated developments, this process is measured by a combination of different indicators, such as educational expansion, tertiarization, individual and general welfare, population, and economic dynamics (see Table 10.1). In order to prevent an identification problem resulting from highly correlated time series, confirmatory factor analysis is used on the fifteen time series (Kolenikov 2009; Harrington 2009). The factor, modernization, is the result of the main component method and orthogonal factor rotation. The factor explains 96 per cent of the variance in the different time series (last row in Table 10.1). The change in the

Table 10.1 Factor loadings (pattern matrix) and unique variances

Variables	Factor: Modernization	Uniqueness	Kaiser-Meyer-Olkin scores
Educational spending	0.9824	0.0348	0.8162
No. of students eligible for university	0.9862	0.0273	0.9569
No. of students in universities	0.9944	0.0112	0.9106
No. of PhD	0.9754	0.0486	0.8344
No. of employees	0.9851	0.0295	0.8811
Share of employees in tertiary sector	0.9817	0.0362	0.8099
Labor volume	0.9759	0.0477	0.8859
Index of real income (1939 = 100)	0.9304	0.1344	0.7842
Consumer price index of private households	0.9885	0.0299	0.9279
No. of employees in public and private banks	0.9653	0.0682	0.8812
Population	0.9747	0.0499	0.8205
Gross domestic product (GDP; 1990 = 100)	0.9897	0.0204	0.9268
Private consume	0.9931	0.0137	0.8806
Public consume	0.9882	0.0234	0.8793
Investments	0.9852	0.0294	0.8892
Overall			0.8876
Eigenvalue	14.4023		
Variance	0.9602		

Source: Federal Office of Statistics; Historical statistics of Switzerland online – own calculation

period-specific factor scores is shown in Fig. 10.1 (right side) from 1946 to 2015. The trend of modernity levels is monotonic and almost linear. The level of modernity at the time of graduation is an indicator of the second cohort effect, while the changing modernization levels in the period between graduation and entering the first job reflects the second period effect.

Statistical Procedure

The time dependent process of entering the labor market is modeled using survival (or event history) models. More specifically, we estimate the propensity of an event (labor market entry) in a given time interval $(t, t + \Delta t]$ using an exponential proportional hazards model of the form $h(t_i) = h_0(t) \exp[\boldsymbol{X\beta}]$, where $\boldsymbol{X}$ is a $n \times p$ matrix of covariates and $\boldsymbol{\beta}$, a $p \times 1$ column vector of parameters. However, in order to consider the time-varying covariates, namely, cohort and period effects in terms of modernization and unemployment after graduation and prior to labor market entry, we make use of the well-established procedure of episode splitting (Blossfeld et al. 2007). As a result, the process of entering the labor market is modeled as a stochastic and time-varying function of individual resources (micro level) and as the change of the modernization process and labor market conditions of business cycles (macro level).

Results

Before presenting the results of the multivariate analyses, we briefly discuss the temporal patterns of educational attainment and labor market entry against the background of the educational expansion in Switzerland. In line with previous research (R. Becker and Zangger 2013; Zangger and Becker 2016), the respondents demonstrate a gradual increase in the level of qualification across birth cohorts in the twentieth century–especially women. With regard to the purpose of this study, Fig. 10.2 depicts the education of the respondents before their entry into the labor market. By comparing this figure to the well documented higher qualification across birth cohorts, it is apparent that successive birth cohorts differ less in terms of their education when entering the labor market than what would be expected from the general trend of an increasing higher qualification as a result of the educational expansion in Switzerland (Becker and Zangger 2013; Zangger and Becker 2016). This suggests an early labor market entry for younger cohorts since they rarely postpone their entry until they complete their highest education. While this pattern might be the result of different processes (e.g., high costs of continuing education

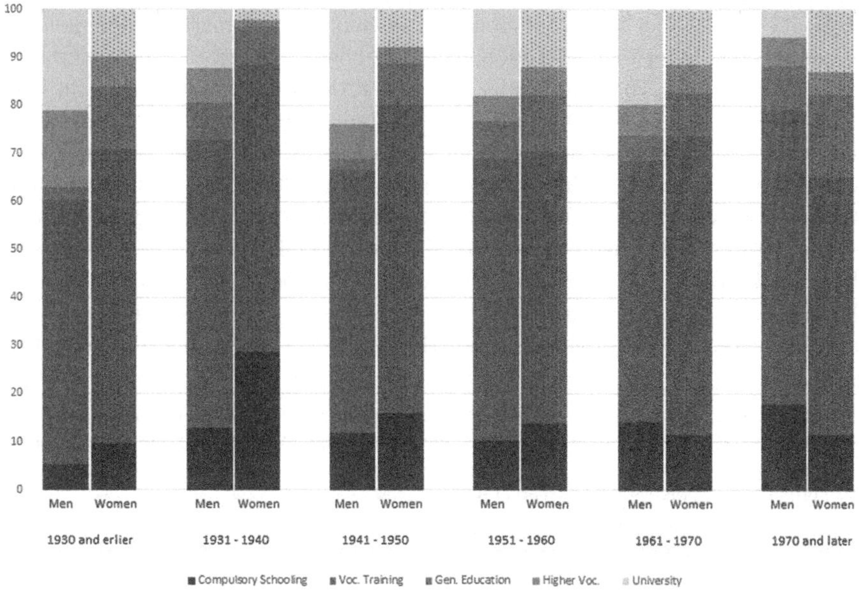

Fig. 10.2 Education prior to labor market entry by birth cohort and sex

makes it necessary to work alongside), it suggests that we need to introduce a control for further education in the multivariate analyses.

Turning to the multivariate results, we focus on three different outcomes: (1) The propensity of entering the labor market (as opposed to being unemployed/ not being part of the labor market), (2) the likelihood of being in the highest, and (3) the likelihood of being in the lowest quartile. Regarding the individual characteristics of interest–education of the individual before entering the labor market and that of the main income earner at the age of 15 years–the expected results were obtained, which is a higher probability of entering the labor market and being in the highest quartile of the status distribution with higher levels of educational achievement.[1] Besides this, there is also evidence of the impact of one's social background, especially with respect to the propensity of entering the highest and the lowest quartile (increasing likelihood of respondents from a higher social status background entering the highest quartile and a decreasing propensity of the same group entering the lowest quartile).

Focusing on the parameters of main interest, first, we observe that the probability of entering the labor market increases monotonically with the level of modernity at the time of graduation. This is the first cohort effect (first three columns of Table 10.2). Thus, younger cohorts are more likely to enter the labor market. On the other hand, the labor market conditions, in terms of unemployment at that time, do not seem to have an effect. Regarding period effects, the opposite result is indicated: With the increasing level of modernity in the years after an individual's graduation, its likelihood of entering the labor market seems to decrease (second and third column). However, this unexpected effect is most likely a methodological artifact. The biographical data used in this analysis only allow the identification of years with distinct events. About ¾ of all respondents entered the labor market within the first year after completing their education; therefore, cohort and period effects overlap in these observations. This collinearity is revealed by the stunning increase in both effect size and standard error of the cohort effects after controlling the period effects. Furthermore, since modernization increases linearly with time, the negative effect of modernity levels after entering the labor market might reflect longer search duration for those who did not directly enter the labor market.[2] Finally, further education (indicated by the positive effect of the dummy variable "Further education after labor market entry") also seems to increase the likelihood of entering the labor market. However, contrary to the impression from the descriptive analysis above, significant interaction of the cohort measure (level of modernity) with further education

[1]Additional analyses (available on request) further illustrate the dependence of one's own education prior to entering the labor market on the education and, to a lesser extent, the social status of the main income earner at the age of 15 years. This suggests a strong indirect effect of one's social background on respondents' labor market performance.

[2]This interpretation is strengthened by the fact that on controlling for search duration (negative impact), the period effect of the level of modernity completely disappears. For the very same reason we do not include search duration in any of the models. Due to the collinearity of search duration and the aggregated time dependent process of modernization, measured in years, it is therefore not possible to model an independent age effect.

Table 10.2 The dynamic process of entry into the labor market and status attainment

	Labor market entry			Highest quartile			Lowest quartile		
Education prior to entry (*Ref.: Compulsory Schooling*)									
(Some) Vocational education	2.009*** (0.132)	1.775*** (0.120)	1.768*** (0.120)	3.018*** (0.658)	2.942*** (0.660)	2.944*** (0.661)	1.042 (0.108)	0.994 (0.108)	0.983 (0.107)
General education & maturity	1.130 (0.111)	1.098 (0.107)	1.095 (0.107)	4.023*** (0.997)	4.055*** (1.010)	4.067*** (1.012)	0.382*** (0.084)	0.376*** (0.083)	0.371*** (0.082)
Higher vocational education	1.852*** (0.203)	1.676*** (0.185)	1.671*** (0.184)	11.775*** (2.841)	11.521*** (2.836)	11.544*** (2.842)	0.153*** (0.070)	0.146*** (0.067)	0.144*** (0.066)
University (of applied sciences)	1.695*** (0.153)	1.538*** (0.140)	1.516*** (0.139)	14.636*** (3.292)	14.385*** (3.303)	14.306*** (3.287)	0.157*** (0.047)	0.151*** (0.045)	0.144*** (0.043)
Social origin (*Ref.: Compulsory Schooling*)									
(Some) Vocational education	1.186** (0.076)	1.141* (0.073)	1.139* (0.073)	1.454* (0.251)	1.455* (0.251)	1.451* (0.250)	0.773* (0.085)	0.760* (0.084)	0.754* (0.083)
General education & maturity	1.210* (0.116)	1.158 (0.111)	1.158 (0.111)	1.478 (0.322)	1.467 (0.320)	1.465 (0.320)	0.696 (0.137)	0.687 (0.135)	0.681 (0.134)
Higher vocational education	1.146 (0.092)	1.113 (0.090)	1.110 (0.089)	1.821** (0.343)	1.827** (0.345)	1.821** (0.344)	0.580*** (0.095)	0.572*** (0.094)	0.568*** (0.093)
University (of applied sciences)	0.974 (0.095)	0.965 (0.094)	0.967 (0.095)	1.487* (0.292)	1.497* (0.294)	1.495* (0.293)	0.367*** (0.099)	0.364*** (0.100)	0.371*** (0.102)

(continued)

Table 10.2 (contined)

	Labor market entry			Highest quartile			Lowest quartile		
Further education after labor market entry	1.254*** (0.058)	1.215*** (0.057)	1.167** (0.059)	1.021 (0.100)	1.012 (0.099)	1.017 (0.100)	0.995 (0.102)	1.268* (0.119)	1.240* (0.118)
Cohort effects									
Modernization	1.098* (0.050)	6.337*** (2.099)	6.521*** (2.163)	0.922 (0.086)	1.037 (0.673)	1.053 (0.684)	1.494*** (0.141)	2.904* (1.445)	3.179* (1.591)
Unemployment	0.997 (0.024)	1.067 (0.063)	1.061 (0.062)	1.108* (0.048)	1.263* (0.132)	1.256* (0.132)	0.937 (0.049)	0.928 (0.113)	0.917 (0.112)
Period effects									
Modernization		0.177*** (0.058)	0.180*** (0.059)		0.916 (0.585)	0.932 (0.596)		0.512 (0.253)	0.541 (0.269)
Unemployment		0.919 (0.053)	0.925 (0.053)		0.866 (0.089)	0.871 (0.089)		1.009 (0.118)	1.023 (0.120)
Cohort (modernization) * further education			0.856* (0.060)			0.879 (0.132)			0.673** (0.094)
Number of sub-episodes	3834	3834	3834	3582	3582	3582	3582	3582	3582
Number of events	2247	2247	2247	564	564	564	536	536	536
Log-likelihood	−2705.25	−2685.64	−2683.19	−1180.89	−1179.75	−1179.38	−1264.54	−1263.51	−1259.51

N: 2344; Exponentiated coefficients; additionally controlled for gender and citizenship; standard errors in parentheses; * $p < 0.05$, ** $p < 0.01$, *** $p < 0.001$

suggests a decreasing likelihood of entering the labor market for younger cohorts in cases where they have pursued further education in later stages in their lives. Including additional higher order terms (especially a three-way interaction of the cohort measure with education prior entry and further education) shows an increasing likelihood of being employed for higher educated graduates who are pursuing further education across time (not reported). Thus, the result in Fig. 10.2 is confirmed: Younger cohorts, who subsequently attain higher education, enter into the labor market earlier than older cohorts do.

While the evidence presented so far is in line with the hypotheses in the theoretical section, the results with regard to entering the highest quartile are puzzling. There is no evidence to support the linear cohort effect in terms of modernization. However, there is a higher likelihood of entering the most favorable labor market positions with an increasing unemployment rate in the year of completing education: With a one percent increase in the unemployment rate, the likelihood of entering the highest quartile increases by about 25% (5th and 6th column in Table 10.2). However, a closer examination of this effect suggests that it is caused by the group of people who graduated between 1992 and 2000. This is by no means surprising since Fig. 10.1 suggests low variation in the unemployment rate in the reference period–with an exception of the 1990s.[3] Thus, it is disputable whether this result reflects the effect of the higher unemployment rate in this period or the (dichotomous) difference between younger and older cohorts, which would be in line with the hypotheses. However, based on the data, we cannot exclude either of the explanations.

Finally, we focus on the third outcome under study, the risk of entering the lowest quartile in the status distribution. Similar trends are observed as reported earlier in the case of entering the labor market. The positive and significant cohort effect of modernization, which are again inflated once controlling for subsequent period effect due to the mentioned collinearity, suggests an increasing hazard of entering the lowest quartile for younger cohorts. Importantly, further examination of the negative cohort-further education-interaction does not provide any evidence in line with the descriptive evidence presented in Fig. 10.2 when including higher order terms. However, the increasing risks for younger cohorts need explanation. The analysis only focuses on those entering paid employment; therefore, the increasing risk of entering the lowest quartile might barely reflect the increase in number of jobs in this segment. This interpretation is supported by the data where we find–although rather weak–evidence for an increasing share of the lowest quartile segment across birth cohorts (Table available on request from the authors). However, the absence of any significant interaction effect (not reported) of the cohort measure and respondents' education prior to labor market entry rejects a polarization hypothesis: Thus, in our analysis we find no evidence for an increasing risk over time of entering the lowest quartile for a particular group (e.g., the lower educated).

[3] We remind the reader that as the data was collected in 2002; therefore, the high increase in the unemployment rate post 2002 does not enter the analysis.

Conclusion

This study aimed to analyze the impact of the level of modernity and the labor market conditions on the school-to-work transition in Switzerland for the historical period from 1946 to 2002. Based on our knowledge, this is the first analysis on the time dependency of the labor market entry across cohorts in Switzerland. In addition, we addressed the direct effects of social background and educational qualification across cohorts on their entry into professional life and whether the institutional arrangement of the education system and its linkage to the labor markets will provide "safety roads" to employment. In order to address these questions, we used data from the life calendar collected in 2002 as part of the Swiss Household Panel, along with administrative data to control for changing labor market conditions (unemployment rate) and constructed a scaling variable that represents the level of modernity. An event-history analysis was conducted on the school-to-work transition of a sample of 2344 individuals born between 1912 and 1986. The aim was to determine the effect of the level of modernity and labor market conditions for different cohorts on: (a) the propensity to enter the labor market, (b) the likelihood to be in the highest quartile, and (c) the probability of being in the lowest quartile of the status distribution in the first job.

While a strong and consistent link has been observed between educational qualifications and labor market outcomes, there was also considerable evidence for a continuous and independent effect of respondents' social background, especially with respect to entering the highest or lowest quartile of the status distribution. Furthermore, we find support for the suggested positive linear influence of the level of modernity at the time of graduation on the likelihood of entering the labor market (cohort effect). However, the corresponding cohort effect of the unemployment level is not statistically significant in most of the models. This could be due to the minor variation in the covered period. On the other hand, the period effects in terms of subsequent levels of modernity between graduation and entrance into employment are of the opposite sign. Instead of describing a true period effect, this result most likely reflects the negative impact of a longer search duration as the level of modernity is a (almost strictly) positive linear function of the underlying time axis. Finally, there is little evidence to support the interaction effects between respondents' prior education and the cohort measures on any of the outcomes under study. Thus, in line with findings of Oesch (2013), there is no evidence for a polarization or displacement at the time of transition into the first job within the covered time window. Although the empirical results emphasize the effects of persistent social inequality on entering the highest or lowest quartile of the status distribution across cohorts, the institutional arrangement of the education system and its linkage to the labor markets seems to protect the majority from precarious employment conditions. However, these concluding remarks are restricted to the school-to-work transition. Factors in the professional careers of people such as further occupational mobility and access to further education and prestigious jobs have not been considered in this analysis. Thus, the afore mentioned outcomes need to be considered in order to draw conclusions related to the long-term consequences of period and cohort effects on people's life chances.

Finally, there are several concerns regarding the validity of our results. First, the data on events is available in years only; therefore, an accurate identification of the period and age effects is not possible. Furthermore, the sample size considerations impede the identification of the hazards of unemployment across time. These considerations are particularly problematic in the present case of the labor market entry since three-quarters of all cases entered the labor market within the first year after graduation.

Appendix

Variable	Observations	Mean	SD	Min.	Max.
First job (Dependent variable)					
Unemployed/Not working	2344	0.041	0.120	0	1
First (lowest) quartile	2344	0.229	0.420	0	1
Second quartile	2344	0.228	0.420	0	1
Third quartile	2344	0.262	0.440	0	1
Fourth (highest) quartile	2344	0.241	0.428	0	1
Gender	2344	1.529	0.499	1	2
Year of birth	2344	1955.516	12.987	1912	1986
Education prior to labor market entry					
Compulsory schooling	2344	0.139	0.346	0	1
(Some) Vocational education	2344	0.587	0.493	0	1
General education	2344	0.084	0.278	0	1
Higher vocational education	2344	0.056	0.230	0	1
University (of appl. Sciences)	2344	0.134	0.341	0	1
Citizenship					
Swiss	2344	0.826	0.379	0	1
Northern & Western Europe	2344	0.015	0.121	0	1
South & Southwestern Europe	2344	0.023	0.149	0	1
Central & (South) Eastern Europe	2344	0.026	0.161	0	1
Rest of the world	2344	0.110	0.313	0	1
Social origin (Education)					
Compulsory schooling	2344	0.159	0.365	0	1
(Some) Vocational education	2344	0.527	0.499	0	1
General education	2344	0.080	0.271	0	1
Higher vocational education	2344	0.143	0.350	0	1
University (of appl. Sciences)	2344	0.091	0.288	0	1
Education after entering labor market	2344	0.348	0.476	0	1
Modernization (cohort effect)	3834	−0.354	0.663	−1.373	1.071
Labor market (cohort effect)	3834	0.680	1.142	0	5.2
Modernization (period effect)	3834	−0.301	0.661	−1.373	1.071
Labor market (period effect)	3834	0.758	1.245	0	5.2

References

Allmendinger, J. (1989). Educational systems and labor market outcomes. *European Sociological Review, 5*(3), 231–250.

Becker, G. S. (1964). *Human capital. A theoretical and empirical analysis with special reference to education*. New York: Columbia University Press.

Becker, R., & Zangger, C. (2013). Die Bildungsexpansion in der Schweiz und ihre Folgen. Eine empirische Analyse des Wandels der Bildungsbeteiligung und Bildungsungleichheiten mit den Daten der Schweizer Volkszählungen 1970, 1980, 1990 und 2000. *Kölner Zeitschrift für Soziologie und Sozialpsychologie, 65*(3), 423–449.

Blau, P. M., & Duncan, O. D. (1967). *The American occupational structure*. New York: Wiley.

Blossfeld, H.-P. (1985). Berufseintritt und Berufsverlauf: Eine Kohortenananlyse über die Bedeutung des ersten Berufes in der Erwerbsbiographie. *Mitteilungen aus der Arbeitsmarkt- und Berufsforschung, 18*(2), 177–197.

Blossfeld, H.-P. (1987). Entry into the labor market and occupational career in the Federal Republic: A comparison with American studies. *International Journal of Sociology, 17*(1/2), 86–115.

Blossfeld, H.-P., Golsch, K., & Rohwer, G. (2007). *Event history analysis with Stata*. New York: Lawrence Erlbaum.

Buchmann, M., & Sacchi, S. (1998). The transition from school to work in Switzerland: Do characteristics of the educational system and class barriers matter? In Y. Shavit & W. Müller (Eds.), *From school to work: A comparative study of educational qualifications and occupational destinations* (pp. 407–442). Oxford: Oxford University Press.

Buchs, H., Müller, B., & Buchmann, M. (2015). Qualifikationsnachfrage und Arbeitsmarkteintritt in der Schweiz. *Kölner Zeitschrift für Soziologie und Sozialpsychologie, 67*(4), 709–736. https://doi.org/10.1007/s11577-015-0342-5.

de Lange, M., Gesthuizen, M., & Wolbers, M. H. J. (2013). Youth labour market integration across Europe. *European Societies, 16*(2), 194–212. https://doi.org/10.1080/14616696.2013.821621.

DiPrete, T. A., Goux, D., Maurin, E., & Tåblin, M. (2001). Institutional determinants of employment chances. The structure of unemployment in France and Sweden. *European Sociological Review, 17*(3), 233–254. https://doi.org/10.1093/esr/17.3.233.

Franzen, A., & Hangartner, D. (2005). Soziale Netzwerke und beruflicher Erfolg: Eine Analyse des Arbeitsmarkteintritts von Hochschulabsolventen. *Kölner Zeitschrift für Soziologie und Sozialpsychologie, 57*, 443–465.

Gangl, M. (2002). Changing labour markets and early career outcomes. Labour market entry in europe over the past decade. *Work, Employment & Society, 16*(1), 67–90. https://doi.org/10.1177/09500170222119254.

Gebel, M. (2009). Fixed-term contracts at labour market entry in West Germany: Implications for job search and first job quality. *European Sociological Review, 25*(6), 661–675. https://doi.org/10.1093/esr/jcp005.

Harrington, D. (2009). *Confirmatory factor analysis*. Oxford: Oxford University Press.

Imdorf, C., & Hupka-Brunner, S. (2015). Gender differences at labor market entry in Switzerland. In *Gender, education and employment. An international comparison of school-to-work transitions* (pp. 267–286). Cheltenham: Edward Elgar Publishing, Inc.

Jann, B., & Combet, B. (2012). Zur Entwicklung der intergenerationalen Mobilität in der Schweiz. *Swiss Journal of Sociology, 38*(2), 177–199.

Kerckhoff, A. C. (1995). Institutional arrangements and stratification processes in industrial societies. *Annual Review of Sociology, 21*, 323–347.

Kolenikov, S. (2009). Confirmatory factor analysis using confa. *Stata Journal, 9*(3), 329–373.

Kramarz, F., & Skans, O. N. (2014). When strong ties are strong: Networks and youth labour market entry. *The Review of Economic Studies*. https://doi.org/10.1093/restud/rdt049.

Lindbeck, A., Snower, D., & Assar Lindbeck, D. S. (1988). *The insider-outsider theory of employment and unemployment*. Cambridge, MA: Cambridge University Press.

Müller, W., & Kogan, I. (2010). Education. In S. Immerfall & G. Therborn (Eds.), *Handbook of european societies. Social transformations in the 21st century* (pp. 217–289). New York: Springer.

OECD. (2015). Switzerland. In *Education at a glance 2015: OECD indicators*. Paris: OECD Publishing.

Oesch, D. (2013). *Occupational change in Europe. How technology and education transform the job structure*. Oxford: Oxford University Press.

Oesch, D., & Rodríguez Menés, J. (2010). Upgrading or polarization? Occupational change in Britain, Germany, Spain and Switzerland, 1990–2008. *Socio-Economic Review, 9*(3), 503–531. https://doi.org/10.1093/ser/mwq029.

Raaum, O., & Røed, K. (2006). Do business cycle conditions at the time of labor market entry affect future employment prospects? *The Review of Economics and Statistics, 88*(2), 193–210.

Shavit, Y., & Müller, W. (Eds.). (1998). *From school to work. A comparative study of educational qualifications and occupational destinations*. Oxford: Clarendon Press.

Shavit, Y., & Müller, W. (2000). Vocational secondary education, tracking, and social stratification. In M. T. Hallinan (Ed.), *Handbook of the sociology of education* (pp. 437–452). Boston: Springer US.

Sørensen, A. B. (1986). Theory and methodology in social stratification. In U. Himmelstrand (Ed.), *The sociology of structure and action* (pp. 69–95). London: Sage.

Thurow, L. C. (1975). *Generating inequality: mechanisms of distribution in the U.S. economy*. New York: Basic Books.

Wolbers, M. H. J. (2007). Patterns of labour market entry: A comparative perspective on school-to-work transitions in 11 European countries. *Acta Sociologica, 50*(3), 189–210. https://doi.org/10.1177/0001699307080924.

Zangger, C., & Becker, R. (2016). Die Bildungsexpansion in der Schweiz – eine Reanalyse unter besonderer Berücksichtigung geschlechtsspezifischer Bildungschancen. *Schweizerische Zeitschrift für Soziologie, 42*(3), 429–441.

Chapter 11
Wealth, Savings and Children Among Swiss, German and Australian Families

Laura Ravazzini and Ursina Kuhn

Introduction

The accumulation of wealth is an important aspect when evaluating the economic situation of families. For many years, the lack of wealth information in survey data in general, particularly longitudinal data, has restrained the research on this topic. Recent demographic changes such as delays in fertility and population ageing, rising female labour force participation and insecure future retirement pensions make the relationship between children and wealth accumulation a particularly relevant topic.

The overall effect of children on net worth is ambiguous because children may influence parents' wealth accumulation through different paths. On the one hand, parents might save more for their financial protection, in anticipation of future income losses, or out of a bequest motive. On the other hand, children might bring higher expenses and lower income (e.g., through reduced labour force participation) and, therefore, reduce the capacity to save. To the best of our knowledge, the link between children and wealth has never been specifically investigated in a comparative perspective. A comparative study using panel data will therefore provide useful insights about the ability of families to save in different settings.

In this contribution, we analyse data from the Swiss Household Panel (SHP), the German Socio-Economic Panel (SOEP) and the Australian Household, Income and Labour Dynamics (HILDA) Survey. We chose these databases because of their panel structure. Germany has been selected as another continental European

L. Ravazzini (✉)
University of Neuchâtel, Neuchâtel, Switzerland & FORS, Lausanne, Switzerland
e-mail: laura.ravazzini@fors.unil.ch

U. Kuhn
FORS-Swiss Centre of Expertise in the Social Sciences, Lausanne, Switzerland
e-mail: ursina.kuhn@fors.unil.ch

R. Tillmann et al. (eds.), *Social Dynamics in Swiss Society*, Life Course Research and Social Policies 9, https://doi.org/10.1007/978-3-319-89557-4_11

country, and both Germany and Australia act as references because of previous literature on the link between children and wealth in these countries.

Our empirical strategy has the following three aims: first, we establish the effect of children on net worth and saving behaviour. Second, we disentangle the effects of income changes from consumption changes by controlling for earned income and labour supply. Third, we use a comparative perspective to indicate whether results are general or country specific.

This chapter is organised as follows. We first provide a brief literature review on the theoretical and the empirical relationships between children and wealth. We then continue with the description of the data, the sample and the methodology. The results are presented separately for short-term effects and long-term effects. The conclusion summarises our findings and points to possible further research.

The Role of Children in Wealth Accumulation

There are different potential effects of children on wealth. Among the motives for wealth accumulation (Keynes 1936; Browning and Lusardi 1996), several might be reinforced through the presence of children. First, parents might save more to protect themselves and their children from financial risks. Second, future parents might save more before the arrival of a child in anticipation of future income losses (e.g., due to reduced labour force participation) or higher expenses. Third, the accumulation of capital necessary to buy houses, cars or other durable goods and finally the bequest motive might be more important for fathers and mothers than for childless individuals.

The increased incentives for wealth accumulation are paired with income losses and higher expenses for children (e.g., for food, accommodation, child-care, education or insurances) (Bradbury 2014). This aspect is also considered in the life-cycle model of Modigliani and Brumberg (1954), which assumes that people choose to maintain stable lifestyles. In its simplest form, people are expected to save during their mature active life and to dissave when young and during retirement. An addition to this theory highlights that the presence of children reduces current savings and the future level of accumulated net worth (Modigliani 1986).[1] Dockery and Bawa (2015) question the expenditure part of this framework and claim that expenditures for children might substitute other expenditures. For example, instead of long distance travels to exotic destinations or visits to fancy restaurants, parents engage in inexpensive activities such as walks in the park, nights at home or visits to close relatives. In addition to this, home production might also increase if activities

[1] "The amount of net worth accumulated up to any given age in relation to life resources is a decreasing function of the number of children and that saving tends to fall with the number of children present in the household and to rise with the number of children no longer present" (Modigliani 1986, pp. 160).

such as cooking, gardening and do-it-yourself become more frequent. Lower expenses in other areas might therefore compensate the additional expenses resulting from having children. Furthermore, the impact of children on wealth accumulation also depends on institutional characteristics, such as child allowances, availability and costs of child-care, the tax system, special programmes targeting children and other programmes of this type (Grinstein-Weiss et al. 2006).

A final point to mention is the potential endogeneity of the relationship between fertility and wealth. Debt and financial instability have been shown to delay marriage (Addo 2014) and are therefore likely to delay or cancel the decision to have children. We know from Dockery and Bawa (2015) that fertility in Australia is inversely related to income, but we do not know its relationship with wealth.

Previous Findings on the Effect of Children on Wealth and Savings

The few studies on the subject focused mainly on Anglo-Saxon countries and show a weak negative effect of children on wealth. Scholz and Seshadri (2009) found that each additional child reduces the average net wealth of US-American families by $6384. In Australia, a recent study estimated that each dependent child reduces couples' wealth by approximately $2000 per year (Dockery and Bawa 2015). Contrary to this, the presence of children benefits savings in the long-run. A simulation study by Love (2010) using the Panel Study of Income Dynamics in the USA indicates that households with children accumulate substantially less wealth during the working years, but, probably out of a bequest motive, save more during retirement and end with more savings than households that have never had children. The effects might be different for some family types, particularly for single parents (Austen et al. 2014). Controlling for other factors, the results from Switzerland indicate that single mothers have 17,890 CHF less in non-housing wealth than childless single women (Ravazzini and Chesters 2018). This difference is large, but single mothers are not representative of the overall population and constitute a particularly disadvantaged and vulnerable group (Grinstein-Weiss et al. 2008). In Germany, having children under five years old was found to have a negative, but insignificant, impact on net worth (Sierminska et al. 2010). A recent study found that parenthood is associated with lower wealth accumulation for women but not for men. This effect can be explained by discontinuous employment experiences (Lersch et al. 2017). Additionally, for Germany, Rottke and Klos (2016) found that overall household consumption drops after a child moves out of the household, but at the same time, adult-equivalent consumption significantly increases. After all children are gone, parents are found to upgrade their personal lifestyle to a level approximately equal to childless peers and save only a small proportion of their resources. Therefore, the saving behaviour in Germany seems quite different from that in America, where savings increase when children leave the households.

Data and Sample

Our analysis is based on three Household Panels of the Cross National Equivalent File (CNEF), namely, the Swiss Household Panel (SHP), the German Socio-Economic Panel (SOEP) and the Household, Income and Labour Dynamics Survey in Australia (HILDA). The main advantage of these databases is that they provide a longitudinal perspective following the same households over time. A disadvantage for an analysis on wealth with survey data is that people at the top – and in some cases at the bottom – of the distribution are underrepresented. To at least partially correct for this problem, the SOEP oversamples high-income households by including a high-income sample since 2002. In the HILDA, wealth variables are top-coded using an average value for all the cases that exceed a given threshold. We decide not to top-code wealth in the SHP and in the SOEP because this would present a loss of information.

There are some important differences between surveys regarding the main variables of interest. The HILDA and the SHP collect wealth at the household level, whereas household wealth in the SOEP is aggregated from information at the individual level. In contrast to the HILDA and the SOEP, which contain detailed information on different assets,[2] the SHP provides only basic information about wealth and does not include negative wealth. More specifically, the SHP distinguishes only between family home wealth and other wealth. In terms of frequency of data collection, the Australian panel offers wealth information for four time points (2002, 2006, 2010 and 2014) and the German panel for three (2002, 2007 and 2012). Currently, a longitudinal analysis on wealth is not possible with the SHP because information about wealth has been collected only in 2012. More information about the quality of the wealth variables in the Swiss panel can be found in Kuhn and Crettaz (2015).

Our analytic sample consists of single adult and couple households with and without children. Other household types have been excluded because, with the exception of the SOEP, we do not know how income and wealth are pooled inside the household.

In addition to wealth variables, the three panel surveys collect information on saving behaviour. The SHP contains a yearly categorical variable at the household level (household can save, household spends what it earns, households eats into wealth, household goes into debt). A similar variable is present in the HILDA in 9 waves of 14, but the question is asked at the individual level. We therefore consider the information given by the main earner of each couple but also comment on findings including the partner's saving behaviours. In two waves, the HILDA additionally provides the reasons why people save. Among these reasons,[3] there are two

[2]The HILDA is the only panel that includes complete information about pension savings from employer's pension plans.

[3]People can choose between 16 well-defined reasons plus one undefined reason. Multiple answers are allowed.

specific answers on descendants (*Education for children or grandchildren, To help children or other relatives*) and three possible answers about home-related expenditures (*Pay off mortgage on home, To buy a home (other than present one), Home improvements / extensions / repairs*), which might still be related to children's needs. The SOEP contains a yearly variable with the amount that households can save for wealth creation and for precautionary savings.

Methodology

Our empirical analysis focuses on the following two dependent variables: the probability to save and net worth. For the first model, we compare households that are saving with those that are not saving. Because a binary variable has been observed in (almost) all panel waves, we can exploit the variance within households over time with a fixed effects (FE) regression. The main advantage of this method is that it excludes any unobserved heterogeneity bias. Even though we have a dichotomous dependent variable, we estimate a linear probability model.[4] As main independent variables, we include the number of dependent children living in the household by age groups (0–4 years, 5–9 years, 10–14 years or 15–24 years). Children older than 15 years are considered as dependent if they are in education and do not work full-time. In addition, we include a binary variable for planning/wanting a child to test whether anticipating a child increases motivation for saving. This variable has not been collected in the German SOEP, however. To test the mediating effect of income on savings, we include household income (yearly earnings adjusted to household size)[5] and working hours (mean working hours for couples). We control for the following variables that have been revealed to be important in previous studies (Finke and Pierce 2006; Pericoli and Ventura 2011; Vespa and Painter II 2011): age and its squared term (of the household head), civil status, years of cohabitation of the couples and home ownership. Despite its possible endogeneity, we also include an indicator about home ownership because repayment of a mortgage might not be considered as savings and because home ownership might increase the money available for non-housing consumption.

[4] For the following reasons, logistic FE models (conditional logistic models) are not a good option for our research design: First, logistic FE models exclude households with a stable saving behaviour (those that always save or never save). Second, it is not possible to compute effect sizes in terms of marginal effects or predicted probabilities. Third, coefficients cannot be compared across models. This last point is crucial for our analysis because we want to compare different model specifications and countries. Nevertheless, we have also estimated FE logistic models as a sensitivity analysis and find consistent conclusions.

[5] Following the modified OECD equivalence scale, we divide the income of a couple's household by 1.5. We do not correct for the number of children, as this effect should be captured by our specific variables about the number of children. Income has been corrected for inflation using the consumer price indexes.

The main advantage of the FE models is that they capture the causal effect of dependent children on the probability to save. As these models have two important limitations, we complement the analysis with an OLS regression on net worth. First, FE models can only analyse changes that occur within the duration of the panel (e.g., maximal until children are 25 in the SOEP). Accordingly, FE models measure the impact of having dependent children in the household compared to the situation of no dependent children in the household. Second, the dependent variable indicates the presence of savings but not the amount saved (this information is available only for Germany). The OLS regression can capture long-term effects of children (once children left the household) on wealth accumulation and will reveal the size of the effect. Net worth is defined as the sum of all assets minus the level of accumulated debts. For couples, we split the amount of household wealth in half. As each country is analysed separately, we use national currencies and adjust for inflation. As a method of analysis, we use (pooled) linear regressions.[6] To address individuals without wealth or debts and to limit the influence of extremely high values, we apply an inverse hyperbolic sine transformation (hereafter IHS) on total net worth (see Friedline et al. 2015 for details). Because we are interested in the effect of children on wealth accumulation in the long term, we need to consider children irrespective of their age and of whether they live in the household. Following Dockery and Bawa (2015), we compute a variable that we call child-years. This variable multiplies the number of children by their age with a maximum of 18 years per child. Lacking more precise information, the maximum of 18 is set as the average age for independency. This maximum considers that children pursuing professional training might become independent before and that children enrolled in university might finish their education later. As in the FE model, we estimate a separate model controlling for income and labour supply. Income refers here to permanent household income, which we define as the average of all available previous earnings and pensions. In addition to the variables included in the FE model (age, civil status, years of cohabitation and home ownership), we control for variables' stable characteristics. The educational level (three levels with the highest educational level of the couple) is included as a proxy for wiser choices in saving and investing behaviours. Living in a city centre is included because it might imply not only higher living costs but also higher property values. We also take into account the number of siblings (in Switzerland the presence of siblings) and a measure for parental socioeconomic status to capture possible effects of inheritances on the accumulation of wealth over the life-course. Other control variables are country specific. In Australia, we include a binary variable for the English mother tongue because non-native speakers find difficulties in terms of integration, whereas we identify foreign-born individuals in Switzerland and in Germany. In Switzerland, we include a variable for the linguistic region, and in Germany we distinguish the Western from the Eastern part. For age, nationality, siblings and parental socio-economic status of couple households, we consider the information provided by the main earner.

[6]We cannot exploit the panel character with the SHP, as we currently have only one wave of data on wealth.

When comparing models of different countries and different surveys, we have to pay attention to different sample sizes and differences in the definition of the variables. We commented on these differences whenever necessary.

The Short-Term Effect of Children on Savings

Using FE models, we first address the probability to save. The first model in Table 11.1 (M1 for Switzerland, M3 for Australia and M5 for Germany) shows that households are less likely to save when they have children in the household. A first general finding is that children older than ten years have a weaker effect on saving propensity than younger children. In Switzerland and Germany, pre-school children (between 0 and 4 years) have, with 5.7% and 2.2%, the strongest negative effect on savings, whereas in Australia, children from 5 to 9 years of age reduce the probability to save most strongly (by 1.8 percent). To test whether lower income or higher consumption are responsible for the lower saving propensity, models M2, M4 and M6 in Table 11.1 control for the mediating effects of income and working hours. In Switzerland, the coefficients for children in the household become only slightly weaker (M2 compared to M1), which means that income and labour supply explain only a small part of the negative effect of small children. Rather, high expenses for children, and most likely high childcare costs, are responsible for the lower saving probability.[7] The same holds for 5- to 9-year-old children in Australia. In Germany, the entire negative effect of pre-school children disappears once we control for income and working hours (M6). This means that households with small children can save less because labour and income drops after childbirth.[8] A second general finding is that expenditures reduce saving propensity considerably for children between 15 and 24 years old. After controlling for income and labour supply, older children reduce the probability to save by 3.5% in Switzerland, by 1.2% in Germany and by 1.9% in Australia.[9] This result is in line with previous findings on consumption for children in other countries (Bonke and Browning 2011). As a cautionary note, we must say that we might underestimate the negative effect of children on

[7] According to the OECD Family Database, childcare fees amount to 67.3% of the average wage. This is the highest proportion among 36 OECD countries. For middle-class double earners, this corresponds to 23.6% of their net income.

[8] Results for Australia become slightly weaker when the saving behaviour of the partner, if present, is included. Without mediating effects (M3), the only significant coefficients results are for dependent children 15–24 years old (−0.10*). Once income and labour supply are excluded (M4), two of the three significant coefficients remain, namely, the positive effect of small children (0.011*) and the negative effect of older children (−0.013**). The effect for children between 5 and 14 years old becomes insignificant.

[9] In Germany, it is possible to estimate the amount saved. Children between 15 and 24 lower savings by 21 euro per month. Interestingly, younger dependent children also make parents save less money (between 12 and 14.5 euro per month).

Table 11.1 FE regression on the probability to save

	CH (M1)	CH (M2)	AUS (M3)	AUS (M4)	D (M5)	D (M6)
Children aged 0–4 years	−0.057**	−0.041**	−0.005	0.014*	−0.022**	0.007*
	(−8.43)	*(−6.06)*	*(−1.13)*	*(2.94)*	*(−6.68)*	*(2.03)*
Children aged 5–9 years	−0.049**	−0.039**	−0.018**	−0.009*	−0.005	0.005
	(−8.51)	*(−6.73)*	*(−3.75)*	*(−1.97)*	*(−1.74)*	*(1.76)*
Children aged 10–14 years	−0.038**	−0.031**	−0.011*	−0.007	−0.001	0.002
	(−7.03)	*(−5.69)*	*(−2.51)*	*(−1.63)*	*(−0.50)*	*(0.93)*
Children aged 15–24 years	−0.034**	−0.035**	−0.015**	−0.020**	−0.006**	−0.012**
	(−7.78)	*(−8.15)*	*(−2.85)*	*(−3.68)*	*(−2.91)*	*(−5.94)*
Yearly earnings/pension		0.000**		0.032**		0.002**
		(8.90)		*(5.37)*		*(32.85)*
Weekly working hours		0.004**		0.004**		0.000**
		(17.04)		*(23.30)*		*(37.75)*
Planning to have a child	0.012	0.018	0.048**	0.048**		
	(1.26)	*(1.95)*	*(7.00)*	*(7.11)*		
Age	0.000	−0.001	0.004**	0.005**	−0.001**	0.001**
	(−0.24)	*(−1.49)*	*(7.95)*	*(9.96)*	*(−7.52)*	*(5.25)*
Years of cohabitation	−0.000	−0.000	0.023*	0.020*	0.015**	0.015**
	(−1.81)	*(−2.10)*	*(2.50)*	*(2.25)*	*(3.00)*	*(3.04)*
Single (ref.)						
Married	0.038*	0.036*	−0.012	−0.001	0.100**	0.074**
	(2.16)	*(1.97)*	*(−1.21)*	*(−0.12)*	*(14.21)*	*(10.62)*
Unmarried couple	0.056**	0.069**	0.053**	0.059**	0.105**	0.092**
	(4.53)	*(5.31)*	*(4.79)*	*(5.40)*	*(16.61)*	*(14.65)*
Separated/divorced	−0.026	−0.038	−0.030*	−0.029*	0.046**	0.021*
	(−1.31)	*(−1.87)*	*(−2.38)*	*(−2.35)*	*(5.36)*	*(2.47)*
Widowed	0.044	0.096**	−0.038	−0.027	0.061**	0.042**
	(1.69)	*(3.63)*	*(−2.45)*	*(−1.76)*	*(5.60)*	*(3.84)*
Ownership	0.006	−0.005	−0.005	−0.003	−0.029**	−0.040**
	(0.70)	(−0.59)	*(−0.93)*	*(−0.65)*	*(−7.41)*	*(−10.34)*
Number of observations	63,022	63,022	66,969	66,969	223,465	223,465
Number of households	12,246	12,246	18,202	18,202	28,801	28,801

Sources: SHP 1999–2014, HILDA 2001, 2002, 2003, 2004, 2006, 2008, 2010, 2012, 2014, SOEP 1992–2014

** $p < 0.01$, * $p < 0.05$. Notes: T-stats in parenthesis. Information on the intention to have a child is not available for Germany. Children refer to dependent children

savings because we consider only the effect of children living in the household and neglect the effects on parents who do not live with their children.

The models in Table 11.1 test also whether planning to have a child increases the probability to save. This hypothesis is supported in Australia, where planning to have a child increases the probability to save by 4.9%. An additional analysis on Australians who save in 2002 and in 2006 (the only waves with information about the reasons for saving) shows that 13% of them declare to save for their children and 28% for home-related expenditures. In Switzerland, planning to have a child has no significant impact on the saving propensity. The coefficient is close to statistical significance, but the effect, even when significant, would be very small.

More generally, the FE analysis on saving behaviour confirms the life-cycle hypothesis. Children slow wealth accumulation because of both lower income and higher expenditures. We are confident that we measured a causal effect because these models analysed only the variation within households over time and not the variation between different household types.[10]

The Long-Term Effect of Children on Net Worth

So far, the analysis was based on children living in the household and was not aimed at establishing the long-term effects that children have on wealth. We now look at net worth to estimate the magnitude of the coefficients in real economic terms and use the variable child-years to capture long-term effects.

Figure 11.1 gives an overview of wealth accumulation over the life course in the three countries and shows average net worth by the age of the household head. Note that absolute wealth levels cannot be compared directly because wealth is measured in national currency. In Australia, the accumulation of wealth is almost linear before 65 years of age, and dissaving starts after retirement.[11] In Germany, dissaving after retirement is much less pronounced. The analysis with Swiss data shows no dissaving directly after retirement, but only later in life. This finding is in line with Moser (2006), who analysed wealth levels by age groups using tax records from the canton of Zurich.

Because this descriptive figure does not distinguish the accumulation of wealth for parents and households without children, we now move to the results of the regression models shown in Table 11.2. In all countries, parents are less wealthy than childless individuals, although the effect is weak.[12] In Switzerland, one child-year reduces net worth by 377 CHF, which amounts to 6714 CHF per child in the long term. This estimation increases slightly (374 per child year) when permanent income and years in paid work are included. Higher expenditures rather than durable income losses explain therefore why parents in Switzerland have lower wealth than childless households. In Australia, children have a slightly stronger negative

[10] Logistic FE models give very similar results in terms of the significance and the direction of the effect.

[11] Including superannuation (2nd and 3rd pillar for retirees and for the active population) to the Australian wealth measure does not change the Australian curve.

[12] In Australia and in Germany, the effects remain significant but become smaller (−0.05 in Germany (M5 and M6) and – 0.10 (M3) and – 0.09 (M4) in Australia) if we apply a bottom-code for negative net worth, and we recode negative values to zero as in Switzerland. This means that the wealth loss associated to children in Switzerland might be underestimated because of censoring of negative values of net worth.

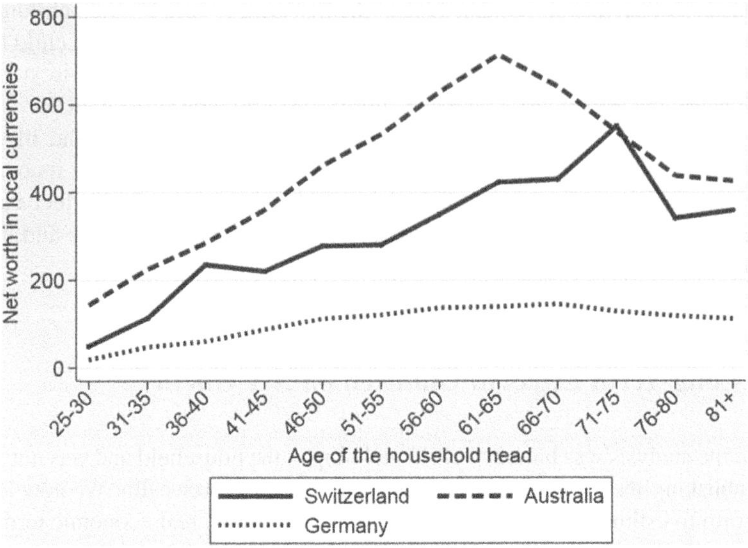

Fig. 11.1 Wealth over the life-cycle in Australia, Germany and Switzerland (Sources: SHP 2012, HILDA 2006, 2010, 2014, SOEP 2002, 2007, 2012. Note: Local currencies represent 2011 AUS$000 s, 2012 CHF000s and 2011 EUR000s. Wealth of couple households has been divided by 2. Weighted data)

impact on net worth (859 AU$ per child-year, 15,462 AU$ for children up to 18 years old). Lost years in paid employment or permanent income losses explain a small part of this effect (118 AU$ per child-year explain 14% of the total negative impact of children on net worth). In Germany, children have an almost negligible impact on the total amount of accumulated wealth (34 EUR per child-year and 619 EUR for children up to 18 years old). This effect is not affected by permanent income or years in paid work. These differences between countries might be generated by institutional contexts or by saving behaviours.

We briefly comment on an additional test that we do not report in tables because of limits of space. When we constrain the analysis of Table 11.2 to retirees, wealth differences between parents and childless households disappear in Switzerland and decrease in Germany and in Australia (−0.005**). A possible explanation for this interesting finding would be that individuals in retirement spend less than childless individuals probably out of a bequest motive.

We also tested whether wealthier individuals are more likely to have children. In Switzerland and in Australia, neither home-ownership nor wealth is significant in simple fertility models. This leads us to conclude that a selection bias is very unlikely in these two countries. In Germany, however, richer parents seem to have more children. This endogeneity constitutes a bias that might underestimate the importance of children on wealth in the OLS regression, but not in the FE model, which takes into account only the variation within households over time.

Table 11.2 OLS regression with IHS transformation on net worth

	CH	CH	AUS	AUS	D	D
	(M1)	(M2)	(M3)	(M4)	(M5)	(M6)
Total child-years	−0.012**	−0.013**	−0.013**	−0.011**	−0.007**	−0.007**
	(−3.47)	*(−3.72)*	*(−11.77)*	*(−10.66)*	*(−4.92)*	*(−4.87)*
Permanent income		0.000**		0.018**		0.027**
		(5.49)		*(23.63)*		*(8.11)*
Years in paid work		0.000		0.026**		0.033**
		(0.05)		*(10.34)*		*(7.42)*
Owner	4.507**	4.418**	3.919**	3.639**	5.786**	5.550**
	(33.80)	*(33.99)*	*(57.04)*	*(55.29)*	*(68.06)*	*(64.22)*
Age	0.043	0.042	0.241**	0.172**	0.149**	0.014
	(1.63)	*(1.45)*	*(22.06)*	*(14.06)*	*(9.27)*	*(0.75)*
Age squared	−0.000	−0.000	−0.002**	−0.001**	−0.001**	0.000
	(0.39)	*(−0.22)*	*(−17.97)*	*(−10.92)*	*(−6.48)*	*(1.57)*
Single (ref.)						
Married couple	−0.681**	−0.990**	0.758**	0.622**	0.316*	0.243
	(−3.01)	*(−4.26)*	*(12.50)*	*(6.62)*	*(2.21)*	*(1.70)*
Unmarried couple	−0.134	−0.405*	0.541**	0.520**	0.707**	0.663**
	(0.58)	*(−1.71)*	*(7.15)*	*(3.70)*	*(3.98)*	*(3.74)*
Separated/divorced	−1.056**	−1.025**	0.493**	0.447**	−1.511**	−1.476**
	(−4.55)	*(−4.43)*	*(4.25)*	*(4.01)*	*(−7.91)*	*(−7.87)*
Widowed	0.221	0.206	0.850**	0.927**	0.149	0.233**
	(0.76)	*(0.71)*	*(5.15)*	*(7.69)*	*(0.38)*	*(1.37)*
Years of cohabitation	0.015	0.016	−0.315	−0.377*	0.010*	0.013**
	(1.88)	*(1.93)*	*(−1.84)*	*(−2.15)*	*(2.36)*	*(3.31)*
Lower secondary (ref.)						
Upper secondary	1.209**	1.182**	0.527**	0.408**	1.626**	1.447**
	(5.98)	*(5.86)*	*(8.17)*	*(6.37)*	*(11.98)*	*(10.79)*
Tertiary	2.040**	1.905**	0.499**	0.056	3.014**	2.510**
	(9.18)	*(8.55)*	*(6.30)*	*(0.68)*	*(20.41)*	*(16.41)*
Living in an urban centre	−0.067	−0.077	0.071	−0.094	0.205*	0.112
	(−0.51)	*(−0.59)*	*(1.34)*	*(−1.78)*	*(2.46)*	*(1.34)*
(Number of) siblings	−0.092	−0.022	0.024	0.003	−0.278**	−0.155
	(−0.60)	*(−0.14)*	*(0.40)*	*(0.05)*	*(−2.51)*	*(−1.41)*
Parental socio-eco status	0.371*	0.315*	0.117**	0.026	0.134**	0.091*
	(2.34)	*(1.98)*	*(3.50)*	*(0.75)*	*(3.53)*	*(2.37)*
Foreign born	−0.621**	−0.637**			−1.475**	−1.350**
	(−4.81)	*(−4.95)*			*(−10.54)*	*(−9.78)*
Native English speaker			0.422**	0.178*		
			(5.33)	*(2.20)*		
French linguistic region	−0.599**	−0.601**				
	(−4.38)	*(−4.39)*				

(continued)

Table 11.2 (continued)

	CH (M1)	CH (M2)	AUS (M3)	AUS (M4)	D (M5)	D (M6)
Italian linguistic region	0.564*	0.638*				
	(2.24)	*(2.54)*				
Eastern Germany					−0.714**	−0.575**
					(−7.21)	*(−5.58)*
Number of observations	3907	3907	30,092	30,092	33,117	33,117
R2	0.322	0.327	0.269	0.287	0.301	0.314

Sources: SHP 2012, HILDA 2006, 2010, 2014, SOEP 2002, 2007, 2012. Notes: T-stats in parenthesis. Standard errors in Australia and in Germany are adjusted for clustering
** $p < 0.01$, * $p < 0.05$. † Foreign born means non-native English speaker in Australia

Conclusions

This study has illustrated how children affect the probability to save and accumulate wealth. The analysis has been run on Swiss, Australian and German panel data using the longest possible time span. Although the selected countries differ in several aspects, this analysis has brought to light some similarities. Dependent children older than 15 are the most expensive and make savings more difficult in all contexts. Pre-school children in Switzerland, who are even more costly than older children, present an exception that is most likely due to high costs for child care. Moreover, small children considerably reduce the propensity to save in Germany and in Switzerland because women tend to drastically reduce their labour supply and, therefore, their income after the arrival of children. The effect of young children on saving is rather small in Australia.

Over the entire life course, the effects of children on wealth and savings show a brighter picture. The accumulated level of net worth is hardly compromised by child rearing. Each child reduces wealth by 6714 CHF in Switzerland, 15,462 AU$ in Australia and 619 EUR in Germany. When we look at the wealth of retirees, the effect wanes or even disappears. This suggests the importance of the bequest motive for wealth accumulation. Therefore, in the long term, children do not seem to be a major financial risk.

The analysis has also highlighted some interesting differences between countries, which merit further investigation. Parents in Germany do not seem to have considerably lower wealth than childless individuals. This could be due to either endogeneity (wealthy individuals tend to have more children), to small costs associated with children (subsidised childcare and public schools) or to particularly thrifty lifestyles. Higher costs of children in terms of wealth accumulation in Switzerland and in Australia could be explained with a more contained family policy. Frequent private schooling and high costs for university in Australia might be an element that hinders positive savings of parents in this country. More generally, the role of institutions and legislations deserves a closer look. Other interesting aspects for future studies are the distinction between the ability to save and the willingness to save and the longitudinal dynamics of net worth. This last analysis will be possible when more waves of data of the SHP become available.

Acknowledgements This contribution is based on the project "Wealth Distribution in Switzerland and Germany: Evidence from Survey data" financed by the Swiss National Science Foundation (Project FNS – D-A-CH-10001AL_166319).

References

Addo, F. R. (2014). Debt, cohabitation, and marriage in young adulthood. *Demography, 51*(5), 1677–1701.

Austen, S., Jefferson, T., & Ong, R. (2014). The gender gap in financial security: What we know and Don't know about Australian households. *Feminist Economics, 20*(3), 25–52.

Bonke, J., & Browning, M. (2011). Spending on children: Direct survey evidence. *The Economic Journal, 121*(554), F123–F143.

Bradbury, B. (2014). Child costs. In B.-A. Asher, F. Casas, I. Frønes, & J. E. Korbin (Eds.), *Handbook of child well-being* (pp. 1483–1507). Dordrecht: Springer.

Browning, M., & Lusardi, A. (1996). Household saving: Micro theories and micro facts. *Journal of Economic Literature, 34*(4), 1797–1855.

Dockery, A. M., & Bawa, S. (2015). The impact of children on Australian couples' wealth accumulation. *Economic Record, 91*(S1), 139–150.

Finke, M. S., & Pierce, N. L. (2006). Precautionary savings behavior of maritally stressed couples. *Family and Consumer Sciences Research Journal, 34*(3), 223–240.

Friedline, T., Masa, R. D., & Chowa, G. A. N. (2015). Transforming wealth: Using the inverse hyperbolic sine (IHS) and splines to predict youth's math achievement. *Social Science Research, 49*, 264–287.

Grinstein-Weiss, M., Wagner, K., & Ssewamala, F. M. (2006). Saving and asset accumulation among low-income families with children in IDAs. *Children and Youth Services Review, 28*(2), 193–211.

Grinstein-Weiss, M., Yeo, Y. H., Zhan, M., & Charles, P. (2008). Asset holding and net worth among households with children: Differences by household type. *Children and Youth Services Review, 30*(1), 62–78.

Keynes, J. M. (1936). *The general theory of unemployment, interest and money*. New York: Harcourt, Brace and World.

Kuhn, U., & Crettaz, E. (2015). *Wealth variables in the Swiss Household Panel: Imputation and first results*. FORS Working Paper 1_15. http://ohs-shp.unil.ch/workingpapers/WP1_15.pdf. Accessed 20 Sept 2016.

Lersch, P. M., Jacob, M., & Hank, K. (2017). Parenthood, gender, and personal wealth. *European Sociological Review, 33*(3), 410–422.

Love, D. A. (2010). The effects of marital status and children on savings and portfolio choice. *Review of Financial Studies, 23*(1), 385–432.

Modigliani, F. (1986). Life cycle, individual thrift, and the wealth of nations. *The American Economic Review, 76*(3), 297–313.

Modigliani, F., & Brumberg, R. (1954). Utility analysis and the consumption function: An interpretation of cross-section data. In K. K. Kurihara (Ed.), *Post Keynesian economics* (pp. 388–436). New Brunswick: Rutgers University Press.

Moser, P. (2006). *Einkommen und Vermögen der Generationen im Lebenszyklus Eine Querschnitts-Kohortenanalyse der Zürcher Staatssteuerdaten 1991–2003*. Statistisches Amt des Kantons Zürich. statistik.info 01/2006. http://lehraufsicht.ch/internet/de/ktzh/leben_arbeit/alter/wirtschaftliche_situation/_jcr_content/contentPar/downloadlist_4/downloaditems/einkommen_der_genera.spooler.download.1326986286982.pdf/si_2006_01_einkommen_vermoegen.pdf. Accessed 20 Sept 2016.

Pericoli, F., & Ventura, L. (2011). Family dissolution and precautionary savings: An empirical analysis. *Review of Economics of the Household, 10*(4), 573–595.

Ravazzini, L., & Chesters, J. (2018). Inequality and Wealth: Comparing the Gender Wealth Gap in Switzerland and Australia. *Feminist Economics*. in press.

Rottke, S., & Klos, A. (2016). Savings and consumption when children move out. *Review of Finance, 20*(6), 2349–2377.

Scholz, J. K., & Seshadri, A. (2009). *Children and household wealth*. Working paper University of Wisconsin – Madison. https://pdfs.semanticscholar.org/8e65/2c168e4381b8611fb26d9e3441db35bc34d0.pdf. Accessed 20 Sept 2016.

Sierminska, E. M., Frick, J. R., & Grabka, M. M. (2010). Examining the gender wealth gap. *Oxford Economic Papers, 62*(4), 669–690.

Vespa, J., & Painter II, M. A. (2011). Cohabitation history, marriage, and wealth accumulation. *Demography, 48*(3), 983–1004.

Chapter 12
Homeownership and Wealth in Switzerland and Germany

Ursina Kuhn and Markus Grabka

Introduction

Although wealth is a central dimension of social inequalities, scientific attention to wealth inequality is relatively recent (e.g., OECD 2015). Several studies have pointed out that wealth inequality is particularly high in countries with low homeownership rates (Kaas et al. 2015; Mathä et al. 2014).

In this contribution, we focus on homeownership and wealth in Switzerland and Germany, which show the lowest proportion of owner-occupiers in Europe with about 40% and 50% of households, respectively. Other European countries have ownership rates of more than 90%, for example, in Romania, Lithuania or Hungary (Eurostat 2015). Nevertheless, real estate represents the most important wealth component, even in Switzerland and Germany (Grabka 2014; Swiss Federal Statistical Office 2014).

Homeownership is not only related to wealth inequality but also to average net worth. There are different explanations for the relationship between homeownership and wealth. First of all, only relatively wealthy households might be able to purchase their own home. Because real estate is typically the most valuable asset category, low ownership rates translate into low values for net wealth at the individual and the country level (Kaas et al. 2015). Secondly, house ownership has shown to have a positive effect on saving behaviour (e.g., Di et al. 2007) and thus contributes to higher wealth levels and lower wealth inequality. The forced repayments of mortgages are an important driver for regular savings. Thirdly, lower

U. Kuhn (✉)
FORS-Swiss Centre of Expertise in the Social Sciences, Lausanne, Switzerland
e-mail: Ursina.Kuhn@fors.unil.ch

M. Grabka
DIW Berlin, Germany
e-mail: mgrabka@diw.de

R. Tillmann et al. (eds.), *Social Dynamics in Swiss Society*, Life Course Research and Social Policies 9, https://doi.org/10.1007/978-3-319-89557-4_12

wealth inequality may result from rising values of real estate. Usually, investment in property yields higher returns than the money in bank accounts. Fourth, property wealth enables an owner to borrow on a mortgage to finance, e.g., a formation of an enterprise or other economic activities, which will pay off later. Having said that, fifth, one can also argue that wealth levels and wealth inequality depend on the extent of the social security system, particularly for old age and health. The necessity for private wealth accumulation tends to be smaller in countries with a comprehensive social security system, as is the case in Germany and Switzerland. Compulsory levies impair wealth accumulation and the investment in housing and leave a large part of the population with a small net worth.

Some of these mechanisms present a causal effect of homeownership on wealth accumulation. Owning a home provides financial security and produces (additional) wealth. This implies that wealth inequality could be lowered by encouraging homeownership. However, there have been doubts on the financial and social benefits of owning for low-income households (Shlay 2006). The housing burst in several countries (e.g., US, Spain or Ireland), and the numerous foreclosures in particular, have raised awareness about the risks of homeownership. Homeownership is particularly risky for low-income households that finance their property with a high level of debt. In a financial crisis, market values decline, while the debt remains unchanged, thus leading to indebtedness. For example, in the US, the median net worth dropped by 44% between 2007 and 2010, and the share of owner-occupiers shrank by nine percentage points (Wolff 2016). In sum, it is controversial whether facilitating access to property to households with little wealth is a means to fight social inequalities.

Homeownership in Switzerland and Germany

Switzerland's ownership rate is low from a comparative perspective but has increased in the last decades from 31% in 1990 to 37% of all households in 2010. This increase is somewhat surprising considering that owning has become more expensive relative to both renting and to the average income (OECD.Stat 2016). Since 2000, prices for private real estate have risen by 159%. The high prices due to the scarcity of land and high construction quality standards present the most frequently mentioned reason for the low ownership rate. Other explanations are a well-functioning rental market with protection for renters (restrictions on rent increases and eviction), a restrictive mortgage system and high down-payment requirements.[1] There is a wide variation in ownership rates within Switzerland, with low ownership in urban areas and ownership rates over 50% in rural areas.

[1] Requirements are an amortisation over 15 years to 65% of the house value, annual costs of owning a house must not exceed 33% of the gross household income and there is a minimum of 20% deposit for the purchase (second and third pillar assets can be used for this) and a ca. of 4% for close costs.

The legislation that is relevant for ownership varies strongly between cantons and municipalities, but there is no general political promotion of homeownership (Thalmann 1999). Despite different taxes for homeowners (wealth tax, income tax on imputed rents, transfer taxes, property taxes), owners have a small tax advantage over renters (Bourassa and Hoesli 2008).[2] However, also taxes vary strongly among cantons and municipalities.

In Germany, the share of owner-occupiers was 46% in 2010 (Statistisches Bundesamt 2013). However, there are significant differences between East and West Germany. While the respective share is almost 50% in the West, only about a third of all East-German households are owner-occupiers (Grabka 2014). Since reunification, the share of owner-occupied households increased by eight percentage points in both parts of the country.

In East Germany, the low share of owner-occupied households can be explained by the socialistic economic system in the GDR, which did not promote the possession of property. In West Germany, the respective share is still rather low because of the vast demolition during the World War II. In addition, about 14 million displaced persons fled between 1945–1950 from formerly German regions in the East to the GDR and FRG. Thus, there was a significant shortage of living space after World War II (Kesternich et al. 2014). The government in West Germany reacted with housing programmes, particularly through social housing.[3] Private housing construction was promoted by the tax deductibility of construction costs or mortgage interest. From 1996 to 2006, this has been replaced by a direct monetary value. Since then, there has been no nation-wide programme that promotes homeownership in Germany. Another reason for the low share of owner-occupied housing in Germany is its long tradition of a well-developed rental market with a comprehensive rent control, thus leading to rather low rental prices. When comparing the costs for renting compared to an acquisition of owner-occupied housing, Voigtländer (2014) finds that for nearly three-fourths of German counties, renting was superior to buying in 2009.[4] Since 2009, there has been a strong increase in property prices, particularly in city regions. Sales prices for condominiums have increased by 55% between 2009 and 2016 (Kholodilin and Michelsen 2017).

Until 1982, the acquisition of owner-occupied property was burdened by a real estate transfer tax of 7%. Between 1982 and 2006, a reduced nationwide tax of 3.5% was established. Since then, every federal state can set its own tax rates that vary

[2] The reasons for the tax advantage are that the taxed value of owner-occupied housing for wealth tax is clearly below market prices, the fact that interests for mortgages and costs for the maintenance of the house can be deducted from taxable income and that capital gains tax rates when a house is sold decrease with tenure in most cantons and taxes are postponed if a new property is bought.

[3] To give an example, between 1961 und 1990, 90% of all new dwellings were built with the aid of social housing programmes in Berlin (Holm 2007).

[4] Restrictions in the access to mortgages and rather high down-payment requirements and high transaction costs play an additional role preventing or dissuading many young households from buying a property at the beginning of their careers (Chiuri and Jappelli 2003).

between 3.5% in Bavaria and 6.5% in Brandenburg. A property tax must be paid by owner-occupiers, but the taxable value is—like in Switzerland—clearly below market values. There are no other owner-specific taxes.[5]

In sum, house ownership in Germany and Switzerland shares many similarities: low share of homeownership, high (and rising) house prices, a well-developed renter market, a restrictive mortgage system and high down-payment requirements. The main differences are the high population growth combined with the limited land in Switzerland, while population is shrinking in rural areas in Germany but growing in cities.

Data

For Switzerland, we use data of the Swiss Household Panel (SHP) from 2012 that include two questions on wealth. A first question asks homeowners to estimate the value of their property after deducting mortgages. In a second question, respondents are asked to estimate the amount of the remaining wealth. Wealth information is available for 4467 households; values for 812 have been imputed. Because of these general questions, wealth estimates are approximate. It is therefore important to compare data of the SHP with other available data sources, even if true values are unknown.

For two reasons, the average levels of net worth are likely to be underestimated in the SHP. First, general questions yield typically lower values than when information is collected for different wealth components separately. Second, surveys in general do not adequately cover the very top of the wealth distribution. Because wealth is extremely concentrated, outliers have an enormous impact on the average measures. According to tax records, 1% of Swiss residents hold 40% of the total wealth (Foellmi and Martínez 2017). Because this study focusses on comparisons between groups rather than wealth concentration, we are however not interested in the top wealth holders.

As an indication for data quality, one can compare the wealth levels in the SHP with national accounts. Net worth per capita in the SHP amounts to 200,548 CHF, while the respective figure from the national accounts shows an average net worth of 263,466 CHF per person (Swiss National Bank, net worth corrected for pension funds). Wealth in the SHP therefore amounts to 76% of the national accounts.[6] Another test of the SHP data is a comparison with CH-SILC 2015, which included a relatively detailed wealth module. The average net worth per person in SILC 2015 was 254,139

[5] When selling, owner-occupied property taxes on capital gains were only raised if the time period between acquisition and sale was less than 10 years.

[6] National accounts also present the value of real estate. The value for real estate per capita in the SHP is very close to one of the national accounts (101,561 CHF vs. 119,923 CHF). However, because the variable in the SHP refers only to primary residence, the two values cannot be perfectly compared.

CHF, which was slightly higher than in the SHP 2012.[7] But considering the general wealth increases between 2012 and 2015, the values seem relatively close. Overall, the SHP seems well suited to study differences between owners and renter households.

For Germany, we make use of the Socio-Economic Panel (SOEP). The SOEP started in 1984 and expanded to East Germany in 1990. As the SHP, the survey is representative for the population and is conducted every year. We also use the survey year 2012 with more than 10,000 households, where information about ten different asset and debt components had been collected.

In the following we analyse data at the household level. Wealth is measured as per capita net worth, which is the sum of all assets less the value of debts. Wealth is however censored at 0 in Switzerland (no negative values).[8] The wealth measure does not include occupational pension plans and promised entitlements to public retirement payments or household effects.

Results

House Ownership, Wealth and Age

We start with descriptive characteristics of the average wealth and wealth inequality.[9] First of all, Table 12.1 shows that Swiss residents are much wealthier than German residents. Secondly, owner households are much wealthier than renter households (five times in Switzerland, seven times in Germany). Even if owner households are a minority (46% in Germany, 37% in Switzerland) they own as much as 86% of the total wealth in Germany and 75% in Switzerland. Thirdly, Table 12.1 shows the decomposition of wealth inequality for the Squared Coefficient of Variation (SCV). Only 3.6% of the inequality in Switzerland and 6.7% in Germany are due to differences between groups. Thus, wealth inequality occurs mainly within owners and renters. Forth, the SCV and the Gini index by group reveal that inequality within renter households is considerably higher than inequality within owner households. Not the wealth gap between owners and renters but the lower inequality within owner households is the main reason that low homeownership rates are associated with high wealth inequality. An increasing share of homeowners implies a lower wealth inequality.

We next look at the relationship between age and wealth. Homeownership has shown to be most beneficial for wealth accumulation when houses are bought at a young age. Households have a longer period to accumulate wealth and to repay mortgage debt, respectively. Figure 12.1 predicts the nonlinear relationship between wealth and age of the household head (main income earner in Switzerland, reference person

[7] The SILC data are not well suited for an analysis on homeownership because 34% of respondents have not indicated the current market value but the taxable or purchase value of the house, which are considerably lower. As a consequence, the wealth difference between owners and renters is likely to be underestimated in SILC.

[8] In SOEP, the share of households with a negative net worth is 7.5%.

[9] Weights provided by the SHP have been calibrated to match the official rate of homeowners.

Table 12.1 Inequality decomposition by ownership status 2012

	Population share (%)	Mean net worth (CHF/€)	Wealth Share (%)	SCV	Gini
CH					
Renter	62.8	83,625	24.8	11.941	0.800
Owner	37.2	429,072	75.2	4.741	0.592
All	100	212,131	100.0	8.691	0.750
Within inequality				8.381	
Between inequality				0.310	
DE					
Renter	54.5	24,246	14.2	43.343	0.936
Owner	45.5	168,619	85.8	1.699	0.545
All	100.0	91,450	100.0	4.627	0.747
Within inequality				4.317	
Between inequality				0.310	

Note: Net worth per capita in 2012, national currencies. Analyses are at the household level. Source: SHP, SOEPv32, private households only

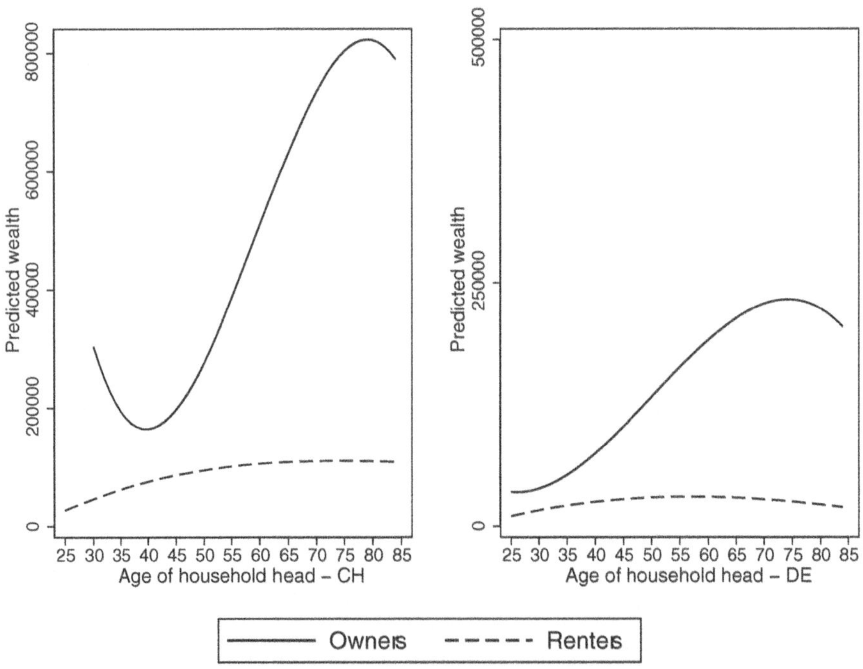

Fig. 12.1 Age wealth profiles by ownership status 2012. Note: Predicted wealth refers to national currencies. Information for owners in Switzerland below 30 years of age is not presented due to a small number of observations. Source: SHP, SOEPv32, private households only

in Germany) using linear regression. The figure shows that house owners are wealthier than renter households but that the gap widens substantially over the life cycle. While the difference between the average wealth of owners and renters is rather small for household heads up to 40 years, it increases quickly thereafter.

There are different possible explanations for this pattern (see also Alik-Lagrange and Schmidt 2015). A first is that young renters also include future property buyers. They might either be saving to buy their own property or even possess the necessary assets but are waiting for a good opportunity to buy a home. At older ages, there are fewer households that prefer owning over renting and can afford buying at the same time. While this effect arises mainly through self-selection into homeownership, more savings of owner-occupiers are a second explanation for the increasing wealth gap between owner and renter households. Thirdly, owner-occupiers, who have been owners for a longer time, may have profited more strongly from rising property's values than younger owners. Fourthly, the probability for significant inheritances is higher at higher ages. Wealth differences between renters and owners in precursor generations can insofar carry forward. Finally, the differences between ages might also be driven by cohort effects. But considering the similarity from Germany and Switzerland, it is unlikely that major historical events like the World War II and the German reunification are main explanations for the rising wealth gap between owners and renters with age in Germany.

Nevertheless, and considering that renting is a viable option in Switzerland and Germany, it is surprising that renters hardly accumulate wealth over the life cycle. Thus, other forms of self-selection might be relevant to explain the wealth difference. For example, if hedonists, who prefer current consumption over savings, are more prevalent among renters, this selection could explain the lower wealth levels of renters.

Another remarkable finding of Fig. 12.1 is the shape of the curve for owners at older ages. While the German households start dissaving at around age 65, the average wealth of owner-occupiers and to a smaller extent of renter households continues to rise to about 80 years of age in Switzerland. One possible explanation for this diverging pattern is the lack of care insurance in Switzerland compared to Germany, which encourages wealth accumulation even after retirement to finance care costs.[10] In contrast, intergenerational wealth transmissions might play an important role for the observed dissaving effect in Germany (Westermeier et al. 2016).

Explaining the Ownership Wealth Gap

To better explain the differences between renters and owners, we use decomposition methods, which are widely used for other group differences, most frequently for the gender–wage gap. The most widely used method is the Oaxaca-Blinder decomposition. Juhn et al. (1993) expanded this approach beyond the mean to different quantiles of the distribution and suggested decomposition into three components: characteristics, coefficients and residuals. More recently, counterfactual distributions are used to explain the differences between groups (see Fortin et al. 2010 for a review on decomposition methods). Here, we adopt the method proposed by

[10] A similar age pattern can be found for the US, where an obligatory nursing care is not implemented either (Grabka et al. 2016).

Chernozhukov et al. (2013), which uses conditional quantile regression. Estimates have been obtained with the Stata command cdeco (for quantiles) and jmpierce (for the mean). The conditional wealth distribution of renters is used as the benchmark. This nonparametric decomposition method is advantageous because it not only focusses on the mean but also does not require assumptions about the underlying distribution.

To mitigate the influence of outliers in the wealth distribution, we apply the inverse hyperbolic sine transformation (Johnson 1949) of net worth for the conditional distribution. Explanatory variables encompass age, household type, gender, permanent income and its square term, educational levels, urban municipality, migration background, wealthy parents, bad health, the presence of siblings and received inheritances and bequest.

Results in Table 12.2 show that differences in these observable characteristics (column 2) explain only a small part of the wealth differences between renters and owners. At the mean, different socioeconomic characteristics explain 16% of the wealth differences in Switzerland and 32% in Germany, respectively. Looking at quantiles, we can see that composition effects become more important if one moves up in the wealth distribution. In Switzerland, the different characteristics of owners and renters explain 16% of the wealth gap at the 25th percentile and 29% at the 90th percentile. In Germany, the composition effect increases from 9% at the 10th percentile to 67% at the 90th percentile. The higher permanent income of

Table 12.2 Results of JMP-decomposition of wealth difference by ownership status

	Total (for information only: absolute difference in CHF/ Euro) (1)	Observed Quantities (2)	Observed Prices (3)	Unobserved Prices and Quantities (4)
CH				
Mean	100% (378,529)	16%	84%	0%
P10	100% (49,780)	0%	27%	73%
P25	100% (113,168)	16%	43%	41%
P50	100% (228,329)	12%	90%	−2%
P75	100% (405,314)	19%	109%	−29%
P90	100% (667,994)	29%	137%	−65%
DE				
Mean	100% (144,076)	32%	68%	0%
P10	100% (19,057)	9%	22%	70%
P25	100% (50,184)	25%	35%	42%
P50	100% (101,248)	35%	62%	3%
P75	100% (174,490)	42%	89%	−30%
P90	100% (290,743)	67%	121%	−89%

Source: SHP, SOEPv31, per capita net worth was transformed using the inverse of the hyperbolic sine

owners compared with renters is the most important driver for the composition effect. However, the effects of observed characteristics (price effects in column 3) are much more important for wealth differences. For example, being an owner and having the exact same characteristics as a renter will lead to a higher net worth in both countries. Rising values of properties and more regular savings of house owners compared to renters are possible explanations for this finding. The impact of unobserved price and quantities is more relevant at the lower and the upper end of the wealth distribution. This indicates that other factors not considered in the regression analyses may play a role.

Summary

This chapter addressed the wealth inequality and wealth differences between owner and renter households in Switzerland and Germany. We have found that owner-occupiers hold on average five or seven times more per capita net worth than renters. Only a small part of wealth inequality can be explained with the wealth gap between owners and renters. In addition, wealth inequality is much lower in the group of owners. The high wealth inequality among renters is an important explanation for wealth inequality in Germany and Switzerland.

If one would like to reduce the high wealth inequality in Switzerland and Germany, promoting homeownership is a possible starting point. Results from a decomposition analysis show that so-called price effects rather than differences in characteristics explain the different wealth levels between owners and renters. There are two main explanations why becoming a homeowner is likely to increase wealth accumulation. Firstly, the rise in the value of property may lead to a higher net worth for owners. Secondly, owners on a mortgage are forced to save on a regular basis and thus accumulate wealth faster than usual tenant households (see also Grabka and Westermeier 2015). Owners might be more homogenous than renters in terms of wealth because rising prices and forced savings due to mortgage repayments affect a large majority of owners in the same way. A central challenge when considering ownership promotion programmes is, on the one side, enabling low-income households to become homeowners and avoiding a "lock-in phenomenon" on the other side, i.e., providing financial aid to affluent persons who would become owners anyway. Furthermore, ownership promotion programmes that alleviate the access to mortgages can bear the risk of creating a bubble, as has been seen in Spain or in the US; thus, well-considered policy reforms must be made.

Acknowledgements This contribution is based on the project "Wealth Distribution in Switzerland and Germany: Evidence from Survey data" financed by the Swiss National Science Foundation (Project FNS – D-A-CH-10001AL_166319).

References

Alik-Lagrange, A., & Schmidt, T. (2015). *The pattern of home ownership across cohorts and its impact on the net wealth distribution: Empirical evidence from Germany and the US* (Discussion Paper No. 11/2015). Deutsche Bundesbank, Research Centre.

Bourassa, S. C., & Hoesli, M. (2008). Why do the Swiss rent? *The Journal of Real Estate Finance and Economics, 40*(3), 286–309.

Chernozhukov, V., Fernández-Val, I., & Melly, B. (2013). Inference on counterfactual distributions. *Econometrica, 81*(6), 2205–2268.

Chiuri, M. C., & Jappelli, T. (2003). Financial market imperfections and home ownership: A comparative study. *European Economic Review, 47*(5), 857–875.

Di, Z. X., Belsky, E., & Liu, X. (2007). Do homeowners achieve more household wealth in the long run? *Journal of Housing Economics, 16*(3–4), 274–290.

Eurostat. (2015). *Wohnstatistiken*. http://ec.europa.eu/eurostat/statistics-explained/index.php/Housing_statistics/de. Accessed 18 Oct 2016.

Foellmi, R., & Martínez, I. Z. (2017). Volatile top income shares in Switzerland? Reassessing the evolution between 1981 and 2010. *The Review of Economics and Statistics, 99*, 793–809.

Fortin, N., Lemieux, T., & Firpo, S. (2010). Decomposition methods in economics. In O. Ashenfelter & D. Card (Eds.), *Handbook of labor economics* (Vol. 4A, 1st ed.). Amsterdam: Elsevier.

Grabka, M. M., (2014). Private Vermögen in Ost- und Westdeutschland gleichen sich nur langsam an. DIW Wochenbericht Nr. 40/2014, S. 959–964.

Grabka, M.M., & Westermeier, C. (2015). Real net worth of households in Germany fell between 2003 and 2013. Economic bulletin 34/2015, p. 441–450.

Grabka, M.M., Boenke, T., Wolff, E.N., & Schroeder, C. (2016). A comparative analysis of augmented wealth in Germany and the United States. Paper presented at the IARIW conference 2016, Dresden.

Holm, A. (2007). Der schwindende Rest. Sozialer Wohnungsbau in Berlin. In: MieterEcho 323/ August 2007.

Johnson, N. L. (1949). Systems of frequency curves generated by methods of translation. *Biometrika, 36*, 149–176.

Juhn, C., Murphy, K. M., & Pierce, B. (1993). Wage inequality and the rise in returns to skill. *Journal of Political Economy, 101*(3), 410–442.

Kaas, L., Kocharkov, G., & Preugschat, E. (2015). Wealth Inequality and homeownership in Europe. University of Konstanz, Working Paper Series 2015–18.

Kesternich, I., Siflinger, B., Smith, J. P., & Winter, J. K. (2014). The effects of world war II on economic and health outcomes across Europe. *The Review of Economics and Statistics, 96*(1), 103–118.

Kholodilin, K., & Michelsen, C. (2017). Keine Immobilienpreisblase in Deutschland – aber regional begrenzte Übertreibungen in Teilmärkten. *DIW Wochenbericht Nr., 25*, 503–513.

Mathä, T., Porpiglia, A., & Ziegelmeyer, M. (2014). Household wealth in the European area: The importance of intergenerational transfers, homeownership and house price dynamics. ECB Working Paper 1690, European Central Bank.

OECD. (2015). In it together: Why less inequality benefits all. Paris.

Shlay, A. (2006). Low-income homeownership: American dream or delusion? *Urban Studies, 43*(3), 511–531.

OECD Stat. (2016). Price to rent ratio. Stats.oecd.org. Accessed on 20 Oct 2016.

Statistisches Bundesamt. (2013). Zensus 2011: 80,2 Millionen Einwohner lebten am 9. Mai 2011 in Deutschland. Pressemitteilung Nr. 188 vom 31.05.2013.

Swiss Federal Statistical Office. (2014). *Vermögenslage der privaten Haushalte*. Neuenburg: BFS.

Thalmann, P. (1999). Which is the appropriate administrative level to promote home ownership? *Swiss Journal of Economics and Statistics (SJES), 135*(I), 3–20.
Voigtländer, M. (2014). Mieten oder Kaufen – Eine Analyse für die deutschen Kreise. IW-Trends 2/2014,
Westermeier, C., Tiefensee, A., & Grabka, M. M. (2016). Erbschaften in Europa: Wer viel verdient, bekommt am meisten. *DIW Wochenbericht Nr., 17*, 375–386.
Wolff, E. N. (2016). Deconstructing household wealth trends in the United States 1983–2013. NBER working paper nr. 22704.

Part III
Politics & Attitudes

Chapter 13
Dynamic Political Attitudes in Partisan Context

Jennifer Fitzgerald and Christopher Jorde

What explains changes in political attitudes? We consider the ways in which partisan choices relate to attitude change. While most studies of the partisan-attitude nexus use attitudes to explain party choices, we flip the script and consider the ways that partisan choices shape attitudes over time. The Swiss Household Panel Survey (SHP) provides an opportunity to evaluate shifts in individuals' views on immigration, government spending and the environment over 16 years. This survey makes it possible to establish how stable these views and party choices are from year to year. It also allows us to model attitudinal changes to identify their chief predictors. These are essential inquiries if we are to understand the ways in which Switzerland has changed and remained the same since the turn of the century.

After decades of stability in Swiss electoral politics, recent elections have become less predictable. Notably, National Council elections are increasingly competitive. Notably, the Swiss People's Party (SVP) has attracted hundreds of thousands of new supporters. Fig. 13.1 displays various parties' electoral fortunes over the last two decades. The full, black line marks the ascent of the SVP across elections. The Greens have also grown in popularity, though more modestly. The remaining main parties, the Social Democrats, Christian Democrats and the Radical Democrats, weakened across these six elections (Swiss Federal Statistical Office 2016).

J. Fitzgerald (✉) · C. Jorde
Department of Political Science, University of Colorado at Boulder, Boulder, CO, USA
e-mail: jennifer.fitzgerald@colorado.edu; Christopher.jorde@colorado.edu

R. Tillmann et al. (eds.), *Social Dynamics in Swiss Society*, Life Course Research and Social Policies 9, https://doi.org/10.1007/978-3-319-89557-4_13

These aggregate electoral patterns demonstrate that Swiss politics have changed significantly in recent years. Yet they do not offer much insight into shifts in people's political views at the individual level. Our objective is to gain a better understanding of how (un)stable key political attitudes are for the Swiss. We also unpack the relationship between partisan choices and views on salient political issues over time.

Theoretical Framework

The partisan shifts depicted in Fig. 13.1 may indicate that people's attitudes are changing and that parties' electoral fortunes are shaped by these changes. For instance, it is possible that as anti-immigration attitudes rise in popularity, the SVP gains new voters over time as a result. But another interpretation is that increasingly competitive campaigns have attitudinal implications. In other words, it may be that parties shape the opinions of their supporters. Per this narrative, the SVP's messaging influences its supporters' views on immigration. Given the disjuncture between the post-war stability and more recent changes in Swiss politics, it is important to unpack these dynamics over time. It is imperative for our understanding of Swiss democracy to ask whether parties actively shape or passively reflect public opinion.

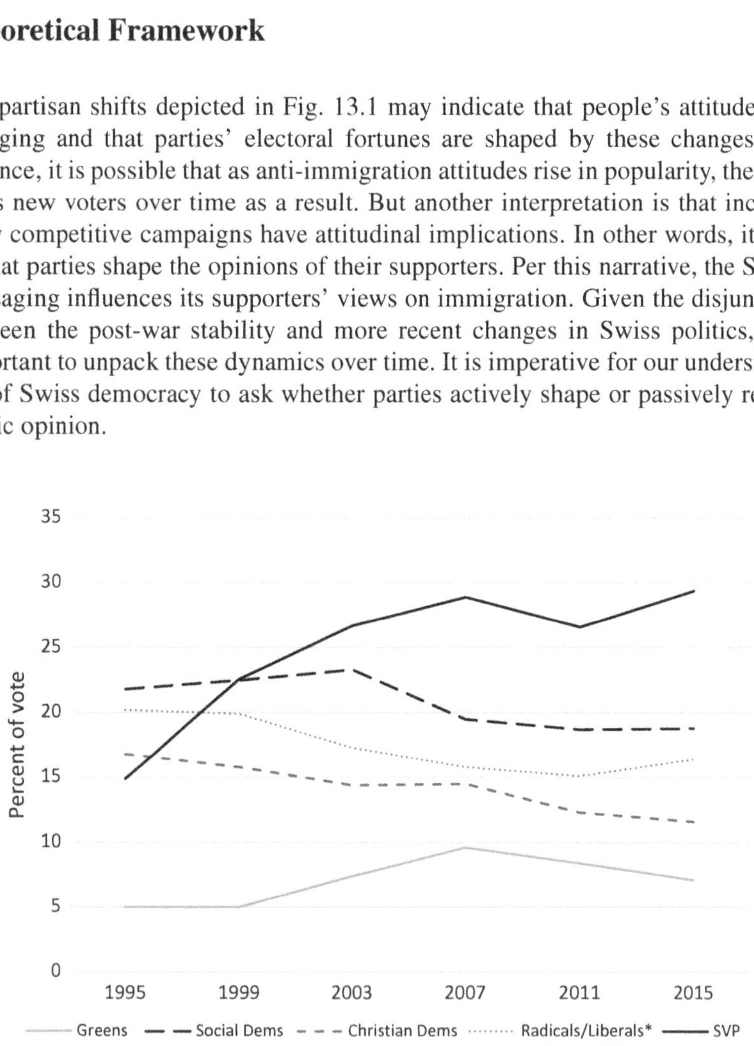

Fig. 13.1 Swiss parties' shares of National Council election votes
Source: Swiss Federal Statistical Office 2016
*As of 2011 election, Radicals' (Free Democrats) share of votes includes Liberals: they merged in 2009 into FDP.The Liberals

Political scientists debate the nature of the relationship between parties and attitudes. Classical theories of democracy and political behavior depict a citizen who decides which party to vote for based on his or her attitudinal preferences (Downs 1957; Campbell et al. 1960). This instrumental model of electoral choice puts policy preferences in the driving position; a citizen arrives at a party selection based on a sense of which party will deliver his or her optimal policies. Yet a contrasting view paints an image of electoral politics in which parties, themselves, shape public opinion. According to this psychological account, voters will shift their views in response to partisan cues. In order to remain consistent with a chosen party's platform, voters will update their attitudes over time (Lodge and Taber 2000, Miller 2000, Sniderman and Levendusky 2007). These two narratives depict very different images of political behavior in democratic settings. We leverage the Swiss case to contribute to this big-picture debate. Given the high level of dynamism evident in Swiss politics over the past decade and a half, it presents an unusually propitious opportunity to test these accounts.

We focus on three attitudes in our analysis: views on immigrants, preferences for social spending levels, and opinions on environmental protection. We are specifically interested in understanding particular points of view on these subjects: choosing native Swiss advantage over immigrants with respect to opportunities, preferring support for decreased federal spending on social programs, and desiring more protection of the environment. These opinions relate directly to issues salient in recent Swiss elections. They are also central issues for particular parties and so they are well suited to testing ideas about the connection between certain attitudes and certain partisan preferences. The SVP, for instance, has made issues of immigration a central feature of its political platform (McGann and Kitschelt 2005). The Radicals' ideology is economic liberalism with a preference for diminished government regulation and spending, and the main raison d'être of the Green party is to promote environmental protection (see Hug and Schulz 2007; Kriesi and Trechsel 2008). If parties are indeed shaping attitudes, the SVP, Radicals and Greens should be most closely affiliated with shifts toward anti-immigrant, anti-spending and pro-environment views, respectively.

With respect to attitude stability across issues, existing work leads us to expect that different kinds of attitudes should display different patterns. The most stable, according to existing research, should be views on immigrants. Studies of lifelong stability in attitudes point to the unusually static nature of racial and ethnic attitudes, which tend to form and crystallize early in life (Sears and Funk 1999). As a core value, environmentalism should be the next most stable over time at the individual level (Inglehart 1997). The least stable of the three should be spending ideas. Economic preferences such as support for government social programs, are the most likely to be updated over time (Brooks and Manza 2008). But given the high level of electoral volatility that characterized the years of the SHP survey, we expect a significant instability for all three issue areas from year to year.

Data and Methods

In most waves of the survey, the SHP asks individuals about their views on several important political issues. These waves are 1999–2009 (annual), 2011 and 2014. The relevant questionnaire items read as follows. The initial primer is: "A number of political goals are questioned; I would be interested to hear your opinion on some of them…".

Anti-immigrant "Are you in favour of Switzerland offering foreigners the same opportunities as those offered to Swiss citizens, or in favour of Switzerland offering Swiss citizens better opportunities?" The response options are: in favour of equality of opportunities, in favour of better opportunities for Swiss citizens. We code this 1 if the final option is selected, 0 otherwise.

Anti-spend "Are you in favour of a diminution or in favour of an increase of the Confederation social spending?" The response options are: in favour of a diminution, neither, in favour of an increase. We code this 1 if the first option is selected, 0 otherwise.

Pro-environment "Are you in favour of Switzerland being more concerned with protection of the environment than with economic growth, or in favour of Switzerland being more concerned with economic growth than with protection of the environment?" The response options are: in favour of stronger protection of the environment, neither, in favour of stronger economic growth. We code this 1 if the first option is selected, 0 otherwise.

For each variable, through our coding we isolate one specific response to highlight while collapsing the other categories. We do this to gain precision in our analysis by examining only one particular stance. The drawback is that we lose information on the other side of the spectrum. To be sure that this choice does not influence our findings, we replicate each analytical step with variables that reflect the full spectrum of response options. The patterns we present below are not substantively changed. Importantly, the collapsed, dichotomous coding that we use in the presented analysis yields conservative estimates of instability because they do not capture shifts within the "0" category over time. We interpret them with this in mind.

We also examine patterns in party support over time. In each annual wave (1999–2014) the SHP records party preference through the question, "If there was an election for the National Council tomorrow, for which party would you vote?" From this item we create a series of dichotomous variables to indicate support for each of the five main parties in modern Swiss federal elections. These are (roughly from left to right): the Green Party, the Social Democratic Party, the Christian Democratic People's Party, the Radical Party,[1] and the Swiss People's Party.

[1]In 2009 the Radical party merged with the smaller Liberal party (technically now FDP-the Liberals). The SHP provides separate support for each party even after the merge. We find that combining these parties' followers into one group as of 2009—as opposed to keeping Radicals

We also include a number of control variables in our models to offer a more detailed and precise analysis. These are *Education level*, *Age* and *Female*. These variables are derived from literature on attitude change in general and attitudes on immigration, spending and the environment more specifically. For instance, young people are more unstable than their elders in their political views (Alwin and Krosnick 1991). Women and the highly educated are most likely to hold anti-immigrant views (Fetzer 2000; Hainmueller and Hiscox 2007). Older citizens are less concerned about the environment (Inglehart 1997), and women tend to be more supportive of social spending than men (Blekesaune and Quadagno 2003; Funk and Gathmann 2006). While these studies provide guidance, little work examines shifts in these attitudes over time; our analysis provides uncommon insight into how these viewpoints develop.

Because we conduct this analysis with an eye toward isolating the impact of partisan preferences on attitude shifts, we include a lagged dependent variable in each model. To further subject the partisan thesis to a tough test, we include a left-right political ideology variable, *Ideology*. The highest values represent the most right-leaning position. These steps set up a high hurdle for partisan effects to appear in the results. Finally, we include a dummy variable for each canton to address the highly decentralized nature of the Swiss party system (Ladner 2001), and we cluster the observations by household number to address the non-independence of observations inherent in a household survey.[2]

With respect to our methods, the descriptive correlations we report below are simple bivariate phi coefficients (in Stata 11), which are suitable for estimating the ways that two bivariate variables relate to each other. The statistical models are logit models that include a one-year lag of the dependent variable. This makes it possible to establish the factors predicting attitudinal position net their attitudinal position in the previous year. Functionally, this captures individuals who adopt the specific attitude of interest during the course of a particular year (since the previous wave of the survey). It also captures individuals who move away from a particular point of view. These models provide insight into the factors that distinguish individuals who hold a particular opinion (about immigration, the environment or social spending) from those who do not, net their previous year's choices. They are therefore between-group (or inter-individual) comparisons that incorporate a dynamic component from 1 year to the next.

Descriptive Findings

From year-to-year, these three attitudes show different levels of stability. For this step in our analysis we utilize all respondents who answer the relevant questions in two consecutive years of the survey. This gives us approximately 50,000

supporters separate—does not influence the results of statistical models. Therefore, for the sake of consistency across waves, we do not include in the statistical analysis support for the much smaller Liberal Party or for the combined partisan entity.

[2] The results we report below are robust to inclusion of additional covariates. These include: occupation, income, religion and political interest.

observations.[3] The waves represented are 1999 through 2009. Later waves are not captured in this step of the analysis because the attitudinal questions become less regularly asked in the most recent waves of the survey. The correlation (phi) between support for Swiss advantage over immigrants at time *t* and the same variable at time *t*-1 is .54. The parallel correlation for environmental protection is .46; for anti-spending attitudes it is .44. These numbers point to a rather high level of instability overall, and in relation to each other they align with the expectations drawn from past work on attitudinal stability. Immigration attitudes are the most stable over time, environmentalism is the next most stable, and economic preferences are the least stable. With respect to individual-level shifts from year to year, the Swiss change their minds rather frequently, but they do so in predictable ways.

How does this compare to stability or instability in party choice? For our investigation into partisan preference over time, we use the same respondents (about 50,000 observations) from the same waves as we did to estimate year-to-year correlations in attitudes. Moving from left to right, the year-to-year correlation is .49 for the Greens (to refresh the memory, this is the correlation between Greens at time *t* and Greens at time *t*-1), .66 for the Social Democrats, .59 for the Christian Democrats, .59 for the Radicals and .63 for the Swiss People's Party (see also Kuhn 2009). These figures reveal more stability in partisan preference as compared to the attitudinal stances. The exception is the Green party, which is the least stable partisan choice, and it is less stable over time than are immigration attitudes.

Another consideration is whether the prevalence of people changing their minds on key issues is increasing. Given the high level of electoral flux in Swiss politics, it is important to establish whether instability is rising or declining. For this step, it makes sense to examine only those respondents who participated in the survey in all sixteen available waves of the survey.[4] Fig. 13.2 details the patterns for the three attitudes of interest over time using the 1999–2009 waves and those 1580 individuals in the full panel. Each dot on the figure represents the phi correlation between a particular variable at time *t* and that same variable at *t*-1 (for instance Anti-immigrant in 2000 and Anti-immigrant in 1999). Over time we see that for each of these issues, people's views are stabilizing across the years of the survey. This relative stability in the later 2000s (decade) as compared to the early 2000s continues into the later waves of the panel. Though we cannot establish year-to-year correlations for years since 2009, we fill in the blanks a bit using the 2011 and 2014 survey waves. For Anti-immigrant views the correlation between 2011 and 2009 is .61; between 2014 and 2011 it is .60. For anti-spending attitudes the correlation between 2011 and 2009 is .47; between 2014 and 2011 it is .43. And for pro-environmental views the correlation between 2011 and 2009 is .53; between 2014 and 2011 it is .51. These are the same individuals as those represented in Fig. 13.2, so we can say that atti-

[3] Observations throughout this analysis are person-years.

[4] If we open this up to include all individuals from all waves who participated in two consecutive waves of the survey, the basic longitudinal patterns are the same. Though the level of year-to-year stability in general is slightly lower.

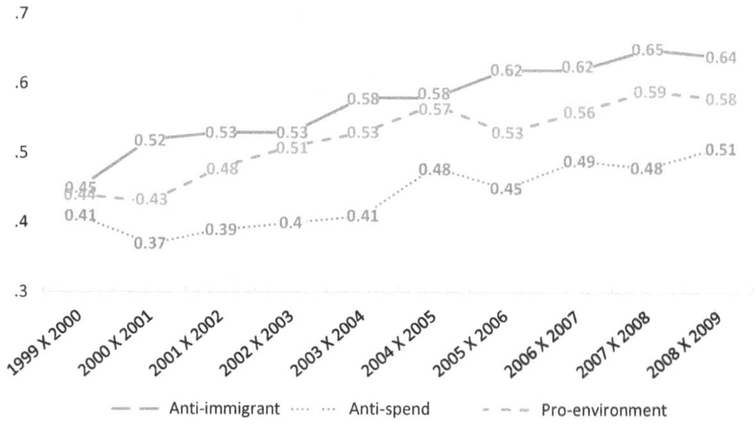

Fig. 13.2 Year-to-year correlations in attitudes

tudes toward immigrants and to a lesser extent the environment in recent years are much more stable than they were at the start of the survey.[5] The outlier is spending attitudes. The year-to-year stability gained in this issue area from 1999 to 2009 seems to have weakened more recently. If there is one attitude that is still in flux at the individual level, it is spending opinions.

Models

What factors account for attitudinal change over time? In other words, who is most likely to shift to a position of anti-immigrant, pro-environment or anti-spending? Furthermore, what is the role of partisan preference in promoting adoption of these attitudes? Table 13.1 presents six models of partisanship and political attitudes: models 1 and 2 focus on the effects of SVP partisanship on anti-immigrant attitudes, models 3 and 4 focus on the impact of Green party support on pro-environment attitudes, and models 5 and 6 focus on Radicals support and anti-spending attitudes. Each model includes canton fixed effects. Odds ratios represent relationships of interest: values less than one indicate a negative relationship, greater than one a positive relationship. An even 1 indicates no impact at all.

[5] Support for each of the major parties in Switzerland also proves to be stabilizing throughout the course of the survey. Replicating the descriptive presentation for attitudes displayed above in Fig. 13.2, we find that the year-to-year stability at the end of the sixteen waves (2013 X 2014) is approximately .10 higher than it was in the earliest waves for three of the parties (1999 X 2000): SVP, Christian Democrats and Social Democrats. Stability in support for the Greens and the Radicals increased only about half as much as for the other parties. This is for those individuals who were in the survey in all waves, just as described for Fig. 13.2. All difference in year-to-year stability from the earliest to the latest waves of the survey are statistically significant. Results available from authors.

Table 13.1 Partisanship and political attitudes: Logit models with lagged dependent variables

	(1) *Anti-Immigrant*	(2) *Anti-Immigrant*	(3) *Pro-Environment*	(4) *Pro-Environment*	(5) *Anti-Spend*	(6) *Anti-Spend*
Lagged DV	11.06* (68.06)	10.81* (67.30)	6.592* (64.73)	6.469* (64.13)	8.283* (54.32)	7.804* (53.00)
SVP	1.780* (12.59)	1.709* (11.36)		0.915* (−1.97)		1.652* (10.31)
Greens		0.669* (−5.04)	2.151* (13.46)	2.244* (13.58)		0.591* (−5.93)
Radicals		0.961 (−0.83)		0.693* (−8.40)	1.284* (5.42)	1.348* (6.23)
Social Democrats		0.657* (−8.98)		1.181* (4.69)		0.507* (−11.82)
Christian Democrats		0.952 (−0.89)		0.984 (−0.34)		0.997 (−0.05)
Education	0.914* (−16.03)	0.917* (−15.38)	0.987* (−2.74)	0.987* (−2.66)	0.955* (−7.63)	0.964* (−5.91)
Age	1.005* (5.80)	1.005* (5.87)	0.996* (−4.54)	0.997* (−4.39)	0.993* (−7.13)	0.993* (−7.14)
Female	1.115* (3.58)	1.109* (3.38)	1.248* (8.74)	1.242* (8.49)	0.883* (−4.00)	0.895* (−3.51)
Ideology	1.184* (20.70)	1.143* (15.11)	0.870* (−20.46)	0.898* (−14.27)	1.276* (27.36)	1.170* (15.84)
Intercept	0.0652* (−36.36)	0.0863* (−31.28)	0.701* (−5.49)	0.613* (−7.24)	0.0636* (−32.75)	0.0989* (−26.21)
N	45666	45666	46197	46197	44428	44428

Exponentiated coefficients; t statstics in parentheses, * $p<0.05$

Fixed effects by canton. Observations clustered by household

The first two models estimate the impact of support for the SVP on a desire for Swiss advantage over foreigners – net their desire for Swiss advantage over foreigners in the previous year. We find that the odds of shifting from 0 to 1 on this variable are nearly doubled for those who support the SVP as compared to those who do not. This corroborates an account of attitudinal change that is guided by partisanship. In model 2 we also see that Social Democrats and Greens are less likely to adopt anti-immigrant attitudes, though substantively the effect is weaker than that of SVP preference.[6] There is no effect of Christian Democrat or Radical partisanship on shifting toward an anti-immigrant position. Education keeps people from adopting a preference for Swiss; age, female and rightist ideology promote this change.

Models 3 and 4 present the results for pro-environment attitudes. Green party supporters are substantially more likely to adopt pro-environment views – the odds of moving from a 0 to a 1 double for Green partisans compared to others. Unlike

[6]The reference category for partisanship in models 2, 4 and 6 are supporters of parties not listed in the model, those who would prefer a particular candidate instead of a party, those who "don't know" who they would vote for, and those who would not vote if an election were tomorrow.

other attitudes, the effect of partisanship is much weaker for the other parties and only supporters of the Radicals are slightly less likely to adopt pro-environment views. This makes sense given than economic growth is put forth as the opposing goal in the survey question about environmental protection. While Social Democratic and SVP partisanship are statistically significant, the effects are substantively minimal. Overall, these models point to a strong influence of the Green party on pro-environment attitudes. Education, age and rightist ideology make this shift less likely; female makes it more likely.

Models 5 and 6 present the results for aversion to social spending by the government. These attitudes offer the clearest divide along ideological lines with conservative party supporters more likely to favor a reduction in social spending and liberal parties less likely to favor a reduction in social spending. Nevertheless the expectation that the Radicals would exert the strongest effect on economic attitudes is not borne out – while the odds of Radical partisans favoring a reduction in spending is about 35% greater compared to the others, the odds of SVP partisans favoring a reduction is about 65% greater.[7] This result surprises us. We discuss it in our concluding section below. Green and Social Democrat supporters are much less likely to adopt an anti-spending perspective. Rightist ideology increases the odds of shifting to an anti-spending position; being well-educated, older and female reduces the odds of this shift.

Interestingly once prior attitudes and partisanship are accounted for the effect of ideology is modest in all of the models. For ideology to have an impact similar to SVP partisanship on anti-immigrant attitudes an individual would need to become substantially more conservative, moving about 3–4 positions on the left-right scale. Similarly, for pro-environment attitudes an individual would need to move at least 5 positions to the left to have an effect comparable to Green partisanship. Even on attitudes toward social spending, which arguably maps closest to the left-right scale of all the attitudes, the effect of ideology remains modest compared to partisanship. This supports the role of political parties in shaping attitudes on specific issues and suggests that those attitudes are not simply extensions of an individual's ideological leaning.[8]

We take one additional step in this analysis. Interaction models enable us to establish the age at which people's attitudes are most shaped by partisanship. This is important to examine for two main reasons. First, it serves as a robustness check. If in our models we are, indeed, capturing influence by parties, then this effect should be strongest for young people. Young citizens are the most malleable; their entry into the electoral system takes place during "impressionable years." As such, our narrative stands to be further refined by considering whether this is the case.

[7] Dropping the ideology variable only widens the impact gap between the SVP and Radicals.

[8] One might suspect that these models do not capture stable partisanship's effects; perhaps one changes one's views and then adopts the relevant partisan preference. To be more confident in our interpretation of partisan effects on attitudes, we tried a number of different configurations such as introducing lagged partisan variables and controlling for supporting the same relevant party in both t and t-1. None of these changes resulted in substantively different findings.

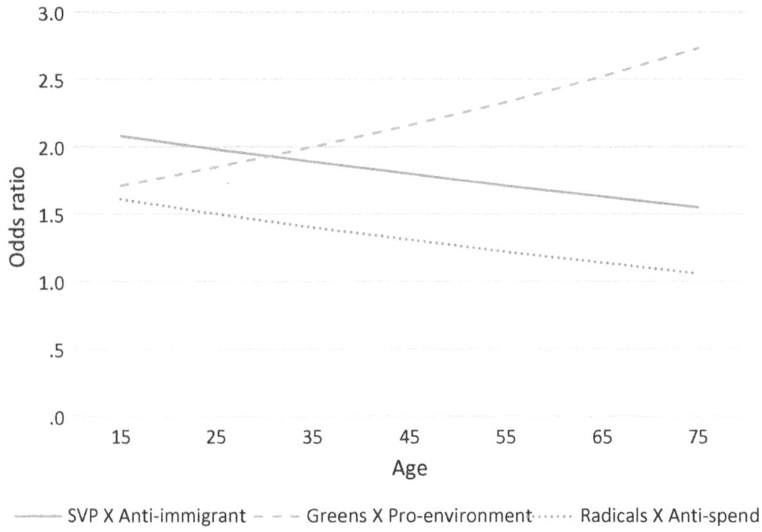

Fig. 13.3 Interaction effects: impact of partisan choice on attitude at different ages

Second, an interest in stability and change should consider not only past trends but likely future ones. Examining how Swiss citizens at different ages respond to partisan cues can help to predict future patterns in political behavior.

Three lagged dependent variable logit models provide the relevant evidence. They parallel models 1, 3, and 5 in Table 13.1 with the addition of an interaction between SVP support and Anti-immigrant attitudes, Greens support and Pro-environment attitudes and Radicals support and Anti-spend attitudes, respectively. We use lincom in Stata to estimate interactive effects. Full models are available from authors.

Figure 13.3 presents the identified patterns for party influence on shifts in key attitudes across ages. Each interaction coefficient is statistically significant at the .05 level. Starting with views on immigrants, we see that the impact of SVP support is strongest among those who are young. The odds of shifting to an anti-immigrant position are about doubled for SVP supporters who are twenty-five and younger. They are increased by 50% among those in their seventies. The same slope is identified for spending attitudes as they are shaped by support for the Radicals, though the effect over all is weaker.[9] For the youngest of respondents, the odds of preferring less social spending are 50% higher among those who choose the Radicals as compared to those who do not. But at the highest age range this effect is about null and is not statistically significant. The outlier in this figure is environmental attitudes. The impact of Green party support on a preference for environmental protection

[9] In response to Table 13.1, Model 6's finding that SVP support is the chief predictor of shifting to an anti-spend position, we also tested the interactive effect of SVP and age on spending views. The effect is not statistically significant.

actually strengthens across age groups. This implies that environmental opinions develop quite differently than do immigration and spending attitudes. We consider this below.

Discussion

Our theoretical point of departure for this chapter was contrasting narratives about partisan choice and attitudes. The classic model of electoral behavior in a democracy depicts a partisan choice motivated by policy preferences. A competing view posits that parties shape people's views on key issues. While each plot likely tells part of a valid give-and-take story of citizen behavior in democratic systems, we pursue a better understanding of how the latter process works. By studying political behavior at the individual level in Switzerland, where the electoral system has been in relative disarray for over a decade, we gain new insights into the relationships between partisanship and attitudes. In this concluding section we summarize our findings and consider the extent to which previous research did or did not prepare us for various aspects of our results.

We find that there has been a great deal of instability from 1 year to the next in people's views on immigrants, the environment and spending. The disorder of the electoral system previewed this finding. But these attitudes vary with respect to how stable they have been. Existing research predicted the relative patterns: immigration attitudes are the most stable, followed in succession by environmental attitudes and then spending preferences. For all three of these issues, attitudes appear to be stabilizing across the years of the survey; most of all for immigration attitudes, least of all for spending views.

We also find evidence that partisanship shapes people's stances on key political issues. The most convincing account can be drawn from our findings on immigration attitudes. Supporting the SVP is strongly associated (more than any other party) with a shift to preferring Swiss advantages over opportunities for immigrants. As attitudinal change theories would predict, the most influence-able are the young. We interpret our models to mean that a person who likes the SVP will adopt key aspects of the party program into their own set of policy preferences over time. The rise of the SVP, therefore, can be at least partly attributed to the party's ability to persuade voters to agree with them on matters associated with immigration. This is an important contribution to our understanding of electoral change in Switzerland, specifically the rise of the SVP.

The account of shifts in environmental and spending attitudes is less clear-cut. For the environment, the Green party plays a chief role, but its influence does not operate as attitudinal change theories would predict. Notably, the impact of Green party support on a pro-environment stance is strongest among the oldest, as opposed to the youngest respondents. Inglehart's value change thesis posits that environmental attitudes (among other post-materialist values) are strongest among younger generations due to the conditions under which they were raised. Young people's for the environment, therefore, would pre-date their entrance into the electoral process. Elder citizens may be the ones who need persuading, and the Green party picks things up from there.

As for opinions on spending, the Radicals have a strong effect on the choice to desire less social spending, but the SVP's effect is—unexpectedly—greater. We suspect that the stronger impact of SVP than Radicals support on anti-spending views is a function of SVP rhetoric about government spending on immigrants. Past work shows that European publics consider immigrants to be particularly undeserving of welfare spending (van Oorschot 2006). This result might also be a function of SVP preference for devolved spending at the cantonal and communal levels since the survey question specifically asks about confederation spending. Both possible interpretations signal that the issue of spending may have morphed over the years in the public dialogue and the public mind.

Overall, our analysis tells a story of significant change but increased stability in recent years. Looking ahead, we predict greater tumult in citizen views on public spending. We also anticipate that the youngest voters will continue to be influenced by the SVP on immigration attitudes. In terms of theory building in political science, our findings signal that greater attention to the socializing role of political parties will enhance our understanding of democratic citizens' political behavior.

References

Alwin, D. F., & Krosnick, J. A. (1991). Aging, cohorts, and the stability of sociopolitical orientations over the life span. *American Journal of Sociology, 97*(1), 169–195.

Blekesaune, M., & Quadagno, J. (2003). Public attitudes toward welfare state policies: A comparative analysis of 24 nations. *European Sociological Review, 19*(5), 415–427.

Brooks, C., & Manza, J. (2008). *Why welfare states persist: The importance of public opinion in democracies*. Chicago: University of Chicago Press.

Campbell, A., Converse, P. E., Miller, W. E., & Stokes, D. E. (1960). *The American voter*. New York: Wiley.

Downs, A. (1957). *An economic theory of democracy*. New York: Harper and Row.

Fetzer, J. S. (2000). *Public attitudes toward immigration in the United States, France, and Germany*. Cambridge, UK: Cambridge University Press.

Funk, P., & Gathmann, C. (2006). What women want: Suffrage, gender gaps in voter preferences and government expenditures. Available at SSRN: http://ssrn.com/abstract=913802 or https://doi.org/10.2139/ssrn.913802 . Accessed on 5 Sep 2016.

Hainmueller, J., & Hiscox, M. J. (2007). Educated preferences: Explaining attitudes toward immigration in Europe. *International Organization, 61*(2), 399–442.

Hug, S., & Schulz, T. (2007). Left-right positions of political parties in Switzerland. *Party Politics, 13*(3), 305–330.

Inglehart, R. (1997). *Modernization and post-modernization*. Princeton: Princeton University Press.

Kriesi, H., & Trechsel, A. H. (2008). *The politics of Switzerland: Continuity and change in a consensus democracy*. Cambridge, UK: Cambridge University Press.

Kuhn, U. (2009). Stability and change in party preference. *Swiss Political Science Review, 15*(3), 463–494.

Ladner, A. (2001). Swiss political parties: Between persistence and change. *West European Politics, 24*(2), 123–144.

Lodge, M., & Taber, C. S. (2000). Three steps toward a theory of motivated reasoning." Ch. 9 in. In A. Lupia & M. D. McCubbins (Eds.), *Elements of reason: Cognition, choice, and the bounds of rationality* (pp. 182–213). New York: Cambridge University Press.

McGann, A. J., & Kitschelt, H. (2005). The radical right in the alps: Evolution of support for the Swiss SVP and Austrian FPÖ. *Party Politics, 11*(2), 147–171.

Miller, W. E. (2000). Temporal order and causal inference. *Political Analysis, 8*(2), 119–146.

Sears, D. O., & Funk, C. (1999). Evidence of long-term persistence of adults' political predispositions. *Journal of Politics, 61*(1), 1–28.

Sniderman, P. M., & Levendusky, M. S. (2007). Chapter 23: An institutional theory of political choice. In R. J. Dalton & H. Klingemann (Eds.), *The Oxford handbook of political behavior* (pp. 437–456). Oxford: Oxford University Press.

Swiss Federal Statistical Office. (2016). Available at http://www.bfs.admin.ch. Accessed Feb 2016.

Van Oorschot, W. (2006). Making the difference in social Europe: Deservingness perceptions among citizens of European welfare states. *Journal of European Social Policy, 16*(1), 23–42.

Chapter 14
What Explains Increasing Euroscepticism in Switzerland? A Longitudinal Analysis

Oriane Sarrasin, Theresa Kuhn, and Bram Lancee

Switzerland and the European Union

On paper everything—or almost everything—points toward Switzerland being part of the European Union (EU). Indeed, this small but wealthy nation is situated at the heart of continental Europe, speaks three languages[1] of EU members (German, French and Italian) and shares strong economic ties with EU members. Nonetheless the EU has never won Swiss hearts, or at least enough of them. In 1992 the Swiss people voted against joining the European Economic Area (EEA) by a short majority (50.3%) of the voters and a comfortable majority of 18 cantons (Trechsel 2007). The country was clearly divided: Most members of the political and economic elite were in favour to joining the EEA, leading to an endorsement of 67% in Parliament, while the populist right-wing Swiss People's Party (SVP) led the opposition. Among Swiss citizens, those with a tertiary education or with a high income tended to support the EEA (Kriesi et al. 1993). There were strong regional disparities too, with Pro-EEA voters to be found mostly among the Swiss French: all French-speaking cantons voted "yes" with approval rates up to 79%, while almost all German-speaking cantons and Ticino rejected it (Trechsel 2007).

[1] The fourth national language—Rumantsch—is spoken in Switzerland only.

O. Sarrasin (✉)
Faculty of Social and Political Sciences, University of Lausanne, Lausanne, Switzerland
e-mail: oriane.sarrasin@unil.ch

T. Kuhn
Department of Political Science, University of Amsterdam, Amsterdam, Netherlands
e-mail: Theresa.kuhn@uva.nl

B. Lancee
Department of Sociology, University of Amsterdam, Amsterdam, Netherlands
e-mail: B.Lancee@uva.nl

R. Tillmann et al. (eds.), *Social Dynamics in Swiss Society*, Life Course Research and Social Policies 9, https://doi.org/10.1007/978-3-319-89557-4_14

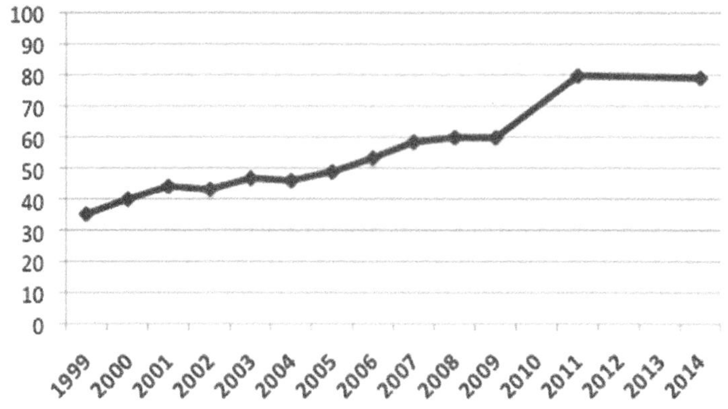

Fig. 14.1 Share of SHP respondents (Swiss citizens, aged minimum 15) who declared being unwilling to join the EU, from 1999 to 2014 (missing years are interpolated)

Reluctance to join the EU has consistently increased since then (see Fig. 14.1, based on the data used in the present chapter). In 2001, following an initiative launched by a pro-European movement (i.e., the European Movement Switzerland), Swiss people clearly voted against (76.8%) opening the negotiations in sight of a potential adhesion to the EU. In 2016, a year after Iceland had withdrawn its application for membership and just days before the United Kingdom voted in favour of a "Brexit", Switzerland officially withdrew its application, which dated from 1992. This was the final step in a gradual decline of the interest of Swiss citizens to be part of the EU. Instead of a full membership to the EU, Switzerland has opted for an 'Alleingang' strategy: staying outside the EU, but maintaining strong economic ties with its members. This "middle way" solution takes the form of bilateral agreements that are very close to the EEA treaty. For instance, Switzerland is part of the Schengen Area, in which the free movement of people is guaranteed. However, even these bilateral agreements have been put into question after the Swiss people decided to limit the free movement of non-Swiss citizens to Switzerland through the so-called "mass immigration" initiative in February 2014 (Ambühl and Zürcher 2015).

While without any doubt there has been a strong decline in the share of Swiss citizens willing to join the EU since the 1990s, there is, to our knowledge, no longitudinal analysis of how changes within individuals affect their attitudes toward the EU. Indeed, while macro factors such as the 2008 economic crisis undoubtedly played a role in explaining the overall decline in support for joining the EU among Swiss citizens, individual life course changes may also explain why many of them withdrew their support for joining the EU at some point in their life. Literature on Euroscepticism in Switzerland (Christin and Trechsel 2002; Skinner 2013; Theiler 2004) has highlighted how, as they do elsewhere (Hooghe and Marks 2005; Hobolt and de Vries 2016), economic and political/cultural factors shape Swiss citizens' reactions to the EU. Extending this examination, we hypothesize that changes in these factors (e.g., a worsening personal financial situation, political ideologies leaning toward the right) may lead to decline in EU support among Swiss citizens that were initially pro-EU. We tested these hypotheses with data from the Swiss Household Panel (1999–2014).

Predicting Unwillingness to Join EU among Swiss Citizens

Economic Factors

Economic factors certainly play a role in influencing Swiss citizens' attitudes toward the EU. Switzerland is one the wealthiest countries of the European continent, with its gross domestic product growing every year despite the various financial crises that have hit its neighbours (Swiss State Secretariat for Economic Affairs—SECO, 2016a). For example, Switzerland has a very low unemployment rate (3.2% in August 2016; SECO, 2016b). In such a prosperous context, Swiss citizens could fear that the country—and/or themselves directly—may lose by joining the EU (Schwok 2010). The fears may be particularly strong among the so-called "losers of globalization" (Kriesi et al. 2008). According to Gabel (1998), to understand who is winning or losing from EU membership, it is necessary to assess individuals' comparative advantage: Low skilled workers (e.g., with low educational attainment, low income or in low status occupations) from high-wage countries such as Switzerland face increased competition from workers from member states with lower wages, while highly skilled citizens of these countries are less affected by international competition. In a similar vein, it has been argued that the withdrawal of economic political borders resulting from EU membership benefits foremost to those who are mobile and connected (e.g., who have transnational ties or networks; Kuhn 2011). These "winners of globalization" possess the resources to cope with their country opening its borders. On the contrary, those depending more on local dynamics may fear that too much is at stake if their country joins the EU.

In line with this argument, European citizens who are worried for their personal as well as the national financial situations (Gabel 1998; Hooghe and Marks 2005) were found to report higher levels of Euroscepticism. Similar results were found in the case of European citizens with a lower income (Lubbers and Scheepers 2007). In addition, European citizens with fewer transnational ties (e.g., who were less likely to have lived abroad or to have socialised with non-nationals) were also found to be more Eurosceptic (Kuhn 2011). In Switzerland, the willingness to join the EEA in 1992 was found to be stronger among Swiss citizens with high income and high educational attainment (Kriesi et al. 1993). Ten years later, Christin and Trechsel (2002) found that Swiss citizens' level of concern about the economy in Switzerland was one of the central factors predicting their reluctance to join the EU. Based on this evidence, we hypothesize that low skilled Swiss citizens (e.g., in low status occupations or with low educational attainment) are less likely to support joining the EU (H1). In addition, Swiss citizens who perceive their personal financial situation as difficult are more likely to be reluctant to join the EU (H2a).

Extending this reasoning, we expect a worsening personal financial situation to be accompanied with more negative attitudes toward the EU (H2b).

Political and Cultural Factors

The bulk of research on Euroscepticism has highlighted that cultural and political factors play a crucial role in predicting individuals' attitudes toward the EU. Indeed, public opinion toward the EU is driven by more than purely rational and utilitarian considerations (see for instance McLaren 2002). Among the numerous political and cultural factors that have been shown to shape individuals' attitudes toward the EU,[2] we focus here on some political ideologies and attitudes that are likely to play a prominent role in the Swiss opposition to the EU.

A first political factor that is expected to drive Swiss citizens' attitudes toward the EU is their political orientation. Most studies on the relationship between political left-right ideology and EU attitudes have provided empirical support for the so-called "horseshoe model": Europeans at the left and right fringes of the political spectrum are more Eurosceptic than voters of mainstream parties (Aspinwall 2002; De Vries and Edwards 2009). While voters on left end are critical of the neo-liberal nature of European economic integration, right-wing Eurosceptics are motivated by the fear that European integration undermines the cultural integrity of their nation (Van Elsas et al. 2016).

By way of contrast the Swiss EU-opposition has been mostly led by right-wing parties, especially the radical right and populist Swiss People's Party (Schweizerische Volkspartei—SVP; Mazzoleni 2016). Constantly on the rise from the 1980s to the early 2010s, the SVP is now the strongest party in Switzerland with more than a quarter of the seats at the Federal Assembly (Swiss Parliament 2016). To a lesser extent, the center-right party Freisinnig-Demokratische Partei (FDP) also opposes EU membership but is generally open to bilateral agreements with the EU (Skinner 2013). Contrary to other non-EU members (e.g., Norway), Swiss left-wing political parties tend to support an adhesion to the EU (Skinner 2013). Because of this right-left divide when it comes to the EU among Swiss political parties, we expect Swiss citizens who subscribe to right-wing ideologies to oppose joining the EU to a greater

[2] Political and cultural factors other than those under consideration here (e.g., national identity, and fears of losing specific Swiss institutions such as neutrality or direct democracy) were shown to shape Swiss citizens' reluctance to join the EU (see Schwok 2010). Since no question about these specific points was asked in the SHP, they cannot be investigated in the present chapter. Regarding national identity, people who exclusively identify with their own country are more likely to be Eurosceptic than individuals who identify (also) as European (Citrin and Sides 2004; Hooghe and Marks 2004) In Switzerland, attachment to the nation is especially high in the German-speaking region (Green et al. 2011), where the strongest opposition to the EU is also found (Theiler 2004). Attitudes toward joining the EU are also more negative in the Italian-speaking region than in the French-speaking region. For this reason and since there is no measure of national identity in the SHP, we account for the linguistic region in our analyses.

extent than Swiss citizens with left-wing political ideologies (H3a). In addition, having one's political orientation moving toward the right should be accompanied with more negative attitudes toward the EU (H3b).

Related to claims at the heart of SVP argumentation, a second political factor that likely plays a role is people's subjective feeling of lack of political influence. Like many other populist parties, SVP often argues that the voice of Swiss citizens are not sufficiently heard by the government and authorities, and that citizens should decide for themselves. Consequently, Switzerland should bypass international regulations. An example is the on-going campaign on "Swiss self-determination", an SVP initiative to make Swiss law prime over international laws and rules (SVP 2016). We thus expect that Swiss citizens who feel that they have no political influence are more likely to oppose joining the EU (H4a). Furthermore, increasing feelings of lack of political influence should result in a stronger reluctance to join the EU (H4b).

Data

The nature of our hypotheses—predicting differences between individuals and within individuals, requires panel data. We therefore analyzed data from the Swiss Household Panel (1999–2014), the only longitudinal survey in Switzerland that contains questions regarding Swiss citizens' willingness to join the EU. We restricted our sample to Swiss citizens, aged at least 15 ($M = 46.26$, $SD = 17.61$). Missing data for the dependent variable were omitted (with the exception of years where the EU item was not included, see below). This resulted in 75,565 observations provided by 14,436 respondents (5.23 observations on average per respondent). There were slightly more female respondents (55.17%). Reflecting the linguistic division of Switzerland, the majority of respondents (70.60%) lived in the German-speaking region (French-speaking region: 25.77%, Italian-speaking region: 3.63%).

Measures

Dependent variable Swiss citizens' reluctance to join the EU was measured with the following item: "Are you in favour of Switzerland joining the European Union or are you in favour of Switzerland staying outside of the European Union?" Possible answers were 1 = "in favour of joining the EU", 2 = "Neither" or 3 = "In favour of staying outside the EU." Because we study *unwillingness* to join the EU, we created a dichotomous variable: 1 = staying outside the EU vs. 0 = else. Note that this item was not included in the survey in 2010, 2012 and 2013. For these years the missing value was imputed with the value of the previous year. Altogether, the share of respondents who favoured staying outside the EU increased from 35.2% in 1999 to 78.9%[3] in 2014 (see Fig. 14.1).

Independent variables First, a set of variables was used to distinguish between the potential winners and losers of globalization. Skills (H1) were measured with respondents' occupational prestige and educational attainment. Occupational prestige was measured with the Cambridge Social Interaction and Stratification Scale (CAMSIS), a continuous instrument that relies on social interactions to estimate individuals' social status (for the Swiss version, see Bergman et al. 2002). Possible CAMSIS scores range from 0 to 100 (in the present data: from 9.50 to 97.15, $M = 56.08$, $SD = 14.32$). Education was measured as the highest level of education; we reduced a 17-category scale to a 6-category one (see Bergman et al. 2009): Primary education (15.05%), secondary without high school diploma (Matura, in Switzerland; 1.31%), secondary with Matura (10.53%), secondary vocational (43.98%), tertiary vocational (16.82%) and university (12.32%).

Respondents' perception of their financial situation (H2) was evaluated with the following item: "Overall how satisfied are you with the financial situation of your household". Possible answers range from 0 = not at all satisfied to 10 = completely satisfied ($M = 7.52$, $SD = 1.94$). We focused on the household's financial situation instead of one's individual finical position because a considerable share of respondents did not work (e.g., housewives, students, minors). Furthermore, finances are most often organised at the household level, rather than at the individual level. In the case of respondents who reported being in employment, we also took into account their perceived risk of unemployment in the next 12 months (from 0 = no risk at all to 10 = a real risk; $M = 1.86$, $SD = 2.37$). When it comes to political factors, respondents were first asked where they placed themselves, from 0 = left to 10 = right (H3; $M = 4.83$, $SD = 2.12$). Their perceived political influence (H4) was measured with scale ranging from 0 = no influence to 10 = a very strong influence ($M = 3.87$, $SD = 2.55$).

Control variables Age and gender (1 = male) were included as younger generations (Down and Wilson 2013) and men (Nelsen and Guth 2000) have been shown to be more supportive of European integration. We also considered whether participants had another citizenship (1 = bi- or tri-national; 10.92%), since those with a transnational background tend to be less Eurosceptic (Kuhn 2011). Respondents' labour force status was tapped with the following categorical scale: working full time (reference; 35.95%), working part time (23.18%), studying (11.80%), being a home carer (9.10%), being retired (16.96%), being unemployed (1.00%), and other occupation (2.00%). We then controlled for respondents' interest in politics, from 0 = not at all interested to 10 = very interested ($M = 5.69$, $SD = 2.71$). Finally, because there are known marked differences in support for joining the EU across the Swiss linguistic regions, we considered where respondents lived: We created two dichotomous variables (Swiss German versus and Swiss Italian versus other, with Swiss French as a reference category).

[3] Please note that all analyses were conducted on unweighted data.

Results

Because of the dichotomous nature of the dependent variable we estimated logit regressions; odd ratios are displayed in the tables. We first estimated random effects (RE) models. RE models use both between-person and within-person variance to estimate coefficients. In a second step, we analyse changes *within* individuals by estimating fixed-effects (FE) models. As FE models only estimate within-individual changes, one cannot include variables for which there were no changes (such as gender or the linguistic region). Finally, because some variables affect only those working (i.e., occupational prestige and probability of losing one's job), we estimated additional RE and FE models including only employed individuals.

Differences between Respondents

Results are displayed in Table 14.1, left column. Confirming our hypothesis (H1), Swiss citizens with higher educational attainment (with a Matura or a tertiary degree compared to those with primary education only) were less likely to be Eurosceptic. Note that respondents with secondary education (without Matura) and secondary vocational education did not differ from those with primary education only. In addition and as hypothesized (H2a), respondents who reported not being satisfied with the state of their household finances were less likely to support joining the EU. When it comes to political and cultural factors, as expected (H3a), self-reported right-wing ideologies were related to a higher probably to reject the EU. Contrary to our expectations (H4a), the more respondents felt that they had a political influence, the more they opposed the EU.

In line with previous literature on Euroscepticism, male and older respondents reported being less willing to join the EU. Students and retired people were more likely to oppose EU membership than citizens working full time, while home carers were less likely. The less interest in politics they expressed, the more respondents were likely to oppose joining the EU. Finally, respondents living in the German- and Italian-speaking regions were more likely to oppose joining the EU than those living in the French-speaking region.

Results of additional analyses performed with respondents in (full or part time) employment are displayed in the right column of Table 14.1. As hypothesized (H1), a higher socsial status was related to a lower probability to oppose joining the EU. Though in the expected direction, the probability to be unemployed within the next 12 months was only marginally significantly related to attitudes toward the EU (H3a).

Table 14.1 Logisitic RE regression predicting unwillingness to join the EU (whole sample and sample restricted to respondents in employment), odd ratios

	Whole sample		In employment	
	OR	(SE)	OR	(SE)
Age	1.05***	(0.00)	1.09***	(0.00)
Male	1.41***	(0.10)	1.53***	(0.16)
Dual citizenship	1.24*	(0.11)	1.14	(0.15)
Education (ref. = primary)				
Secondary w/o Matura	0.75	(0.18)	0.35*	(0.15)
Secondary with Matury	0.60***	(0.06)	0.31***	(0.07)
Secondary vocational	1.03	(0.09)	0.56**	(0.11)
Tertiary vocational	1.22†	(0.13)	0.76	(0.16)
University	0.71**	(0.08)	0.42***	(0.10)
Labour status (ref. = full time)				
Part time	0.92	(0.06)	0.97	(0.07)
Studying	1.84***	(0.16)		
Home carer	0.66***	(0.06)		
Retired	1.28**	(0.10)		
Unemployed	1.27	(0.19)		
Other occupation	1.05	(0.15)		
Satis. With hh finances	0.95***	(0.01)	0.98†	(0.01)
Unemployment risk			1.02†	(0.01)
CAMSIS			0.97***	(0.00)
Political orientation	1.35***	(0.01)	1.43***	(0.02)
Political interest	0.87***	(0.01)	0.84***	(0.01)
Political influence	1.03***	(0.01)	1.03**	(0.01)
Linguistic region (ref. = French)				
German-speaking	6.56***	0.53	8.70***	1.00
Italian speaking	5.43***	0.98	9.17***	2.50
Constant	0.03	0.01	0.05	0.02

*** $p < .001$; ** $p < .01$; two-sided tests
Source: SHP 1999–2014

Changes within Respondents

Results are displayed in Table 14.2, left column. Only a few within-individual changes yielded a significant impact on attitudes toward the EU. Contrary to our expectations, *changes* in economic factors were not accompanied with a change in attitudes toward the EU (H2b). When it comes to political factors, increasingly right-wing political attitudes (H2b) were significantly related to a higher probability to oppose joining the EU (H3b). By way of contrast, changes in feelings of political influence had no impact (H4b). When it comes to the control variables, reaching

Table 14.2 Logisitic FE regression predicting unwillingness to join the EU (whole sample and sample restricted to respondents in employment), odd ratios

	Whole sample		In employment	
	OR	(SE)	OR	(SE)
Age	1.38***	0.01	1.41***	0.01
Education (ref. = primary)				
Secondary w/o Matura	1.18	0.49	0.46	0.45
Secondary with Matury	0.95	0.13	4.56†	3.96
Secondary vocational	0.84	0.13	2.18	1.78
Tertiary vocational	0.88	0.17	3.10	2.56
University	1.09	0.24	3.40	2.97
Labour status (ref. = full time)				
Part time	0.95	0.08	1.03	0.11
Studying	0.95	0.12		
Home carer	0.91	0.12		
Retired	1.35*	0.16		
Unemployed	1.00	0.19		
Other occupation	0.98	0.19		
Satis. with hh finances	1.02	0.01	1.02	0.02
Unemployment risk			0.99	0.01
CAMSIS			0.99	0.01
Political orientation	1.10***	0.01	1.10**	0.02
Political interest	0.95***	0.01	0.94***	0.02
Political influence	0.99	0.01	1.01	0.01

*** $p < 001$; ** $p < 01$; * $p < 05$; † $p < 10$; two-sided tests
Source: SHP 1999–2014

retirement and a decreasing interest in politics were related to more negative attitudes toward the EU. Finally, additional analyses performed on respondents in employment (Table 14.2, right column) show that, contrary to our expectations (H1b and H2b), neither a lower social status nor an increased probability to be unemployed are related to a higher probability to oppose joining the EU.

Conclusion

The analyses we performed on the SHP data (1999–2014) provided results in line with previous literature on Euroscepticism: Both economic and political factors matter in shaping Swiss citizens' attitudes toward the EU. On the one side, the so-called losers of globalization—that is, those who are less likely to benefit from an adhesion to the EU (e.g., individuals with low skills)—were found to be more likely to oppose joining the EU. On the other side, individuals who report right-wing political ideologies reported a stronger opposition than those with left-wing ideologies.

Analyzing changes within individuals—which is rarely done when investigating attitudes toward the EU—sheds further light on the respective weight of economic and political factors. Moving toward the right side of the political spectrum was related to an increased probability to oppose joining the EU. This illustrates the relationship, in Switzerland, between radical right or populist ideologies and the willingness to shut (or remain close) Switzerland's boundaries. In contrast, changes in individual's life course were largely unrelated to changes in attitudes toward the EU. While economic factors explain variation between individual's attitudes towards joining the EU, transitions within individuals could not be related to changes in attitudes. This suggests that the bulk of the overall decline in joining the EU among Swiss citizens may be due to macro-factors (e.g., economic crises). It might also be that joining the EU is not seen as impacting individuals' life, hence the lack of effect from changes in personal financial situation. Overall, this is in line with the argument that apparent divide between the losers and winners of globalization may be more cultural than utilitarian. For instance, when it comes to attitudes toward immigration in Switzerland, it has been found that most of the differences between lowly and highly educated are in place before young people start education (Lancee and Sarrasin 2015). Thus, the impact of education—often attributed to the acquisition of skills–is likely to be explained by the social origins of individuals. A similar mechanism may be at play with regard to attitudes toward the EU.

To sum up, it seems highly unlikely that Swiss citizens will decide to join the EU at any time in the future. Furthermore, the more they will move to the right of the political spectrum, the more they will move away from the EU. For this reason, future research on the topic should concentrate on attitudes toward the bilateral agreements, such as investigated in the SHP in 2012 and 2015. This is all the more relevant since Swiss citizens' decisions—such as limiting immigration to Switzerland—may call into question these agreements.

References

Ambühl, M., & Zürcher, S. (2015). Immigration and Swiss-EU free movement of persons: Question of a safeguard clause. *Swiss Political Science Review, 21*, 76–98.

Aspinwall, M. (2002). Preferring Europe ideology and national preferences on European integration. *European Union Politics, 3*, 81–111.

Bergman, M. M., Lambert, P., Prandy, K., & Joye, D. (2002). Theorization, construction and validation of a social stratification scale: Cambridge social interaction and stratification scale (CAMSIS) for Switzerland. *Swiss Review of Sociology, 28*, 7–25.

Bergman, M., Hupka, S., Joyce, D., & Meier, T. (2009). *Recodification de la formation dans les enquêtes*. Basel: Basel University.

Christin, T., & Trechsel, A. H. (2002). Joining the EU? Explaining public opinion in Switzerland. *European Union Politics, 3*, 415–443.

Citrin, J., & Sides, J. (2004). More than nationals: How identity choice matters in the new Europe. In R. Herrmann, M. Brewer, & T. Risse (Eds.), *Transnational isdentities: Becoming European in the EU* (pp. 161–185). Lanham: Rowman & Littlefield.

De Vries, C., & Edwards, E. (2009). Taking Europe to its extremes: Extremist parties and public Euroscepticism. *Party Politics, 15*, 5–28.

Down, I., & Wilson, C. J. (2013). A rising generation of Europeans? Life-cycle and cohort effects on support for 'Europe'. *European Journal of Political Research, 52*, 431–456.

Gabel, M. (1998). *Interests and integration: Market liberalization, public opinion, and European Union*. Ann Arbor: University of Michigan Press.

Green, E. G. T., Sarrasin, O., Fasel, N., & Staerklé, C. (2011). Nationalism and patriotism as predictors of immigration attitudes in Switzerland: A municipality-level analysis. *Swiss Political Science Review, 17*, 369–393.

Hobolt, S. B., & de Vries, C. E. (2016). Public support for European integration. *Annual Review of Political Science, 19*, 413–432.

Hooghe, L., & Marks, G. (2004). Does identity or economic rationality drive public opinion on European integration? *PS-Political Science & Politics, 37*, 415–420.

Hooghe, L., & Marks, G. (2005). Calculation, community, and cues: Public opinion on European integration. *European Union Politics, 6*, 421–445.

Kriesi, H., Longchamp, C., Passy, F., & Sciarini, P. (1993). *Analyse der eidgenössischen Abstimmung vom 6. Dezember 1992. VOX Nr* (p. 47). GfS and DSP: Adliswil.

Kriesi, H., et al. (2008). *West European politics in the age of globalization*. Cambridge: Cambridge University Press.

Kuhn, T. (2011). Individual transnationalism, globalisation and euroscepticism: An empirical test of Deutsch's transactionalist theory. *European Journal of Political Research, 50*, 811–837.

Lancee, B., & Sarrasin, O. (2015). Educated preferences or selection effects? A longitudinal analysis of the impact of educational attainment on attitudes toward immigrants. *European Sociological Review, 31*, 490–501.

Lubbers, M., & Scheepers, P. (2007). Explanations of political euro-scepticism at the individual, regional and national levels. *European Societies, 9*, 643–669.

Mazzoleni, O. (2016). Between opposition and government: The Swiss People's party. In F. Decker, B. Henningsen, & K. Jakobsen (Eds.), *Rechtspopulismus und Rechstextremismus in Europa: Die Herausforderung der Zivilgesellschaft durch alte Ideologien und neue Medien* (pp. 110–118). Baden-Baden: Nosmos Verlag.

McLaren, L. (2002). Public support for the European Union: Cost/benefit analysis or perceived cultural threat. *Journal of Politics, 64*, 551–566.

Nelsen, B., & Guth, B. (2000). Exploring the gender gap: Women, men and public attitudes toward European integration. *European Union Politics, 1*, 267–291.

Schwok, R. (2010). Suisse – Union européenne : L'adhésion impossible? Lausanne: Presses Polytechniques et Universitaires Romandes,. Collection Le Savoir Suisse.

Skinner, M. S. (2013). Different varieties of Euroscepticism? Conceptualizing and explaining Euroscepticism in western European non-member states. *Journal of Common Market Studies, 51*, 122–139.

State Secretariat for Economic Affairs. (2016a). GDP quarterly estimates. Retrieved from https://www.seco.admin.ch/seco/en/home/wirtschaftslage---wirtschaftspolitik/Wirtschaftslage/bip-quartalsschaetzungen-.html

State Secretariat for Economic Affairs. (2016b). Arbeitslosenquote nach Kantonen [unemployment rate per canton]. Retrieved from https://www.amstat.ch/v2/?lang=de

Swiss Parliament. (2016). *Council members*. Retrieved from https://www.parlament.ch/en/ratsmitglieder?k=*.

Swiss People Party. (2016). *Volksinitiative „Schweizer Recht statt fremde Richter (Selbstbestimmungsinitiative)*. Retrieved from http://www.svp.ch/kampagnen/uebersicht/selbstbestimmungsinitiative/um-was-geht-es/

Theiler, T. (2004). The origins of Euroscepticism in German-speaking Switzerland. *European Journal of Political Research, 43*, 635–656.

Trechsel, A. (2007). Direct democracy and European integration: A limited obstacle. In C. Church (Ed.), *Switzerland and the European Union: A close, contradictory and misunderstood relationship* (pp. 36–51). London: Routledge.

Van Elsas, E. J., Hakhverdian, A., & van der Brug, W. (2016). United against a common foe? The nature and origins of Euroscepticism among left-wing and right-wing citizens. *West European Politics, advance online publication.*

Chapter 15
Economic Context and Attitudes towards the Welfare State: The Relationship between (Perceived) Unemployment Risk and Demand for Social Policy

Nicolas Pekari, Jan Rosset, and Flurina Schmid

Introduction

Preferences regarding the welfare state and redistributive policies have attracted much scholarly attention in the past decades (Lupu and Pontusson 2011; Svallfors 2012). One of the main reasons is that these preferences are expected to influence individuals' electoral choices and thus impact public policy. Therefore, they are seen as crucial for understanding cross-country differences or temporal evolution in the shape or size of welfare states in democracies (Meltzer and Richard 1981; Svallfors 1997). Individual preferences are also expected to be shaped by a potentially changing context. Changing levels of inequality or changing levels of unemployment rates for instance should in theory influence the size and composition of groups potentially benefitting from or contributing to the welfare state and thus shape the incentive of favouring certain type of policy (Meltzer and Richard 1981; Rehm 2009). However, most of the studies on the topic have analysed the influence of the context across countries rather than over time and those that look at the evolution of attitudes towards the welfare state within specific countries have focused mainly on Anglo-Saxon countries. These studies tend to show a rather limited impact of a changing context on preferences, even in times of a dramatic change of economic conditions such as the recent Great Recession (Brooks and Manza 2013; Margalit 2013; Soroka and Wlezien 2014).[1]

[1] See however Rosset and Pontusson (2014) who document a trend for an increased demand for redistribution among middle income groups in those western European countries that were most severely hit by the crisis.

N. Pekari (✉) · F. Schmid
FORS-Swiss Centre of Expertise in the Social Sciences, Lausanne, Switzerland
e-mail: nicolas.pekari@fors.unil.ch

J. Rosset
University of Geneva, Geneva, Switzerland
e-mail: jan.rosset@unige.ch

R. Tillmann et al. (eds.), *Social Dynamics in Swiss Society*, Life Course Research and Social Policies 9, https://doi.org/10.1007/978-3-319-89557-4_15

Although economic conditions have not changed in Switzerland as much as in many other European countries during the Great Recession (Ball 2014; OECD 2013a, b), this case is relevant for the study of the evolution of public opinion regarding the welfare state. Indeed, Swiss direct democratic institutions allow civil society actors to put new topics on the agenda (popular initiative) or to oppose decisions taken by representatives by organising popular votes on specific bills. This means that citizens regularly vote on specific policies and that public opinion is thus likely to be particularly influential. Another interesting factor is the rise, over the last two decades, of a right-wing populist party, the Swiss People's Party (SVP), which has almost tripled its vote share since the early 1990's and moved the position of Swiss representative bodies more towards the right of the political spectrum. While this could itself be a sign of a shift of Swiss public opinion away from the welfare state, the situation might be more ambiguous because this electoral shift is concomitant with an increased importance of non-economic issues in Swiss electoral politics, with notably issues such as immigration or European integration becoming more salient (Bornschier 2015). Given that citizens' preferences on those cultural issues do not correlate with their stances on economic issues (Rosset et al. 2016) and the rise of importance of the former set of issues, it cannot be assumed that economic preferences of the Swiss are directly reflected in their electoral choice. It is therefore particularly interesting to explore how Swiss public opinion has evolved on issues related to social policy since the turn of the millennium.

For the period from 1999 to 2014, the Swiss household panel (SHP) provides individual level data on preferences with regard to several dimensions of the welfare state and include measures of risk perception which is relatively rare for generalist surveys. Making use of this data, the goal of this chapter is, on the one hand, to describe the evolution of political attitudes towards the welfare state of Swiss residents over the 1999–2014 period and, on the other hand, to test some of the theories explaining opinion formation at the individual level.

Our analyses show that overall levels of public support for social policy have not dramatically changed. There has been, however, a shift in the nature of policies that attract more support and meaning that the level of support for social spending and for more progressive taxation is quite different in 2014 as it used to be 15 years earlier. On the one hand there has been an increase in the share of Swiss residents calling for higher taxes on high incomes, but on the other hand, a decrease in support for social spending. The decrease in support for social spending seems at odds with the fact that an increasing proportion of Swiss feel at risk of losing their job. We explain this apparent contradiction to our finding that individual preferences are relatively weakly affected by changing economic conditions.

We focus on attitudes towards unemployment benefits to show that whereas objective levels of risk are associated with preferences towards unemployment benefits, the relationship between one's risk profile and preferences is mainly a result of structural factors such as education or economic status. The role of deeply rooted social structures for the preferences regarding unemployment benefits suggests that changes in economic conditions and unemployment rates in particular are likely to only partially translate into citizen's preferences.

The chapter is structured as follows: the next section discusses the literature on the welfare state and on the Swiss political context. We then turn to an analysis of overall trends in support for levels of taxation for the rich and social spending and relate these trends to changes in the level of perceived economic insecurity. The next section is devoted to an individual-level analysis that focuses on the relationship between objective economic conditions to policy preferences by addressing the link between objective and perceived risk and then perceived risk and preferences for redistribution. The remainder of the chapter discusses the results and concludes.

Preferences for the Welfare State and the Role of the Economic Context

Attitudes towards the welfare state have been extensively studied using various sources of survey data. While early research has mainly focused on general support for the welfare state (or redistribution) and on the role of individuals' economic status in explaining their preferences, recent studies have brought several refinements. First, it appears that preferences towards the welfare state cannot be summarized simply in terms of support or opposition towards the welfare state but that they vary in relation to different dimensions of the welfare state. Being in favour of a specific social policy - say unemployment benefit – does not mean that individuals will also endorse other facets of the welfare state such as for instance health insurance or pensions. In addition to support for specific areas of the welfare state, the public seems to have quite contrasted views on two different but complementary aspects of social policies. These can be primarily understood on the one hand as ways of taking economic means "from the rich" or, on the other hand, as ways of "giving them to the poor" (Cavaillé and Trump 2015). Support for each of these aspects of the welfare state can be explained by different individual characteristics and the study of social policy attitudes needs to take both of these facets into account. Second, it appears that even if self-interest plays a role in the formation of preferences with regard to social policy, the definition of this self-interest is multi-faceted also. To put it simply, individuals do not simply differ in terms of their income levels, but also in terms of for instance the risk of losing their job, the type of private insurance they would get would they lose their jobs and so on. Consequently all those characteristics are to be taken into account in order to understand individuals' rationale to support the welfare state. Whereas previously the political economy literature based its theories on class and income (Esping Andersen 1990; Korpi 1983; Meltzer and Richard 1981) to explain welfare state support, a more recent focus, developed as a counterargument to the first literature, has been on economic risk (Cusack et al. 2008; Iversen and Soskice 2001).

The global financial crisis has made this line of work particularly relevant. At its wake, there is more unemployment, temporary and involuntary part-time work, and financial insecurity (OECD 2013a). However, economic insecurity is not a new concern. As shown by Hacker et al. (2013) for the US, economic insecurity has seen a steady rise starting from the mid-1980s, affecting practically all population groups. Many authors have also commented on the modern labour market bringing increased employment instability and growing job insecurity (Anderson and Pontusson 2007; Dekker 2010). It can also be argued that the welfare state has always been most effective in insuring against risk and that this has been its main objective all along, rather than redistribution (Esping-Andersen 1999). Though lower-income individuals tend to also have a higher risk of becoming unemployed, this correlation depends on the country and the policy domain, and there is a substantial amount of individuals that are cross-pressured (Rehm et al. 2012). Thus income alone cannot satisfactorily resume both the redistributive and insurance aspect of the welfare state.

These changes in the labour-market have also affected Switzerland where the combined share of individuals who are unemployed or precariously employed (temporarily and involuntary part-time) amounted to about 15% already before the financial crisis of 2007–8, which is not much lower than the OECD average at the time (Rueda 2012). While intuitively it seems that high level of insecurity should be associated with a higher demand for an insurance against economic risk and thus demand for social policy, this cannot be taken for granted because of labour market dualization. Some groups (labour market insiders) remain largely unaffected by unemployment risk and might see high levels of insecurity chiefly through the prism of increased social expenses and others, even if they face high level of insecurity, might fall outside of the scope of the traditional instruments of the welfare state and therefore not be particularly supportive of social policies which they see as particularly benefitting the insiders.

The question therefore remains open as to whether employment insecurity is associated with higher demand for social protection. There are indeed a two requirements for structural changes in the labour market to impact demand for social policy. First, it is only if the public actually perceives a higher risk that objective risk can matter for public opinion. Second, this perceived risk needs to translate into policy preferences, which means that individuals update their demand for social policy based on their assessment of risk. The latter implies individual preferences are very flexible.

Ever More *Mittelstand*? Preferences that Reflect an Anti-Rich and Anti-Poor Sentiment

In order to analyse citizens' perception of their economic risk and their preferences for social policy we focus on three different questions asked in the Swiss Household Panel which have been included in the survey since 1999 annually until 2009 and from then on in an interval of 2 or 3 years. The three questions relate to citizen's perception of unemployment risk ("How do you evaluate the risk of becoming personally unemployed in the next 12 months?" on a scale from 0 to 10, where 0 means "no risk at all" and 10 stands for "a real risk"), their preferences with regard to higher taxation of the rich ("Are you in favour of an increase or in favour of a decrease of the tax on high incomes?" With the three answer categories being: „in favour of an increase", "in favour of a decrease" and "neither") , and increased spending for social security ("Are you in favour of a diminution or in favour of an increase of the Confederation social spending?" With again three answer categories). These variables have been recoded in order to obtain the share of respondents who do feel at least some degree of unemployment risk (i.e. have not answered 0 on the scale), and those who favour increased taxation for the rich and increased social spending respectively.[2]

Figure 15.1 shows the development of opinions over time. A striking observation is the concomitant rise of perceived unemployment risk with the decreasing trend of support for social spending. In the three first years about 45% of respondents felt they were to some extent threatened by unemployment and around the same share favoured increased social spending. Since 2001, the two lines follow opposed trends and in the post-financial crisis period the gap between the share of respondents

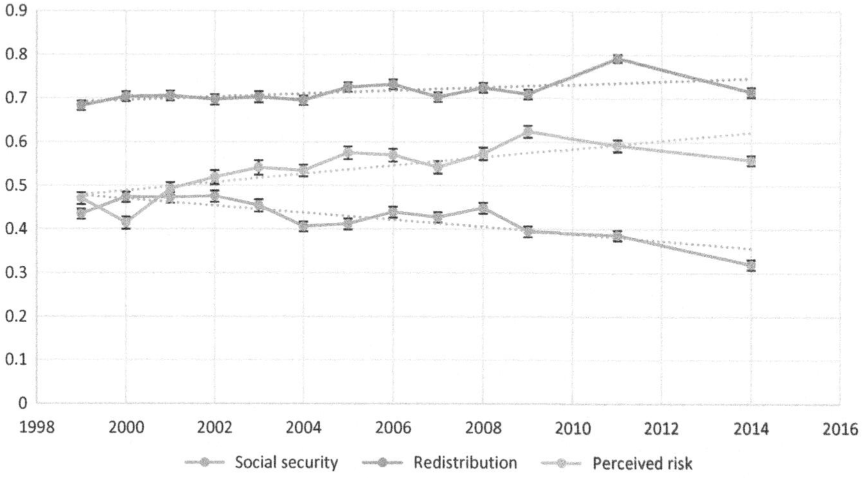

Fig. 15.1 Perceived unemployment risk and attitudes towards redistribution and social security over the 1999–2014 period, based on data from the Swiss Household Panel

[2] In these analyses data from all three SHP samples and cross-sectional weights are used. Note that when restricting the analysis only to respondents who participated in the SHP since 1999 and making use of longitudinal weights similar trends appear suggesting that shifts in the opinions of the Swiss is not merely due to composition effects or generational change.

feeling threatened and those who support increased social protection has amounted to around 20% points. Not only has the perception of risk increased with around 6 in 10 Swiss residents not feeling completely safe about their jobs, but the share of respondents favouring increased social spending has dropped below 40% since 2009.

Interestingly, the level of support for increased taxation of the rich has remained rather stable over the same period or even slightly increased from already very high levels in 1999. The high-point of this shift coincides with the aftermath of the financial crisis. In 2009, almost 80% of SHP respondents favoured increasing taxes for the rich. While the share has slightly decreased afterwards it appears that the general trend in relation to redistribution is a rising one. To borrow Cavaillé and Trump's (2015) terminology "redistribution from the rich" enjoys high and potentially even increasing levels of support while support for "redistribution to the poor" has declined since the end of millennium from already relatively low levels. How to interpret these trends?

The high level of support for increased taxation for the rich might show the inequality-averse preferences of the Swiss. But these opinions seem to be particularly oriented against reducing the post-tax income gap at the top of the income distribution rather than increasing state intervention in favour of those located towards the lower end of the income distribution. This trend is surprising given the overall increase of perceived job insecurity and thus the potential for having to resort to the welfare state. Of course one potential explanation could be that individuals do not feel sufficiently threatened by economic risk to favour increased state intervention from which they will unlikely benefit, but this observed paradoxical trend between overall level of perceived risk and preferences for social protection calls for a closer analysis of the causal chain linking economic conditions to individual preferences. To what extent does the objective economic situation of an individual impact his or her perception of that situation? And to what extent does this perceived situation impact their policy preferences? Studying this relationship is precisely the goal of the next section which proposes an individual-level analysis of attitudes towards unemployment benefits specifically.

Individual-Level Analysis: The Link between Objective Unemployment Risk, Perceived Risk and Demand for Social Protection

In order to analyse the micro-foundations of the link between objective risk of unemployment, the perception of this risk and finally demand for more protection in the specific domain of unemployment benefit, we rely on SHP data from the year 2011 which includes all variables of interest and for which unemployment figures across occupations were available. We focus on objective risk as defined by the level of unemployment in one's occupation - a common measure of objective unemployment risk using data from the Federal Statistical Office. Given our focus on unemployment risk, we restrict the sample to the active population who are the only ones who might be directly impacted.

Our analysis relies on two distinct steps. In a first step, we assess whether the Occupational Unemployment Rate is indeed associated with the perception of unemployment risk. In a second step we analyse the link between occupational unemployment rate and policy preferences regarding unemployment policies. More precisely, we are interested in assessing to what extent this link is mediated by one's perception of risk and to what extent mediated by other factors – in particular education and income – that might also affect the relationship.

Our empirical strategy implies having two dependent variables corresponding to the two stages of the analyses. The first one is perceived unemployment risk which has been measured using the same question as the one presented above[3].

The dependent variable in our second set of models is respondent's preferences with regard to unemployment benefits. Here, we use a specific question on whether spending for unemployment benefits should be increased, decreased or kept at its current level[4]. As is often done in studies on redistributive policies we recode this 3-category variable into a dummy variable distinguishing between those who favour an increase in unemployment benefit spending (coded 1) and those who either support a cut or favour a status quo (both coded 0), the latter de facto corresponding to an opposition of an increase in unemployment benefits.

The focus independent variable in both analyses is the Occupational Unemployment Rate (OUR). This has been created using data from the Swiss Labour Force Survey conducted in 2011 which includes about 30′000 individuals and allows computing average unemployment rates per occupation. We have computed these measures for each of the ISCO-2 digit occupations documented in the survey and matched these OUR measures with individuals based on their occupation. This measure corresponds very closely to what unemployment occupational risk has been operationalized in the literature so far (see Rehm 2009).

Our models further include a series of control variables that can be classified into two main categories: sociodemographic variables and individual characteristics that are associated with the economic self-interest of respondents. Among variables that belong to this second subset, we include the yearly net income at the individual level. We also include a variable measuring relative skill specificity. For this variable, we used data that is made available by Torben Iversen on his website and provides skill specificity measures that have been computed based on the ISSP surveys. This variable measures how specific one's skills are and should therefore

[3] To recall: "How do you evaluate the risk of becoming personally unemployed in the next 12 months?" on a scale from 0 to 10, where 0 means no risk at all and 10 stands for a real risk.

[4] Note that we measure here whether respondents are in favour of increasing spending on unemployment benefits specifically in contrast to the more general question presented in the previous section. The exact wording of the question used in the individual-level analysis is the following: "The government spends money in different sectors. Could you please tell me, for the following sectors, if you wish the government would spend more, less or the same amount? "

capture how difficult it is for a person to find a job that makes use of these specific skills in case of job loss (see Cusack et al. 2006; Iversen and Soskice 2001). Whether one has a temporary or long term working contract, thus whether a person is a labour market outsider or insider (see Rueda 2007), is measured with a dummy variable (0 = unlimited contract; 1 = temporary contract). We further include a control variable that measures previous unemployment experience (coded 1 for all those who reported having been unemployed in the past and zero otherwise). Furthermore, we also control for the number of earners in a household by distinguishing between individuals who are the only wage earners in their household (coded 0) and those who live with at least one other wage earner (coded 1). The underlying idea is that the consequences of unemployment on one's financial situation are tougher if that person is the only wage earner in the household.

The sociodemographic control variables includes age (measured as a metric variable), gender (0 = man; 1 = woman), education (a three category variable in which the reference category is no or only compulsory education; the other two categories being "above compulsory" and "tertiary" education). We also add a dummy variable for region which controls for all the observed and unobserved regional characteristics of the 7 Swiss regions as defined by the Swiss Federal Statistical Office (corresponding to the NUTS-2 level). In some of the models we further include a variable measuring social class. For this we use Oesch's class scheme which includes 8 different categories: Self-employed professionals and large employers, small business owners, (associate) managers and administrators, office clerks, technical professionals and technicians, production workers, socio-cultural (semi-)professionals and service workers. According to its author, this class scheme captures social stratification in modern societies, taking also account of the deindustrialization, the welfare state expansion, and the increased participation of women in the labor market. The focus is not only on hierarchical divisions but also on horizontal cleavages to reflect better the heterogeneity of today's middle class (Oesch 2006).

As the two dependent variables in our models have different measurement levels, we use an OLS regression to model perceived unemployment risk (which is measured with a11 point scale) and a logistic regression for the model in which preferences for unemployment benefits represent the dependent variable coded as a dummy. In addition to these analyses, we perform a product of coefficients test for the second set of models. This enables us to estimate how much of the relationship is mediated by perceived unemployment risk and how much by the socioeconomic factors we focus on: education and income. This test is similar to the Sobel test (Baron and Kenny 1986; Sobel 1982), used to determine mediation effects.[5]

[5] Note, however, two important differences in our approach. First, as our dependent variable is dichotomous, it is necessary to standardize the coefficients before doing the calculations (for more details, see MacKinnon and Dwyer 1993). We use a user written Stata command called binary_mediation to achieve this. Second, we use bootstrapping to calculate standard errors and significance levels, which are not given by the binary_mediation command. This has also been proven to be a superior approach, especially when not working with very large samples (Preacher and Hayes 2008).

Table 15.1 OLS regression models predicting perception of unemployment risk

		Model 1	Model 2	Model 3	Model 4
Occup. Unemp. Rate		0.299***	0.281***	0.238***	0.233***
Skill specificity		0.338***	0.369***	0.421***	0.396***
Contract type	Fixed	−1.157***	−1.432***	−1.541***	−1.521***
Net income (10′000 s)		−0.015	−0.049***	−0.064***	−0.058***
Past unemployment	Yes				0.628***
Number of earners	>1				−0.221**
Region (GE Lake)	Middleland		−0.715***	−0.728***	−0.646***
	North-west		−0.745***	−0.725***	−0.653***
	Zurich		−0.200	−0.209	−0.135
	East		−0.871***	−0.863***	−0.744***
	Central		−0.763***	−0.795***	−0.717***
	Ticino		−0.265	−0.329	−0.324
Gender	Female		0.0389	0.0782	0.0713
Age			0.0282***	0.0300***	0.0307***
Education (low)	Middle			0.282*	0.238
	High			0.196	0.116
Class (self-emp prof)	Small business owners			−1.321*	−1.159*
	Managers and admins			−0.0896	0.0156
	Office clerks			−0.325	−0.175
	Tech professionals			−0.203	−0.0683
	Production workers			−0.441	−0.25
	Socio-cultural profs			−0.739	−0.59
	Service workers			−0.309	−0.154
Constant		3.173***	2.972***	3.263***	3.374***
N		2112	2112	2112	2105
R-squared		0.069	0.106	0.116	0.124

*** $p < 0.01$, ** $p < 0.05$, * $p < 0.1$

In Table 15.1, we find in the first model with only the four objective variables related to the theories on risk: OUR, skill specificity, contract type (insider/outsider status), and income that all except the last are highly significant predictors of perceived unemployment risk with the relationships working in the expected direction. The relationships remain, and become significant for income, when controlling for basic sociodemographics in model 2, social class in model 3, and past unemployment and number of earners in model 4. This seems to show that these objective measures, and namely OUR, do capture something that people are aware of and can be used as a way of measuring the insecurity one feels at her or his workplace.

Table 15.2 Logistic regression models predicting being in favour of increased unemployment spending

		Model 1	Model 2	Model 3	Model 4
OUR		0.115***	0.0935***	0.0591	0.0462
Risk perception			0.105***		0.0855***
Income (10′000 s)				−0.087***	−0.080***
Education (low)	Middle			−0.418***	−0.398***
	High			−0.401**	−0.371*
Region (GE Lake)	Middleland	−0.463***	−0.398***	−0.500***	−0.443***
	North-west	−0.826***	−0.770***	−0.908***	−0.866***
	Zurich	−0.779***	−0.765***	−0.806***	−0.802***
	East	−0.829***	−0.763***	−0.942***	−0.886***
	Central	−0.799***	−0.732***	−0.796***	−0.744***
	Ticino	0.621**	0.616**	0.769***	0.770***
Gender	Female	0.302***	0.293***	0.0342	0.0525
Age		0.0214***	0.0199***	0.0314***	0.0293***
Constant		−2.353***	−2.616***	−1.207***	−1.498***
N		2680	2680	2506	2506
Pseudo R-squared		0.04	0.049	0.06	0.065

*** $p < 0.01$, ** $p < 0.05$, * $p < 0.1$

Depending on the model, the difference in perception of risk between workers in an occupation with the lowest and highest rates of unemployment is of between 1.4 and 1.8 points on an 11-point scale, a similar effect of that of having a temporary versus fixed contract. It should be pointed out that the R-squared, especially in the model with only the objective measures, is very low, indicating that there is much else determining one's perceived risk.

As expected, having been unemployed in the past increases worries among individuals, possibly making unemployment possibilities seem more real for. Not being the only earner in the household does also diminish somewhat the perceived risk, as expected.

There are relatively strong regional effects, which seem to reflect at least in part the fact that unemployment tends to be higher in French and Italian speaking regions, as well as in the canton of Zurich in the German speaking part of Switzerland. Older individuals also show a tendency towards a higher perceived risk, but no gender differences arise. Surprisingly, class, at least as operationalized here with the eight classes of Oesch (2006) has practically no effect, which goes against our suspicion that the OUR might confound somewhat with class differences.

In the second step, we ran four models predicting individual preferences for increasing unemployment spending (see Table 15.2). We find that in the first model with OUR and basic sociodemographic controls, the effect of the first on preferences is highly significant, as predicted by the theory. In the second model, we add risk perception. If OUR was completely mediated by the perceived risk, which seemed already unlikely given our first set of models, we would expect the effect of

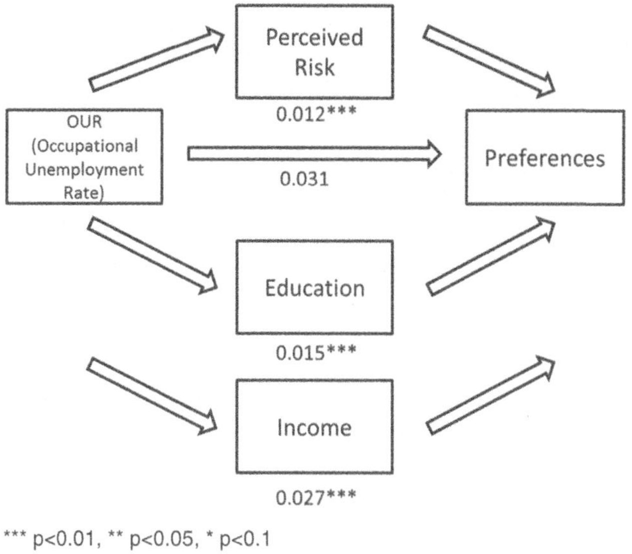

Fig. 15.2 Product of coefficients test: non-standardized direct and indirect effects. *** $p < 0.01$, ** $p < 0.05$, * $p < 0.1$

OUR to become non-significant. This does not happen, which tells us that both measure in part different things and influence individual preferences by different mechanisms.

In Model 3, we test our hypothesis of the effect of OUR on preferences being mediated by income and education, and find strong support. OUR becomes completely non-significant ($p = 0.122$) when these two variables are added, thus hinting at a strong mediation effect. Both education and income are highly significant at predicting one's preferences regarding unemployment spending. Risk perception in turn remains significant with these variables added. Interesting again is the strong effect of regions, showing that expectations towards the welfare state are heterogeneous within Switzerland.

So as to better understand the mediation effects, we present in addition the results of a product of coefficients tests (Baron and Kenny 1986; MacKinnon and Dwyer 1993). In this test, five regression models are run, the resulting coefficients are standardized and, based on the latter, the effects of the different paths are calculated. The regressions comprise the five variables of interest: preferences regarding unemployment spending, OUR, perceived unemployment risk, education, and income. The variables are coded as in the models above. In all five models, we control for age, sex, and region. In Fig. 15.2, we show the resulting unstandardized effects of the three paths of interest. We use bootstrapping to calculate standard errors and the significance of the paths. Table 15.3 shows the rest of the results, namely the proportion of the total effect that is mediated by each of the three variables and the total direct and indirect effects.

Table 15.3 Product of coefficients test: proportion of total effect mediated and total effects

Proportion of total effect mediated: risk perception	0.141
Proportion of total effect mediated: Education	0.180
Proportion of total effect mediated: Income	0.321
Proportion of total effect mediated: All	0.642
Total indirect effect	0.055***
Total effect	0.086***

*** p < 0.01, ** p < 0.05, * p < 0.1

As expected by the theory, we find that perceived risk significantly mediates the relationship between OUR and preferences (p < .01). However, this only represents about 14% of the total effect between OUR and preferences, which is relatively low compared to what we should find were this the main explanation for this effect. The size of the mediation effect by income is the same as that of risk perception but is not significant. Education in turn mediates the effect of OUR on preferences by 18% and is highly significant (p < .01). Income is highly significant and mediates as much as the two others combined, 32%. The combined effect of both sociodemographic variables is 0.042, more than three times that of risk perception. In total, they explain 50% of the total effect between OUR and preferences. A proportion of 64% of the total effect is mediated, the remaining direct effect being non-significant. This means that the two explanations proposed are likely to account for most of the relationship and no crucial component has been omitted from this analysis.

Our results indicate that individuals' perception of unemployment risk is to some extent linked to the unemployment rate in their occupation and that this link in part explains the relationship between the latter and policy preferences. However, we find that a more important explanation is related to the socioeconomic characteristics of individuals in a given occupation. We argue that this is because unemployment tends to be higher among individuals with low income and education levels. Thus occupations with higher unemployment rates tend to also to group together individuals with similar sociodemographic background. This means that belonging to a group more affected by unemployment will make the individual more inclined to support policies that help the unemployed, not so much out of self-interested calculations, but rather through a higher awareness of the issue, identification with those affected, and shared norms or solidarity (Svallfors 2006).

Conclusion

Preferences for social policy are expected to be influenced by a changing economic context. Individuals whose economic conditions or prospects evolve are generally expected to change their preferences because what they have to gain or lose from the welfare state also evolves over time. In line with this reasoning, times of increased economic insecurity should also lead to increased support for social policies because the odds of benefiting from them increases for the majority of the population.

However, in the 1999–2014 period studied here, there is in Switzerland a paradoxical trend of an increased perception of economic risk, but a stable or even declining level of support for social spending, although levels of support for redistribution from taxing the rich more have remained relatively high.

In themselves these macro-level evolutions of public opinion are interesting as they show that there are different and independent components of support towards the welfare state (see e.g. Cavaillé and Trump 2015) and that Swiss residents have perceived a change in the level of unemployment insecurity. However, they also call for a closer examination of the link, at the individual level, between objective and subjective levels of risk subjective and social policy preferences which is at the heart of most theories linking economic conditions with public preferences.

The Occupational Unemployment Rate represents one of the main measures for assessing one's objective risk of unemployment. While previous studies have consistently shown a strong correlation between this indicator and individuals' preferences with regard to the welfare state, the mechanisms that would explain this association have rarely been tested. Yet, we argue, understanding these mechanisms is crucial for appreciating how, within a country or an occupation, changes in the level of unemployment might affect policy preferences. Is the relationship between occupational unemployment rates and preferences mediated via risk perception, in which case we could expect an increased level of unemployment to affect perception of risk and ultimately policy preferences? Or is it linked to the fact that the level of unemployment in one's occupation is itself associated with other more stable individual characteristics that will remain unaffected by shifts in macro-level unemployment in which case little change in public opinion can be expected even at times of rapid changes in levels of unemployment risk?

Based on data from the Swiss Household Panel survey, our individual-level analysis provides a nuanced answer to these pressing questions in the context of rising unemployment in Europe. On the one hand, it seems that individuals' perceived risk is to some extent determined by their objective level of risk of being unemployed (measured by Occupational Unemployment Rate), which provides evidence for the relevance of objective risk measures in the formation of social policy preferences. On the other hand, we find that a larger part of the association between occupational unemployment rate and policy preferences runs via education and income, characteristics that are relatively stable across time. As a result, our findings tend to challenge the view that changes in the level of unemployment rate would affect public opinion regarding social policies in general and unemployment benefits in particular. The recent rise in unemployment across industrialised countries greatly affects individuals' risk of losing their job. This rise might however not be followed by a rise in demand for more unemployment benefits due to the fact that deeply rooted social cleavages seem to account for much of the relationship between subjective evaluations of risk and social policy preferences.

While the findings presented show the relevance of studying the mechanisms that link objective measures of risk with policy preferences, they remain limited in scope and call for further analytical sophistication. By studying a single country, we are able to overcome some of the methodological limitations of previous studies, but at the same time restrict the generalizability of our results. Are the patterns we identify specific to a country with low levels of unemployment? Are they linked to the specific context of a rise of anxiety following the crisis that hit industrialized and particularly European countries after 2007? To answer these questions, more case studies conducted across a variety of nations and especially over time would certainly helpful. But this endeavour is limited by data availability, as few surveys include subjective measures of risk. In addition, the relevance of the research question that is addressed in this article clearly pertains to dynamic changes in the macro-economic context. However, our cross-sectional analysis does not allow to directly study the link between changes in the macro- (country) or meso- (occupation) levels of unemployment with policy preferences. Future research on that topic should ideally make use of longitudinal data at the individual-level in order to analyse how shifts in context affect individuals. Future waves of the SHP including individuals' perceptions of economic risk and their preferences with regard to unemployment benefits should allow for such analyses.

References

Anderson, C. J., & Pontusson, J. (2007). Workers, worries and welfare states: Social protection and job insecurity in 15 OECD countries. *European Journal of Political Research, 46*(2), 211–235.

Ball, L. M. (2014). *Long-term damage from the Great Recession in OECD countries*. NBER working paper no. 20185: National Bureau of Economic Research.

Baron, R. M., & Kenny, D. A. (1986). The moderator–mediator variable distinction in social psychological research: Conceptual, strategic, and statistical considerations. *Journal of Personality and Social Psychology, 51*(6), 1173.

Bornschier, S. (2015). The new cultural conflict, polarization, and representation in the Swiss party system, 1975–2011. *Swiss Political Science Review, 21*(4), 680–701. https://doi.org/10.1111/spsr.12180.

Brooks, C., & Manza, J. (2013). A broken public? Americans' responses to the great recession. *American Sociological Review, 78*(5), 727–748.

Cavaillé, C., & Trump, K.-S. (2015). The two facets of social policy preferences. *The Journal of Politics, 77*(1), 146–160. https://doi.org/10.1086/678312.

Cusack, T., Iversen, T., & Rehm, P. (2006). Risks at work: The demand and supply sides of government redistribution. *Oxford Review of Economic Policy, 22*(3), 365–389.

Cusack, T. R., Iversen, T., & Rehm, P. (2008). Economic shocks inequality, and popular support for redistribution. In P. Beramendi & C. J. Anderson (Eds.), *Democracy, inequality and representation* (pp. 203–231). New York: Russell Sage Foundation.

Dekker, F. (2010). Labour flexibility, risks and the welfare state. *Economic and Industrial Democracy, 31*(4), 593–611.

Esping Andersen, G. (1990). *The three worlds of welfare capitalism*. Princeton: Princeton University Press.

Esping-Andersen, G. (1999). Politics without class: Postindustrial cleavages in Europe and America. In *Continuity and change in contemporary capitalism* (pp. 293–316).

Hacker, J. S., Rehm, P., & Schlesinger, M. (2013). The insecure American: Economic experiences, financial worries, and policy attitudes. *Perspectives on Politics, 11*(01), 23–49.

Iversen, T., & Soskice, D. (2001). An asset theory of social policy preferences. *American Political Science Review, 95*(4), 875–893.

Korpi, W. (1983). *The democratic class struggle*. London: Routledge and Kegan Paul.

Lupu, N., & Pontusson, J. (2011). The structure of inequality and the politics of redistribution. *American Political Science Review, 105*(02), 316–336. https://doi.org/10.1017/S0003055411000128.

MacKinnon, D. P., & Dwyer, J. H. (1993). Estimating mediated effects in prevention studies. *Evaluation Review, 17*(2), 144–158.

Margalit, Y. (2013). Explaining social policy preferences: Evidence from the great recession. *American Political Science Review, 107*(01), 80–103.

Meltzer, A. H., & Richard, S. F. (1981). A rational choice theory of the size of government. *The Journal of Political Economy, 89*(5), 914–927.

OECD. (2013a). *How's life?* Paris: OECD Publishing.

OECD. (2013b). *OECD employment outlook 2013*. Paris: OECD Publishing.

Oesch, D. (2006). *Redrawing the class map: Stratification and institutions in Germany, Britain, Sweden and Switzerland*. London: Palgrave Macmillan.

Preacher, K. J., & Hayes, A. F. (2008). Asymptotic and resampling strategies for assessing and comparing indirect effects in multiple mediator models. *Behavior Research Methods, 40*(3), 879–891.

Rehm, P. (2009). Risks and redistribution: An individual-level analysis. *Comparative Political Studies, 42*(7), 855–881.

Rehm, P., Hacker, J. S., & Schlesinger, M. (2012). Insecure alliances: Risk, inequality, and support for the welfare state. *American Political Science Review, 106*(02), 386–406.

Rosset, J., & Pontusson, J. (2014). The impact of the great recession on public preferences for redistribution in Western Europe. Paper presented at the APSA Washington.

Rosset, J., Lutz, G., & Kissau, K. (2016). Representation of political opinions: Is the structuring pattern of policy preferences the same for citizens and elites? In M. Bühlmann & J. Fivaz (Eds.), *Political Representation. Roles, Representatives and the Represented (pp. 117–134)*. London: Routledge.

Rueda, D. (2007). *Social democracy inside out: Partisanship and labor market policy in advanced industrialized democracies*. New York: Oxford University Press.

Rueda, D. (2012). Dualization and crisis. *Swiss Political Science Review, 18*(4), 523–530.

Soroka, S., & Wlezien, C. (2014). Economic crisis and support for redistribution in the United Kingdom. *Mass Politics in Tough Times: Opinions, Votes and Protest in the Great Recession*, 105.

Svallfors, S. (1997). Worlds of welfare and attitudes to redistribution: A comparison of eight western nations. *European Sociological Review, 13*(3), 283–304.

Svallfors, S. (2006). *The moral economy of class: Class and attitudes in comparative perspective*. Stanford: Stanford University Press.

Svallfors, S. (2012). *Contested welfare states: Welfare attitudes in Europe and beyond*. Stanford: Stanford University Press.

Sobel, M. E. (1982). Asymptotic confidence intervals for indirect effects in structural equation models. *Sociological Methodology*, 13, 290–312.

Chapter 16
Does Commitment Change Worldviews?

Gian-Andrea Monsch and Florence Passy

In this chapter, we examine whether commitment affects participants' worldviews. Worldviews, or meanings,[1] are defined as thinking-feeling tools individuals use to make sense of their social and political environment (Mead 1934; Weber 1978). In the present study, participants are those individuals who join an environmental protection organization, a charitable organization, or a union. Evidence in the literature on biographical consequences of activism is supportive (e.g., Passy and Monsch forthcoming; Giugni 2004): Individuals who join an organization synchronize their worldviews with the cultural scripts that circulate in the community. For example, Blee (2016) shows that women who join far-right organizations experience a critical transformation indebted to a radical shift in their interpersonal network. As one of her interviewee's states: "I made new friends and started to become obsessed with race....I thought about race 24/7" (p.9). Commitment therefore affects people's meanings. Yet, a conflicting argument exists in the literature, one that stresses a reverse causality, that is to say, specific worldviews are required to belong to the so-called mobilization potential eventually leading the individual to engage in joint action (e.g., Cotgrove and Duff 1980; Gamson et al. 1982; Kriesi 1989; Klandermans 1997). With this logic in mind, individuals solely join political or civic organizations if their meanings correspond. Commitment, then, does not change worldviews. Our present contribution aims to shed light on this debate by analyzing the effects of joining a political or civic organization on worldviews over time.

[1] In this contribution, we use the terms "worldviews" and "meanings" interchangeably.

G.-A. Monsch (✉)
FORS-Swiss Centre of Expertise in the Social Sciences, Lausanne, Switzerland
e-mail: gianandrea.monsch@fors.unil.ch

F. Passy
University of Lausanne, Lausanne, Switzerland
e-mail: florence.passy@unil.ch

R. Tillmann et al. (eds.), *Social Dynamics in Swiss Society*, Life Course Research and Social Policies 9, https://doi.org/10.1007/978-3-319-89557-4_16

According to McAdam (2009: 69) "cognitive liberation is sometimes a product rather than a cause of protest." Accordingly, we suggest that the story behind the relation between worldviews and joint action is more nuanced than has previously been stated. Commitment can have a variety of influences on activists' meanings because commitment experiences are particular. For example, we know that life course effects of movement participation in terms of employment, marriage, and childbirth patterns are usually stronger for women than for men (e.g., Van Dyke et al. 2000; Viterna 2013). Yet do we also find group specific variation in terms of effects on worldviews? We advance that there is a *plurality of effects on the meanings* of people who take on a commitment. Some perceive the world as members who sustain the commitment do. Others become members of a political or civic organization without the necessary cognitive tools. For the latter, we assume that synchronization of worldviews will occur once they join a specific organization.

Three questions structure our contribution. First, does commitment generally change the worldviews of new members? Second, does commitment have a group-specific effect, especially when it comes to members who join an organization with dissimilar meanings? Finally, are these effects durable? Before we answer these questions, it is necessary to offer a short overview of the literature on participation in social movements.

Worldviews of New Members: Before and after Commitment

The study of members' worldviews and the relation to commitment is fraught by divisions. Scholars focus either on causes to join an organization, or on effects of participation, rather than treating commitment as what it actually is: a continuum. Individuals who join activism belong to a specific group: The so-called movement potential (Klandermans 1997). Alongside structural factors (biographical availability and social networks), such individuals are internally predisposed toward participation. Indeed, their worldviews lead them to worry about specific social problems or to harness an awareness of certain political conflicts. Joiners possess a specific social anchorage and are equipped with particular values (e.g., Cotgrove and Duff 1980; Gamson et al. 1982; Kriesi 1989; Klandermans 1997; Passy and Giugni 2001). For example, activists within the post-industrial movement commonly belong to the new-middle class, are highly educated, and are part of the post World War generations. In addition, they share post-materialist values, are left wing oriented and highly progressive (e.g., Kriesi 1989; Passy and Monsch 2016). While the literature on the matter highlights the characteristics of a movement's potential, it fails to answer the two following questions: First, what happens to joiners with similar worldviews as those who are already committed? Second, what about people recruited outside the mobilization potential? We have elsewhere shown that the latter is a fairly common phenomenon (Passy and Monsch 2016). Unionists, for instance, often begin their commitment in the wake of a conflictual experience at work and lack the worldviews a typical union member would have. Another example is the widespread practice of street-recruitment, which attracts new members outside the traditional movement potential. Does commitment affect the worldviews of this group of people? And if it does have an impact, is it a durable one?

Studies investigating individuals after they have committed have revealed that activism has multiple and durable impacts on an individuals' life (e.g., McAdam 1988, 1989; Sherkat and Blocker 1997; Giugni and Grasso 2016). In addition to altering activists' social networks and influencing activists' practices, such as orienting personal choices and adopting new lifestyles, commitment shapes activists' worldviews and identity (e.g., Taylor 1989; Beckwith 2016; Whittier 2016). In a study on pro-life activists, Munson (2009) demonstrates that beliefs regarding abortion rarely impel individuals to get involved. By joining pro-life groups, however, activists went through a socializing process during which participant's views became more robust and consistent about abortion, while some converted from pro-choice to pro-life beliefs. Scholarship in social movement and volunteering studies emphasizes that commitment has substantial and durable effects on volunteers' worldviews and lives (Wilson and Musick 2000; Wilson 2012). While these findings are remarkably consistent across studies (McAdam 1989), many of them are beset by methodological problems (Giugni 2004). Among these, causality is without contest the most harmful. Many studies rely on retrospective data and lack a control group. This problem is not specific to social movement studies as scholars investigating biographical outcomes of volunteerism face the same drawback (Wilson and Musick 2000; Wilson 2012). In addition, most studies focus on high levels of commitment and are restricted to a specific type of activists: The New-left contention.

Thanks to the panel design adopted by the Swiss Household Panel (SHP) data, we are able to overcome these shortcomings. First, we take time into consideration and analyze what happens before and after individuals join a civic or political organization. Second, as the SHP is a general population survey, we are in a position to compare members with non-members. With longitudinal data and a control-group we are able to make a causal argument on the consequences of collective action on people's worldviews. Finally, our data set includes both highly committed members as well as the large majority of passive members who support a cause financially.

Malleable Understandings of Common Good and Politics

We define worldviews,[2] or meanings, as a thinking-feeling tool that allows individuals to perceive reality and the world around them, to make sense of their social and political environment, and set their intentionality to act (Jasper 2014, Searle 2004).

[2] Worldviews are neither values nor attitudes. Values are "enduring beliefs" (Rokeach 1973) whereas we know that an individuals' mind changes (see work on mind plasticity, e.g. Macrae and Bodenhausen 2000). Attitudes are orientations towards a positive or negative assessment of something or someone specific. Here, we consider broader worldviews that help individuals make sense of their social and political environment.

Opting for this terminology situates us in the interpretative tradition in sociology (e.g., Mead 1934; Berger and Luckmann 1967; Goffman 1967; Blumer 1969 among many others). Weber (1978), one of the main proponents in this field, conceives of human beings in terms of 'voracious meaning makers'. Hence, worldviews lie at the center of individuals' life: They enable them to perceive social realities, to make sense of them, and to act in their social environment. But meanings are social entities too. Cognitive processes are socially constructed, which means that worldviews are shared within the social sites an individual evolves in (e.g. commitment community, family, workplace, nation). They are constructed through social interactions (e.g., Mead 1934; Blumer 1969; Collins 2004; Fligstein and McAdam 2012): Through talks and disputes, individuals practice cultural scripts which circulate in the social sites they partake in (Mische 2008; Polletta 2008), and this practice shapes their worldviews and orients their action.[3] Correspondingly, moving from one social site to another affects individuals' meanings (Zerubavel 1997; Eliasoph and Lichterman 2003). With this definition in mind, we expect that *joining a political or civic organization has an impact on members' worldviews*.

However, activists join and experience their commitment differently. Therefore, we expect *variation among members regarding the effect of commitment on worldviews*. As we saw in the previous section, some joiners already share their worldviews with members of a given organization. For these individuals, we suppose stability, i.e. joining commitment will not drastically change their meanings. Others engage with dissimilar views compared to those present among members. They encounter a host of new cultural scripts which can be practiced through talks and disputes with fellow members, as well as within informal networks. Commitment is hence expected to affect their worldviews. It remains to be known if changes are durable, as the literature suggests.

In addition, individuals have many worldviews though not all of these are affected by political and civic commitment. We focus on two particular dimensions: Worldviews about common good and politics because they are the ends and means of the joint action taking place within the organizations considered here: Members of organizations of environmental protection use a contentious action repertoire (means) that aims to protect the environment (end). Volunteers of charitable organizations provide support to deprived people (end), and by helping the poor directly, seek to supplement state intervention (means). Unionists, finally, use institutional and contentious politics (means) to protect worker's rights (end).

Activists are supposed to act on a specific *understanding of common good*. Those goods are specific, as they should objectively improve people's well-being and be shared by all community members (Aristotle 1988; Murphy 2005). Who are the beneficiaries of the common good? Is it society as a whole or restricted to specific

[3] While we stress the social construction of worldviews, we nonetheless endorse an agentic conception, with room for idiosyncrasy and an individual capable to resist. Individuals are involved in various social sites and face different and often conflicting worldviews that they have to integrate in their self. This integration and use of their cognitive resources is made with agency (see Swidler 1986; Fligstein and McAdam 2012).

groups? And are members concerned by many common goods or only by the one they commit to? Six indicators allow us to evaluate this dimension: General trust, women's penalization, measures for women, changes for foreigners, environmental protection, and wealth redistribution.[4]

The second dimension is their *understanding of politics*, which is how people perceive and think about actors in the political arena. Are state actors accountable for the common good and should they intervene to enlarge and secure it? Do individuals legitimize state actors and their performances? And what is the role of a citizen in democracy? Should a citizen be interested in, and vigilant about, political processes and decisions? Should a citizen value the importance of taking part in participatory politics? We rely on seven indicators to evaluate this dimension: Opinions on the amount of social expenses, general satisfaction with democracy, trust in the Federal Government, political interest, and the intention to boycott, demonstrate, and strike.[5]

Unfortunately, survey data in general is limited in scope regarding the analyzable nuances of people's worldviews. This is especially visible when one wants to enquire into worldviews provided by a general population survey, as the SHP is mandated to cover a broad range of subjects. As a consequence, some indicators are proxies at best, or are loosely related to our concept. For example, political interest provides only a rough measure for political vigilance. While someone probably has to have some interest in politics in order to be vigilant, one can easily imagine that

[4] For *general trust*, respondents were asked whether they would say that most people can be trusted or if you can't be too careful in dealing with people, where 0 means "Can't be too careful" and 10 means "Most people can be trusted." *Women's penalization* was measured with this item: "Do you have the feeling that in Switzerland women are penalized more than men in certain areas", where 0 means "not at all penalized" and 10 "strongly penalized"? For *measures for women*, we used the following question: "Are you in favor of Switzerland taking more steps to ensure the promotion of women", where 0 means "not at all in favor" and 10 "totally in favor"? Respondent's opinions about *changes for foreigners* is evaluated with the following: "Are you in favor of Switzerland offering foreigners the same opportunities as those offered to Swiss citizens, or in favor of Switzerland offering Swiss citizens better opportunities?" Respondents could be either favorable to equal opportunities, to better opportunities, or neither. Regarding *Opinion about environmental protection,* respondents were asked whether they are favorable to Switzerland being more concerned with environmental protection than with economic growth, and vice-versa. Again, respondents could either be in favor of environmental protection, economic growth, or neither. The question for *wealth redistribution*, finally, evaluates whether the respondent is in favor of an increase or decrease in the taxes on high income, or neither.

[5] For their opinion on *social expenses*, respondents were asked whether they are in favor of a diminution, in favor of an increase of the Confederation social spending or neither of the two. *Satisfaction with democracy* was measured with this item: "Overall, how satisfied are you with the way in which democracy works in our country", if 0 means "not at all satisfied" and 10 "completely satisfied." *Trust in the Federal Government* is based on this question: "How much confidence do you have in the Federal Government" if 0 means "no confidence" and 10 means "full confidence." *Political interest* is measured with the following question: "Generally, how interested are you in politics, if 0 means "not at all interested" and 10 "very interested"? To evaluate the *intention to boycott, demonstrate and strike,* respondents were asked with three items: "If 0 means never and 10 certainly, tell me to what extent, in the future, you are prepared to take part in a boycott/demonstration/strike."

someone is politically interested without being vigilant. As a consequence, the validity of our measures is somewhat limited, making it hard to evaluate the underlying theoretical dimensions. We nonetheless consider the ensemble of attitudinal indicators analyzed a reasonable representation of a worldview. Therefore, the SHP's panel design largely outweighs this drawback, offering a rather unique opportunity to explore the worldviews of members over time.

How to Analyze Changes in Worldviews?

Our analyses investigate worldviews of all the individuals included in the original sample who responded regularly over 11 years (*1999 to 2009*).[6] 1999 is the starting date of the panel and 2009 is the last year when questions on membership were asked annually. From 2009 onwards, the membership questions were put into a rotative module and are now only measured once every 3 years. Membership is obviously crucial for the analyses conducted here as it allows us to attribute respondents to the group of members who sustain commitment, new joiners, and non-members respectively.[7] It was tempting to add the years 2011 and 2014 where the information on membership exists. However, this would have required us making assumptions about individuals' commitment in 2010, 2012, and 2013. To increase the robustness of the findings, we decided to dismiss this time period from our sample.

We then decided to look only at membership for the years 2003, 2004, and 2005 in order to *observe the same group over time*. This decision excludes people who join or leave in other years but brings along two key advantages. First, the worldviews of every joiner can be observed over a substantial amount of time: Four years before and after commitment takes place.[8] Second, an identical group of joiners is observed over time, thereby eliminating any inter-individual differences from the analyses. These tend to erase intra-individual variation, which makes the procedure a valuable one. In terms of age, we include a large age range in our working sample so as to provide respondents with the opportunity for membership unrestricted by age or mobility. In the first year of inquiry (1999) we took individuals from 15 years to 80 years of age for the last year of observation (2009).[9]

---

[6] "Regularly" means that an individual has to take part in every wave where a specific question was asked. However, as not all indicators were measured over the whole timespan, the sample size slightly varies between indicators.

[7] For membership, respondents are asked the following question: "I will now read out a list of associations and organizations. Could you tell me for each of them whether you are an active member, a passive member or not a member?"

[8] Due to data availability, this is not always possible. "Intention to demonstrate", for example, is only available between 1999 and 2008. Hence, for this particular indicator, we provide data for 4 years before but only 3 years after an individual has become a member.

[9] All these decisions are the product of an iterative process during which we tested several possible constructions of the membership variable and ran analyses with and without weights. Overall, the results are very similar and we are confident with the result presented here.

The analyses presented below merge members of environmental organizations, charitable organizations, and unions.[10] In addition, we decided to combine active and passive membership because the number of active members is too small to be analyzed separately. Moreover, we have elsewhere shown that commitment affects worldviews of both active and passive members (Passy and Monsch 2016). Whereas active members enjoy opportunities to practice community specific cultural scripts in their interactions with other members, empirical evidence shows that passive members rely on people in their interpersonal network (friends and relatives) who are favorable or committed to the community in question (see also McAdam 1988; Klandermans 1997). We hence take full advantage of the potential of the SHP panel design. This allows us to observe the same individuals yearly over a long period, both before and after they become members. In addition, as the SHP is a general population survey, it naturally entails a control group of non-members. These characteristics make these data well suited to study biographical consequences.

Specific Worldviews of Members

Before turning to the effects of commitment on worldviews, we need to clarify three points. How important is political and civic commitment as a phenomenon in Switzerland? Is it common for new members to maintain their commitment? And do members hold specific worldviews which depart from non-members? First, commitment is clearly an important and widespread phenomenon in Switzerland. According to the SHP data, more than 40% of all respondents are members of Green contention, unions, or a charitable organization.[11] Commitment in Switzerland is hence a widespread phenomenon including about half of the national population. Given the fact that we do not possess indicators on other types of activism, such as LGBT, human rights, migrants' rights, peace groups, etc., the evidence inevitably underestimates the range and extent of commitment in the country. Another element is the rather stable feature of commitment over time. From 1999 to 2009 the numbers do not change and are quite impressive. What is stressed is that investigating political and social participation, and consequences of commitment on worldviews, is not merely a rhetorical question, especially given the large number of individuals involved. Second, we ask whether members, who have just joined a collective endeavor, are inclined to maintain their commitment. After all, if worldviews are affected by commitment, the effect must occur once activists enjoy social interactions and practice cultural scripts within the given community.[12] We observe such

[10] We do this for three main reasons; first, limited constraints. Second, it allows us to obtain reasonable numbers to analyze subgroups, especially for the group of joiners who possess other understandings. Third, the results are very similar when members of these groups were analyzed separately.

[11] We tested this factor for the years 1999, 2004 and 2009.

[12] About 80% of members under study are passive members who support their respective organization financially. We have shown that passive members are also involved in social interactions and practice the cultural scripts available in their commitment communities (Passy and Monsch 2016).

sustained commitment in the SHP data: Around 80% of all individuals who were committed in 1999 sustain their involvement over time (30% sustain commitment between 2 and 4 years and 50% more than 5 years). Sustained exposure to social interactions within these communities thus offers opportunities to influence members' worldviews at the very least.

Finally, *worldviews of members' depart from those of non-activists*. As shown in Table 16.1, members who sustain participation clearly hold specific meanings when it comes to their understanding of common good and politics.[13] Let us discuss this aspect in more detail. Members' understanding of common good clearly differs from that of non-members. On average, they trust others, perceive women as more penalized than men, and are prone to encourage women promotion more. These worldviews significantly depart from those of non-members (see Eta and Chi-squared coefficients). Additionally, members think foreigners should benefit from the same opportunities than Swiss citizens, environmental protection should be a priority, and taxes for higher income earners should be increased to enable a better distribution of common good. These questions concern members more than non-members.

Members' understandings of *politics* are also specific, especially regarding their political interest and intention to boycott, to demonstrate, and to strike. Meanwhile, differences for their opinions concerning increases in the state's social expenses, their overall satisfaction with democracy, as well as their trust in the Federal Government are statistically significant, but only by a small margin. It is surprising to note that members are more satisfied with democratic procedures and are more inclined to trust politicians. Indeed, we could have expected a more critical stance resulting in less satisfaction and trust because state de-legitimization is considered to constitute an important factor for protest participation (Piven and Cloward 1977). Three elements help clarify this result. First, the Swiss population generally displays a high level of political trust compared to populations of other European countries (Bauer et al. 2013). Second, many types of organizations are included in the member category, entailing that individuals could be members of a typical protest actor or not. For example, the union community is quite fragmented in Switzerland when it comes to sectorial (public vs. private) and ideological (left wing vs. Christian) lines (Kriesi and Trechsel 2008). In turn, this influences the action repertoire deployed and the subsequent conception of politics. Finally, the two indicators used to assess Swiss democracy and its political institutions are rather general. While it is necessary to take these exceptions into account, the overall picture remains clear: Members possess a specific understanding of politics.

However, less is known about the time-span necessary for activists to synchronize their worldviews with their peers. It seems reasonable to expect variation with respect to the participant's level of commitment and the political challenge their mobilization involves. For individuals lightly committed to a mobilization of low level of political challenge, we expect that the process takes longer than for active members involved in challenging contentions.

[13] People in this category were members of either an organization of environmental protection, charity, or union during 2003, 2004, and 2005.

Table 16.1 Comparison between worldviews of members and non-members

UNDERSTANDINGS OF COMMON GOOD			
	Members	**Non-members**	
	Means	**Means**	**Eta**
General trust in people	6.60 (1.7)	6.02 (1.9)	.14***
n	*827*	*1614*	
Women penalized	5.75 (1.8)	5.50 (1.9)	.06**
n	*821*	*1602*	
Measures for women	6.07 (2.5)	5.81 (2.6)	.05*
n	*809*	*1559*	
	%	%	χ^2
Changes for foreigners	83	67	67.8***
n	*781*	*1506*	
Environmental protection	59	48	26.5***
n	*784*	*1454*	
Taxes for high income	82	77	16.0***
	792	*1499*	
UNDERSTANDINGS OF POLITICS			
	Members	**Non-members**	χ^2
Increase in social expenses	50	44	30.2***
n	*779*	*1499*	
	Means	Means	Eta
Satisfaction with democracy	6.30 (1.4)	6.04 (1.5)	.08***
n	*807*	*1563*	
Trust in Federal Government	5.94 (1.6)	5.62 (1.8)	.09***
n	*808*	*1565*	
Interest in politics	6.57 (2.2)	5.45 (2.5)	.22***
n	*814*	*1584*	
Intention to boycott	5.52 (3.0)	3.98 (3.1)	.23***
n	*811*	*1570*	
Intention to demonstrate	5.34 (2.9)	3.70 (3.0)	.25***
n	*810*	*1580*	
Intention to strike	4.79 (3.1)	3.27 (2.9)	.23***
n	*806*	*1562*	

Note: *p < 0.05 **p < 0.01 ***p < 0.001. Eta for interval scaled variables and χ^2 for dummies.
Source: Swiss household panel

Throughout the discussion of Table 16.1, we have shown that *members possess a distinct understanding of common good and politics* when contrasted with non-members. They have a more inclusive vision of society, are more concerned by different common goods, legitimize state actors more, and have a more vigilant and participatory conception of citizenship. As other variables (e.g. education, social class) were not assessed, this is merely correlational evidence which highlights the differences between members and non-members.

Multiple Effects of Commitment: Stable and Malleable Worldviews

Members possess specific worldviews. But when do these meanings become specific? Table 16.2 allows us to investigate whether and under which conditions worldviews of members change. The table is organized in the following manner: The bold vertical line in the middle marks the moment respondents became members. In relation to this moment, the columns before and after the bold vertical line outline the 4 years prior (t-4, t-3, t-2, t-1) and after (t + 1, t + 2, t + 3, t + 4) these individuals began participation. In addition, at the right end of Table 16.2 we have added a column where t-tests between the indicators 1 year before people started commitment (t-1) and 1 year after this event happened (t + 1) are reported. This is so in order to evaluate whether members' worldviews changed. Like in Table 16.1, the rows go through the indicators of joiners' understandings of common good and politics with the exception that each indicator is listed twice: Once for all joiners and once for new members with other worldviews.[14] Accordingly, discussion of the results centers first on all joiners, then turns to the sub-group with other meanings.

What happens to worldviews of joiners? Do they change after they join their respective organization? And if changes occur, are they durable? Overall, we observe a high degree of stability for individuals who enter into participation: *Their worldviews do not change*. Their understanding of common good and of politics remains the same before and after joining a given organization. However, two exceptions contradict this general pattern of stable worldviews: Trust in others and political interest. Both the level of trust and interest in politics increases once individuals join an organization. The literature on volunteerism shows similar results (Eggert and Giugni 2010 for political interest; Sivesind et al. 2013 for social trust). Our result therefore backs these findings. Indeed, commitment affects social trust and political interest in a positive manner.[15] Social trust and political interest set aside, the worldviews of activists do not change. This implies that social interactions which occur after individuals enter activism do not necessarily influence their worldviews. As we see when comparing the results with those reported in Table 16.1, joiners are already close to members before they start participation, and these particular understandings remain stable over time. Hence, scholarship that stresses that activist groups recruit newcomers in their mobilization potential is right: Their worldviews overlap substantially with those of members already committed.[16]

---

[14] We defined benchmarks for new members with other worldviews in relation to the results for the member category in Table 16.1 (see the greater-than signs in Table 16.2). For the interval-scaled indicators, the basis for this decision was the means of members who sustain participation. For nominal-scaled indicators, we have excluded the respective modal value of faithful members.

[15] Measures for women and taxes on high income also show significant changes (see t-test in Table 16.2). However, these difference remain small and tend to vanish over time (see t + 2, t + 3 and t + 4).

[16] Additional analyses show that members also predominately belong to the movement potential in terms of their social characteristics (age, social class, and education).

Table 16.2 Joiner's worldviews of common good and politics over time

UNDERSTANDINGS OF COMMON GOOD									
Time	t-4	t-3	t-2	t-1	t + 1	t + 2	t + 3	t + 4	t-1 vs t + 1
All joiners	Means (SD)	Means (SD)	Means (SD)	Means (SD)	Means (SD)	Means (SD)	Means (SD)	Means (SD)	t-test
General trust in people (n = 983)	–	–	–	6.30 (2.0)	6.62 (1.9)	6.64 (1.9)	6.66 (1.9)	6.67 (1.9)	6.10^{***}
Women penalized (n = 923)	–	5.58 (2.2)	5.66 (2.2)	5.61 (2.1)	5.67 (2.1)	5.67 (2.1)	5.62 (2.0)	5.46 (2.0)	ns
Measures for women (n = 902)	–	5.95 (2.9)	5.92 (2.9)	5.96 (2.8)	6.21 (2.7)	6.09 (2.7)	6.15 (2.7)	5.99 (2.7)	3.68^{***}
Joiners with other worldviews									
General trust in people	–	–	–	2.87 (1.6)	4.48 (2.0)	4.35 (1.7)	4.34 (1.8)	4.40 (2.0)	7.89^{***}
(n = 141) < 5.0	–	3.39 (1.7)	3.54 (1.7)	3.61 (1.5)	3.81 (1.9)	3.82 (1.8)	3.83 (1.8)	3.89 (1.8)	$1.66^{(*)}$
Women penalized (n = 214) < 5.5	–	2.92 (2.0)	2.82 (2.0)	2.91 (2.0)	3.42 (2.1)	3.49 (2.1)	3.31 (2.1)	3.28 (2.1)	3.92^{***}
Measures for women									
(n = 227) < 5.5									
All joiners	%	%	%	%	%	%	%	%	t-test
Chances for foreigners (n = 857)	75	73	74	73	74	75	76	76	ns
Environmental protection (n = 861)	53	53	52	50	50	53	52	53	ns
Taxes for high income (n = 856)	78	79	79	78	81	79	78	78	2.16^{*}
Joiners with other worldviews									
For equal chances for foreigners	0	0	0	0	6	7	3	6	2.91^{**}
(n = 125)	0	0	0	0	6	8	7	7	4.11^{***}
For environmental protection	0	0	0	0	11	5	7	11	3.65^{***}
(n = 286)									
For higher taxes for high income									
(n = 110)									
UNDERSTANDINGS OF POLITICS									
Time	t-4	t-3	t-2	t-1	t + 1	t + 2	t + 3	t + 4	t-1 vs t + 1
	%	%	%	%	%	%	%	%	t-test

(continued)

Table 16.2 (continued)

UNDERSTANDINGS OF COMMON GOOD									
All joiners									
Increase in social expenses (n = 824)	49	49	47	45	46	46	47	45	ns
Joiners with other worldviews									
For an increase in social expenses (n = 322)	0	0	0	0	4	4	5	2	3.82***
All joiners	Means (SD)	Means (SD)	Means (SD)	Means (SD)	Means (SD)	Means (SD)	Means (SD)	Means (SD)	t-test
Satisfaction with democracy	6.23 (1.6)	6.18 (1.6)	6.15 (1.7)	6.18 (1.5)	6.16 (1.6)	6.18 (1.6)	6.20 (1.6)	6.20 (1.6)	ns
(n = 907)	6.02 (1.9)	5.92 (1.8)	5.84 (1.8)	5.68 (1.8)	5.60 (1.8)	5.56 (1.8)	5.63 (1.8)	5.69 (1.8)	ns
Trust in Federal Gov. (n = 913)									
Interest in politic (n = 936)	6.03 (2.4)	6.10 (2.4)	6.16 (2.4)	6.10 (2.5)	6.22 (2.4)	6.19 (2.4)	6.26 (2.3)	6.27 (2.4)	2.62**
Intention to boycott (n = 914)	4.68 (3.4)	4.71 (3.4)	4.99 (3.5)	4.81 (3.4)	4.69 (3.4)	4.64 (3.4)	4.36 (3.4)	–	ns
Intention to demonstrate (n = 926)	4.32 (3.4)	4.44 (3.3)	4.51 (3.4)	4.40 (3.3)	4.42 (3.3)	4.32 (3.3)	4.25 (3.3)	–	ns
Intention to strike (n = 902)	3.81 (3.3)	3.90 (3.3)	4.05 (3.4)	3.93 (3.3)	3.91 (3.3)	3.76 (3.2)	3.72 (3.2)	–	ns
Joiners with other worldviews									
Satisfaction with democracy	4.59 (1.2)	4.47 (1.4)	4.49 (1.4)	4.58 (1.2)	4.67 (1.5)	4.74 (1.4)	4.74 (1.4)	4.70 (1.5)	ns
(n = 211) < 6.0	3.98 (1.4)	3.95 (1.4)	3.80 (1.5)	3.82 (1.5)	3.89 (1.5)	3.83 (1.5)	3.83 (1.5)	3.96 (1.5)	ns
Trust in Federal Gov.	3.22 (1.8)	3.34 (1.7)	3.32 (1.7)	3.14 (1.8)	3.50 (1.9)	3.52 (1.9)	3.62 (1.9)	3.63 (1.9)	3.81***
(n = 230) < 5.5	1.59 (1.7)	1.59 (1.7)	1.61 (1.7)	1.52 (1.7)	1.77 (1.9)	1.69 (1.8)	1.60 (1.8)	–	3.16**
Interest in politic (n = 248) < 5.5	1.41 (1.6)	1.45 (1.6)	1.51 (1.6)	1.41 (1.6)	1.58 (1.8)	1.71 (2.0)	1.54 (1.8)	–	2.56*
Intention to boycott (n = 293) < 5.0	1.24 (1.5)	1.22 (1.5)	1.30 (1.6)	1.32 (1.6)	1.43 (1.8)	1.47 (1.8)	1.43 (1.8)	–	1.91(*)
Intention to demonstrate									
(n = 340) < 5.0									
Intention to strike (n = 389) < 5.0									

Note: (*)$p < 0.10$ *$p < 0.05$ **$p < 0.01$ ***$p < 0.001$. t-tests for dependent samples. Source: Swiss household panel

However, the picture changes once we consider *joiners with other worldviews than those who sustain commitment*. For this group, we observe a significant change once membership has begun. A synchronization process is clearly at work, be it for their understandings of common good, or regarding their understandings of politics. While very few indicators were significant when all joiners are considered together, most of them are affected by commitment for joiners with other worldviews. And these changes are not merely visible a year after membership has occurred (t + 1), but remain stable over time, and do not regress to the level before the organization was joined. As for the dimension of common good, five out of six indicators show a significant change once members with other understandings commence their commitment. While still significant, the question regarding the level of women's penalization departs from this general picture. Joiners with other worldviews than those shared by members of environmental protection groups, charitable organizations, and unions, only increase slightly in their perception that women are disadvantaged. By contrast, they become more favorable to taking measures for the promotion of women. Joiners' with other worldviews see their understandings of politics equally affected by commitment. This group becomes more inclined towards an increase in state social expenses, more interested in politics, and shows a higher protest intention on average. However, satisfaction with democracy, as well as trust in the Federal Government, diverges from this general trend. While satisfaction with democracy grows slowly over time (t + 2, t + 3 and t + 4), trust in the Federal Government is not affected by commitment.

Multiple Effects on Members' Worldviews

This chapter provides evidence for two arguments. On the one hand, many individuals join a political or civic organization with similar worldviews to those held by members of the organization. In that regard, the low numbers for the group of joiners with other understandings is a result in its own right, as only few joiners belong to this group. This group's worldviews is only marginally affected by commitment. On the other hand, *commitment has a durable effect on the worldviews of individuals who join a commitment with other understandings*. Unfortunately, we are limited by very general indicators, as well as by small numbers, when we want to compare subgroups. Further research will be required to investigate the worldviews of members over time.

Throughout this chapter, we argued that commitment changes people's worldviews. The results indicate that commitment has a differential effect on the understandings of common good and politics of individuals who become members of an environmental protection organization, a charitable organization, or a union. The majority of joiners engage with meanings close to those of members who sustain commitment, a result that sustains the argument put forth by movement potential scholars, who claim that, individuals need to hold particular worldviews in order to join an organization. However, a non-negligible part of joiners become members with other worldviews of common good and politics, and this group is clearly affected in the way we suggested: Their worldviews are synchronized and these changes are durable. Thus, stability and changes are not mutually exclusive when it comes to the effects of political and civic participation.

Our major aim consists in taking a first step towards the study of variations among socialization patterns and pointing out that *mental consequences are group specific*. In terms of future research, we should analyze the various effects of commitment according to different groups. We would hence further our knowledge regarding the conditions under which commitment has an effect on members' worldviews, concerning the gendered experience in union activism, for example (Van Dyke et al. 2000). Longitudinal data would be indispensable if we were to undertake such a study. The SHP data has proven valuable in this respect. However, assessing the meanings of members with the sole use of indicators destined to survey a general population has its limits. In the future, an additional task will hence be to develop more refined measurements, which could take the form of a panel study dedicated to analyzing the effects of political commitment, to complement this fascinating dataset. Going down this path will increase our understanding of the role played by political and civic commitment for participant's worldviews in particular, and allow us to examine the effects on their life course more generally.

References

Aristotle. (1988). *Ethica Nicomachea*. Oxford: Oxford University Press.

Bauer, P. C., Freitag, M., & Sciarini, P. (2013). Political trust in Switzerland: Again a special case? SSRN.

Beckwith, K. (2016). All is not lost: The 1984-85 British miners' strike and mobilization after defeat. In L. Bosi, M. Giugni, & K. Uba (Eds.), *The consequences of social movements* (pp. 41–65). Cambridge: Cambridge University Press.

Berger, P. L., & Luckmann, T. (1967). *The social construction of reality: A treatise in the sociology of knowledge*. Garden City: Anchor Books.

Blee, K. M. (2016). Personal effects from far-right activism. In L. Bosi, M. Giugni, & K. Uba (Eds.), *The consequences of social movements* (pp. 66–84). Cambridge: Cambridge University Press.

Blumer, H. (1969). *Symbolic interactionism: Perspective and method*. Englewood Cliffs: Prentice-Hall.

Collins, R. (2004). *Interaction ritual chains*. Princeton: Princeton University Press.

Cotgrove, S., & Duff, A. (1980). Environmentalism, middle-class radicalism and politics. *The Sociological Review, 28*, 333–351.

Van Dyke, N., McADam, D., & Wilhelm, B. (2000). Gendered outcomes: Gender differences in the biographical consequences of activism. *Mobilizations, 5*, 161–177.

Eggert, N., & Giugni, M. (2010). Does associational involvement spur political integration? Political interest and participation of three immigrant groups in Zurich. *Swiss Polit Sci Rev, 16*, 175–210. https://doi.org/10.1002/j.1662-6370.2010.tb00157.x.

Eliasoph, N., & Lichterman, P. (2003). Culture in interaction. *The American Journal of Sociology, 108*, 735–794.

Fligstein, N., & McAdam, D. (2012). *A theory of fields*. Oxford: Oxford University Press.

Gamson, W. A., Fireman, B., & Rytina, S. (1982). *Encounters with unjust authority, the Dorsey series in sociology edition*. Homewood: Dorsey Press.
Giugni, M. (2004). Personal and biographical consequences. In D. A. Snow, S. A. Soule, & H. Kriesi (Eds.), *The Blackwell companion to social movements*. Oxford: Blackwell.
Giugni, M., & Grasso, M. T. (2016). The biographical impact of participation in social movement activities: Beyond highly committed new left activism. In *The consequences of social movements* (pp. 85–105). Cambridge: Cambridge University Press.
Goffman, E. (1967). *Interaction ritual: Essays on face-to-face behavior*. New York: Anchor Books.
Jasper, J. M. (2014). Feeling-thinking: Emotions as central to culture. In B. Baumgarten, P. Daphi, & P. Ullrich (Eds.), *Conceptualizating culture in social movement research* (pp. 23–44). London: Palgrave Macmillan.
Klandermans, B. (1997). *The social psychology of protest* (1st ed.). Oxford and Cambridge: Wiley-Blackwell.
Kriesi, H. (1989). New social movements and the new class in the Netherlands. *The American Journal of Sociology, 94*, 1078–1116.
Kriesi, H., & Trechsel, A. H. (2008). *The politics of Switzerland. Continuity and change in a consensus democracy*. Cambridge: Cambridge University Press.
Macrae, C. N., & Bodenhausen, G. (2000). Social cognition: Thinking categorically about others. *Annual Review of Psychology, 51*(1), 93–120.
McAdam, D. (1988). *Freedom summer*. Oxford: Oxford University Press.
McAdam, D. (1989). The biographical consequences of activism. *American Sociological Review, 54*, 744. https://doi.org/10.2307/2117751.
McAdam, D. (2009). Recruits to civil rights activism. In *The social movements reader. Cases and concepts* (2nd ed., pp. 66–74). Malden: Wiley-Blackwell.
Mead, G. (1934). *Mind, self and society from the standpoint of a social behaviorist*. Chicago: University of Chicago Press.
Mische, A. (2008). *Partisan publics: Communication and contention across Brazilian youth activist networks*. Princeton: Princeton University Press.
Munson, Z. W. (2009). *The making of pro-life activists. How social movement mobilization works*. Chicago: The University of Chicago Press.
Murphy, M. C. (2005). The common good. *The Review of Metaphysics, 59*, 133–164.
Passy, F., & Giugni, M. (2001). Social networks and individual perceptions: Explaining differential participation in social movements. In *Sociological Forum* (pp. 123–153). Springer.
Passy, F., & Monsch, G.-A. (2016). Contentious minds. How ties and talks sustain activism. Book Manuscript.
Passy, F., & Monsch, G.-A. (forthcoming). Personal and biographical consequences of activism. In D. A. Snow, S. A. Soule, H. Kriesi, & H. McCammon (Eds.), *Wiley-Blackwell companion to social movements*. Malden: Wiley Blackwell.
Piven, F. F., & Cloward, R. (1977). *Poor People's movements: Why they succeed, how they fail*. New York: Vintage Books.
Polletta, F. (2008). Culture and movements. *The Annals of the American Academy of Political and Social Science, 619*, 78–96.
Rokeach, M. (1973). *The nature of human values*. New York: Free Press.
Searle, J. R. (2004). *Mind: A brief introduction*. Oxford: Oxford University Press.
Sherkat, D. E., & Blocker, T. J. (1997). Explaining the political and personal consequences of protest. *Social Forces, 75*, 1049–1070.
Sivesind, K. H., Pospíšilová, T., & Frič, P. (2013). Does Volunteering Cause Trust? *European Societies, 15*, 106–130.
Swidler, A. (1986). Culture in action: Symbols and strategies. *American Sociological Review, 51*, 273.
Taylor, V. (1989). Social movement continuity: The Women's movement in abeyance. *American Sociological Review, 54*, 761–775.

Viterna, J. (2013). *Women in war: The micro-processes of mobilization in El Salvador*. Oxford and New York: Oxford University Press.

Weber, M. (1978). *Economy and society: An outline of interpretive sociology*. California: University of California Press.

Whittier, N. (2016). Aggregate-level biographical outcomes for gay and lesbian movements. In L. Bosi, M. Giugni, & K. Uba (Eds.), *The consequences of social movements* (pp. 130–156). Cambridge: Cambridge University Press.

Wilson, J. (2012) Volunteerism research: A review essay. Nonprofit Volunt Sect Q XX:1–37.

Wilson, J., & Musick, M. (2000). The effects of volunteering on the volunteer. *Law and Contemporary Problems, 62*, 141–168.

Zerubavel, E. (1997). *Social mindscapes: An invitation to cognitive sociology*. Cambridge: Harvard University Press.

Conclusion

Marieke Voorpostel, Robin Tillmann, and Peter Farago

This book brings together diverse studies based on longitudinal data from the Swiss Household Panel. Following a large sample of households over a period of almost two decades allows us to give a detailed picture of how life courses have evolved over time. At the same time, such data can also paint a picture of Swiss society over the last two decades. This book illustrates these two types of social dynamics, the changes in individual lives and those at the societal level grouped around three themes: health, wellbeing and life satisfaction; resources, work and living conditions; and politics and attitudes. This chapter brings together the main conclusions from the studies in this book.

Health, Wellbeing and Life Satisfaction

The contributions on health, wellbeing and life satisfaction mainly focus on changes and events over the life course. Lillard contributes a chapter on smoking that incorporates change on both the macro- and micro-level by showing the smoking behaviour of different cohorts of men and women in Switzerland over the life course. He finds that the smoking behaviour of Swiss men and women resembles, to a certain extent, that found in other countries. He shows that older cohorts smoke more than younger ones and that men smoke more than women do, although women behave more like men in younger cohorts. For the younger cohorts, smoking peaks in the early twenties and decreases from the late twenties onward. Peak smoking rates occurred at older ages in the oldest cohorts. For all cohorts and over time, smoking prevalence has generally been decreasing in connection with factors such as advertising bans, the prohibition from smoking in enclosed public areas and at the workplace, and increased taxes on tobacco.

The study by Lucchini and Della Bella assesses the relationship between body mass index (BMI) and health satisfaction, both between and within individuals. They show that men and especially women with a BMI different from normal

R. Tillmann et al. (eds.), *Social Dynamics in Swiss Society*, Life Course Research and Social Policies 9, https://doi.org/10.1007/978-3-319-89557-4

weight had significantly lower levels of satisfaction with their health, with the strongest effects being for obesity and severe obesity. Looking at intra-individual changes, any change from normal-weight BMI to either underweight or overweight decreases satisfaction with health among women but not among men. The fact that women suffer more in terms of satisfaction with their health if they are obese suggests that differences in health satisfaction not only are related to physical health but may also reflect that women face more weight-related stigma than men do. According to recent statistics, obesity rates in Switzerland are low in comparison to in other OECD countries but have been increasing in the last 15 years. Stigmatization may play a more important role in a society where obesity is relatively rare.

Three chapters relate life events in the family domain to life satisfaction, health and wellbeing. The chapter by Wernli and Zella relates changes in life satisfaction to a number of transitions in the family life course. They find that union formation, the transition to marriage and the birth of children all make people more satisfied with their life in general. They find downward trends for divorce and widowhood. An important finding of their study is that changes in life satisfaction are often temporary, and the timing and duration sometimes vary for men and women. For example, whereas women show stronger increases following the transition to marriage, they also seem to suffer more prior to and during a relationship's dissolution. Men, on the other hand, become less satisfied with their lives after a break-up, and their unhappiness lasts longer compared with women.

The chapter by Ryser and Le Goff and that of Hewitt, Voorpostel and Turrell zoom in on the dynamics surrounding single family transitions. Ryser and Le Goff assess what happens to different aspects of wellbeing and attitudes about the family when cohabiting couples marry. Previous studies have shown that cohabiting individuals tend to hold less traditional family values and also show higher levels of depressive symptoms and less happiness. In their study, Ryser and Le Goff assess the extent to which couples that decide to get married are already different prior to this transition, suggesting a process of selectivity, and whether we can observe a change in wellbeing and attitudes as cohabiting couples marry. They show that cohabiting couples hardly show any variation in wellbeing when they become married, supporting the idea of selection. Yet, they also show that although there is little variation in the overall population, the transition to marriage seems to affect some groups more than others: differences in life satisfaction by gender and educational attainment prior to marriage disappeared following the transition.

Hewitt, Voorpostel and Turrell also compare cohabitation and marriage but focus on relationship dissolution. Their main question is whether relationship dissolution affects mental and physical health to the same extent if the couple is married as it does when they are cohabiting. Comparing Australia and Switzerland, they find no strong short-term effect on physical health but show that separation from marriage results in a greater decline in mental health than separation from cohabitation, with only marginal differences between the countries. In line with the findings from Wernli and Zella, they show that on average, individuals return to their prior levels of mental health after a few years.

These three chapters demonstrate a clear link between mental health and wellbeing, and events and transitions in the family domain in the lives of the Swiss resident population in the last two decades. Rather than simply observing trends in marriage, fertility, childbirth and wellbeing, the chapters show how wellbeing and health change in the process of experiencing these events at the individual level, often suggesting that family events affect wellbeing but predominantly showing that higher or lower levels of wellbeing tend to be only temporary.

The last chapter in this section shifts the focus to the relationship between immigration and health. Potarca and Bernardi examine whether there is evidence of a "healthy immigrant effect" in Switzerland, in which migrants report better health than natives do. Although this "epidemiological paradox" is found in several other countries, they find the opposite to be the case in Switzerland: migrants have poorer health compared with Swiss natives, even after adjusting for differences in socio-economic status. They also show that legal status has a significant influence on health disparities between Swiss natives and immigrants. Swiss who are naturalized in later life and non-Swiss show poorer health compared to Swiss natives and those who became Swiss at a young age. By incorporating retrospective information on the timing of naturalization, they demonstrate that a comparison at a single time point between Swiss and non-Swiss is not enough to better understand the relation between migration and health: the timing of naturalization matters.

Resources, Work and Living Conditions

The second part of the book combines six chapters that either address how life course events and trajectories affect various outcomes related to socio-economic resources, work and living conditions or take more of a macro-perspective and show how cohorts have changed over time.

Masia, Budowski and Tillmann link health to poverty outcomes. The longitudinal nature of the SHP data allows them to show how health deterioration of a household's breadwinner increases the risk that the household will enter into poverty and precariousness. Not only do they show that health affects precariousness, indicating a causal relationship between the two, but they also show how the health of the household breadwinner affects the situation of all household members, hence moving beyond the individual level.

The chapter by Gazareth, Iglesias, Crettaz and Suter and the one by Bühlmann both look at life course trajectories to draw conclusions on how Swiss society has changed, in terms of determinants of material deprivation (Gazareth et al.) and in terms of job insecurity and instability (Bühlmann). Gazareth and colleagues show that the majority of households can be characterized by stably non-deprived trajectories over time. Households that experience material deprivation tend to fluctuate in and out of deprivation. Trajectories of durable deprivation are scarce. They conclude further that the classical determinants of social inequality, such as social class, play a larger role than life course transitions. Bühlmann focuses on the increasing levels of precarious employment in the last decades. He first shows that in Switzerland, only a minority held a permanent position and did not perceive their job as insecure in 2010. He then examines the dynamics of vulnerability in the years leading up to 2010. In this period, exclusion from the labour market and precarious employment increased, partly because of changes in social policies. His analysis of the SHP data shows six types of trajectories: stable and secure, stable but insecure (the largest group), increasing insecurity, turbulent entries, out of the work force, and paths to exclusion. In line with the macro-trends, he finds that especially the younger generation has experienced turbulent entries into the labour market. Paths to exclusion are more common among lower-educated older individuals. This study shows how individual trajectories produce macro-outcomes and how some groups are more at risk of trajectories to vulnerability than others.

Zangger and colleagues put the school-to-work transition into context by incorporating the timing of different cohorts entering the labour market and linking this to levels of modernity of Swiss society (by which they mean the combination of educational expansion, the size of the labour force, changes in the occupational structures, and the increase in qualification requirements). They find that timing matters: there is a positive association with the level of modernity at the time of one's graduation on the likelihood of entering the labour market. Younger cohorts are more likely to enter the labour market upon graduation. The authors did not find an increasing risk of entering the lowest status group over time. Education and social background remain important, emphasizing the persistent social inequality in entering at the top or bottom of the status distribution across cohorts.

The final two chapters in this section deal with wealth. Until recently, wealth in Switzerland has received little research attention, mostly because of a lack of available data. With the inclusion of questions on wealth in the SHP in 2012, it has become possible to gain more insight into household wealth in Switzerland. As other household panels have also included measures of wealth, we can compare Switzerland to other nations. Ravazzini and Kuhn compare saving behaviour and wealth in Switzerland, Germany and Australia and assess the role of children in the household. They find for all three countries that older children are the most expensive, limiting families' ability to save. Younger children limit the ability to save in Germany and, even more so, in Switzerland. This may result from the stronger reduction in labour supply as women leave the labour market upon having children. Analysing the data on wealth, the authors find that in the long run, children only have weak negative consequences on wealth accumulation. The second chapter on wealth, by Kuhn and Grabka, looks at the relationship between homeownership and wealth in Germany and Switzerland. In both countries, owners are wealthier than renters are because they save more in paying off their mortgage and because property prices have increased. The authors also find that overall wealth inequality is high in both countries and that wealth inequality is larger among renters than among owners. These analyses complement the chapters on household welfare and material deprivation by adding an important element of social inequality.

Politics and Attitudes

The third part of this volume deals with political parties and (political) attitudes. The first three chapters combine a macro-level change over time with individual-level dynamics. They show that attitudes in Switzerland have changed over time. Between 1999 and 2014, the Swiss have become increasingly anti-immigrant, anti-social spending, sceptical about joining the European Union and concerned with protecting the environment. The contributions then assess intra-individual patterns of change to try to explain these trends.

Fitzgerald and Jorde assess the extent to which individual partisan preferences shape attitudes about immigration, social spending and the environment. Rather than following the classic model of electoral behaviour that assumes policy preferences shape political party choice, they turn this upside down and use longitudinal data from the SHP to show that partisanship also drives changes in political attitudes. They first show that anti-immigration, anti-spending and pro-environment attitudes show significant intra-individual variation, although they have become more stable over time. Linking changes in attitudes to partisanship, the authors find that partisanship shapes people's stances on key political issues. Supporting the Swiss People's Party (SVP) is associated with a shift to supporting opportunities for Swiss citizens over those for immigrants. The authors argue that the rise of the SVP can be at least partly attributed to the party's ability to convince voters on matters associated with immigration. For preferences regarding environmental policies, support for the Green Party is a major driver. Finally, opinions on social spending are driven by a preference for the Radicals or, even more strongly, by a preference for the SVP. The authors link this to the SVP's rhetoric on government spending on immigrants.

Sarrasin, Kuhn and Lancee focus on Euroscepticism. The increasingly critical attitude that the Swiss hold towards the EU implies that at least part of the population has changed their opinion over time. After showing that citizens with a higher socio-economic status are more likely to support joining the EU and those holding right-wing values are less likely to, the authors move on to explain what drives individual changes in attitudes. Their study shows that a move towards the right side of the political spectrum increases the likelihood of opposing joining the EU. In contrast, whereas economic values explain attitudes towards the EU, changes in individual life courses largely unrelated to changes in attitudes. This suggests that mostly macro-factors, such as economic crises, are driving the overall decline in support for joining the EU.

The chapter by Pekari, Rosset and Schmid addresses attitudes towards the welfare state, in particular the support for social spending and for higher taxation of the rich. In the period 1999—2014, there was an increased perception of job insecurity, which we already saw in the chapter by Bühlmann, and simultaneously a slightly declining level of support for social spending. This appears to be a contradiction. Policy preferences are expected to reflect a changing economic context, where increasing risks of unemployment would suggest more support for social spending, such as on unemployment benefits. Fitzgerald and Jorde provided a possible explanation for this trend by linking decreasing support for social spending to the SVP's narrative of government spending on immigrants. Pekari and colleagues go in a different direction and examine this paradox by assessing the relationship at the individual level. They find that the perceived risk of unemployment, which is linked to policy preferences, is related to the actual risk of becoming unemployed (as measured by the Occupational Unemployment Rate). Yet, they find that education and income, which are rather stable over time, are stronger determinants of social policy preferences. The authors conclude that social cleavages, rather than subjective evaluations of risk, drive social policy preferences, which provides a further explanation of why increasing levels of subjective job insecurity can develop in parallel with decreasing support for social spending.

Finally, Monsch and Passy analyse the relations between political and civic commitment and change in worldviews over time. The main question of the chapter is whether and under which conditions becoming a member (of an environmental protection organization, a charitable organization or a union) changes a person's worldviews, which they measure by looking at general trust as well as attitudes on gender equality, immigration, environmental protection, social spending, politics and activism. The authors show that the worldviews of joiners in general do not change after joining a given organization. However, in line with the literature on volunteerism, general trust and interest in politics increase after joining an organization. This suggests that the worldviews of joiners overlap with those of members who are already committed. The picture appears different regarding joiners with worldviews that are different from those of committed members. In this case, the authors argue, a synchronization process is at work as a significant change occurs once membership has begun. Overall, the authors show that political and civic participation is associated with both stability and change in worldviews.

Concluding Remarks

The collection of studies in this volume demonstrates, on the one hand, that individual life courses shape outcomes in various domains at the individual and household level. The experience of certain life events may produce a number of changes, ranging from life satisfaction to wealth accumulation. On the other hand, several studies in this book demonstrate that persistent social inequalities and social cleavages exist in Switzerland for many outcomes. In particular, classical determinants of social inequality such as social class play an important role in terms of trajectories of material deprivation and vulnerability in the labour market. Education and social origin still matter regarding school-to-work transitions, and wealth inequality remains high in Switzerland. These social and socio-economic cleavages continue to shape political attitudes, particularly with regard to the EU and the welfare state. Persistent social inequalities especially put those groups at risk who have limited resources and face increasing instability in their life course.

All in all, the contributions collected in this volume are proof of the wealth of the SHP data for empirical analyses using different theoretical and methodological approaches. Due to the quality of its data, the Swiss Household Panel is a first-class source for scientific work. It is widely being used by Swiss and international researchers, resulting in a plethora of high-quality scholarly publications. It thus achieves the main purpose of a research infrastructure and is successfully in its twentieth consecutive year – and hopefully for many future interview waves to come.

The manufacturer's authorised representative in the EU is Springer Nature Customer Service Centre GmbH, Europaplatz 3, 69115 Heidelberg, Germany. If you have any concerns regarding our products, please contact ProductSafety@springernature.com

Printed and bound by CPI Group (UK) Ltd, Croydon, CR0 4YY
30/09/2026
02225659-0007